DIET
9·1·1

Also by Yolanda Bergman with Daryn Eller

FOOD COP:
Yolanda, Tell Us What to Eat

DIET
9·1·1

Food Cop to the Rescue with
265 New Low-Fat Recipes

Yolanda Bergman
with
Daryn Eller

BANTAM BOOKS
NEW YORK • TORONTO • LONDON • SYDNEY • AUCKLAND

About the nutritional information in this book:

The nutritional information provided with each recipe is derived from the database MasterCook Mac, a software program based on food analysis from the United States Department of Agriculture and various other sources.

DIET 911
A Bantam Book / April 1997

All rights reserved.

Book design by James Sinclair

Library of Congress Cataloging-in-Publication Data

Bergman, Yolanda.
Diet 911 : food cop to the rescue with 265 new low-fat recipes /
Yolanda Bergman with Daryn Eller.
p.   cm.
Includes index.
ISBN 0-553-09992-2
1. Low-fat diet—Recipes.   I. Eller, Daryn.   II. Title.
RM237.7.B45   1997
641.5'638—dc21   96-48488
                                                  CIP

Published simultaneously in the United States and Canada

Bantam Books are published by Bantam Books, a division of Bantam Doubleday Dell Publishing Group, Inc. Its trademark, consisting of the words "Bantam Books" and the portrayal of a rooster, is Registered in U.S. Patent and Trademark Office and in other countries. Marca Registrada. Bantam Books, 1540 Broadway, New York, New York 10036.

PRINTED IN THE UNITED STATES OF AMERICA
BVG   10   9   8   7   6   5   4   3   2   1

I dedicate this book with all my heart to my children, Nolina and Rylan. Also to my best friend, Sue. I am grateful for your presence in my life, and I love you all.

Acknowledgments

I would like to thank all of the clients I have worked with over the past fifteen years. They have allowed me to step into their lives, souls, appetites, and kitchens and lead them on a path to a better life with food. They keep me in tune with the ever-changing world of food, diet, and how we eat, and help me learn as I teach them. They are the ones that make my day when they call and say "I'm in a size six!" or "I really like the way I'm eating now and I don't even miss mayonnaise anymore." It makes it all worthwhile.

Among my clients, there are a few whose loyalty has been an inspiration to me daily: Susan Geliebter, Kimmy Robertson, Hallie Todd, Robin Riker, Anne LeGassick, and Paul Cooper. There are many wonderful clients who love my food service in Los Angeles, but there are a few who have remained on the service regularly and I want to thank them for their long-term patronage: Bob Ferretti, Rylie Ellis, Charlie Matthau and Positive Ray, John Wright, Mary Pattiz, Barry Greenfield, Patricia Snyder, Wendy and Don Woodard, and Elliot Mintz.

I would like to thank Katie Hall, Elise Petrini, and Barb Burg at Bantam for believing in me and supporting me over a period of seven years. A huge thank-you to Gary Bernstein for shooting the best book covers in the world and making me look at least as decent as the food. Also, great thanks to Gary for believing in my work and my message.

There are two wonderful women who have helped me with the ups and downs of writing and creating this book and been very supportive. Thanks to Carla Glasser, my agent, who is always wise, understanding, a great listener, and maintains a great sense of humor. And a very special thanks to Daryn Eller. Daryn and I have worked together for the past seven years on various projects, and I thank her from the bottom of my heart for being a great writing partner. Through it all we have maintained a friendship and understanding. Daryn was one of the first writers to really hear my message about eating well and help me get it out to the public. We have both grown through the years in our careers, and I admire her work and her patience.

Last, but definitely not least, is a big hug and a huge thanks to the executive chef of my home delivery and catering service, Susan Kay. We have worked together for the past decade developing recipes and keeping my Los Angeles–based food business a top-notch service. Sue and her husband, Bob, work hard to make sure the quality of the food is superb and consistent. Sue Kay is creative, hardworking, loyal as the day is long, and patient, and I thank her for everything she has done. Also, great thanks to Mike Bender, my client coordinator, for his loyalty and professionalism.

I thank my Mom and my Pa for their support, wisdom, and understanding. And I thank Richard and my children for being the "testers" of my kitchen creations and for supporting the world of healthy food that I bring to them. My kids are among the next generation of healthy bodies that won't have to fight the battles of food disorders or food-related illnesses. I wish this for you and all of your children as well.

Contents

Introduction

I Want to Help You . . .
And I Want to Tell You the Truth

Every day we read articles about how fat America is. Television ads hawking diet centers or meal replacements remind us that we've got a lot to lose, and magazines reiterate the message month after month. We're overweight, we're unhealthy, we're a mess. Even the former surgeon general C. Everett Koop has declared obesity a national disease. We are in a state of diet emergency.

Yet for all the talk about how Americans are too fat for their own good, everyone seems to be at a complete loss when it comes to explaining why. A lot of people try to blame it on bad genes, but can all our weight problems really be caused by a few errant strands of DNA? Is our eating behavior just a manifestation of being "born that way"?

I don't think so. If that were the case, there would be nothing short of drug or gene therapy that we could do to change our lot in life. But that's simply not the case. There are many, many reasons why Americans are fat. More important, there are just as many solutions to the problem.

I'm frustrated by all the lies—about certain foods and their nutritional value, about what it takes to get lean and healthy. I want to help you get past these falsehoods and get food back into your life as a pleasure. Food has become a burden, but it should be a joy. You should be able to have chocolate, cookies, cheese, bread, wine, and other indulgences. You should be able to celebrate with food when you're happy, use it to nurture yourself when you're sad and to relieve stress when you're tense—and be able to do so without getting fat or sacrificing your health.

The pages of this book are dedicated to helping you accomplish just that. Think of it as your emergency help line—your Diet 911. This help line is here to give you answers, not more lectures on things you already know about how to get thin and stay healthy.

For the past fourteen years I have been a diet consultant to people who want to change the way they eat. As such, it's been my job to know food; there's hardly a product on the market that I haven't scrutinized, a type of restaurant menu I haven't deciphered, a recipe I haven't reworked in order to help my clients get leaner, healthier foods into their lives. So if you want a healthy substitute for the oily pasta sauce you've been using, I've got a list of alternatives. If you want ideas for nonfattening dinners, as easy as slipping a frozen meal into the oven—but much more healthy—I've got plenty of suggestions.

I want you to become an expert on food—healthy, nonfattening food. You may feel like you're already an expert on nutrition; by now we've all been educated to death about things like fat and cholesterol, carbohydrates and calcium. Yet being an expert on nutrition is different from being an expert on food. It's one thing to know the exact number of protein grams you should get daily, quite another to know what to grab for breakfast when you've got only seconds to spare. Or how to order a healthy lunch from the take-out place down the block. Or what's quick to fix for dinner on days when you come home dog tired. You don't need more nutrition data; you need to know how to translate the information you already have into tangible eating solutions.

Lately I've been irked by a television commercial that illustrates my point perfectly. The ad shows a very pretty and sophisticated woman coming home from work, briefcase in hand. Her little daughter is waiting for her with big eyes and a rumbling tummy. Mom, I'm hungry, she says. You then see a moment of anxiety come over the woman's face; she's tired from a long day at work, but doesn't want to disappoint her daughter. Suddenly she smiles. Cut to McDonald's, where the whole family is seen eating fast-food burgers as if they were homemade soup and fresh bread.

The commercial's statement is that to be a loving working mom all you have to do is provide your family with a great McDonald's dinner. Take the kids on over to Mama McDonald's. You can see why this message hits home. When we're hungry, we want food that's easy to prepare and on the table fast, nutrition be damned. Like Scarlett O'Hara, we'll think about it tomorrow.

It doesn't have to be that way. It's time that we took back control of the food in our lives. So many of my clients come to me overwhelmed by the prospect of slimming down, starting another diet, having to contort themselves to fit the latest fashion in weight loss. They feel defensive, anxious, and vulnerable, and they've begun to wonder if there really is a realistic way to eat happily and be fit. There is. There is! You can! You can do this!

I'm not going to give you some convoluted diet with rules that make you feel as though you're living someone else's life. I don't believe you should be calculating calories here and counting fat grams there. Is that any way to live? No, and nobody has to.

What you need are real-life solutions. You need to know how to get the fat out of your life and work more fruits and vegetables, lean proteins, and whole grains into your diet. You need to know how to make food with fresh and natural ingredients that's healthy, nonfattening, great tasting and, most important, no-hassle. No-brainer.

No-brainer. That's a term that you're going to see running throughout this book. It refers to eating ideas—I hate to call them recipes, they're so easy—that require anywhere from one to five steps. Sometimes a no-brainer may be as simple as opening a bottle of something that's nonfattening and satisfying—maybe something you haven't even heard of yet.

I am happy to report that, as we near the end of the century, the health food industry has made great strides. Years ago, health food was boring and brown. Today it's sold in glitzy natural food markets like Whole Foods in Los Angeles, Bread and Circus in Boston, and Alfalfa's in Denver. And it's everything from natural macaroni and cheese you can make with skim milk, to instant cup o' soups you can use a hundred ways, to fat-free chocolate cookies and tortilla chips. I'm also a great believer in ignoring the direction on food packages; that way, you can make healthy food even healthier. Rice mixes that call for oil? Leave it out. Soups that ask you to mix in whole milk? Go for skim. Don't let food manufacturers intimidate you. If you know what to look for and how to prepare it, you'll be in hog heaven (minus the fat, of course).

For times when you have more than a few minutes to spare, you'll find recipes here that are so delicious no one will ever know they're made without a drop of added fat. And even these are simple to make. I'm a proponent of using all the healthy conveniences available, and I've incorporated many of them into these wonderful dishes.

At night, when we sit down to scrumptious, healthy, nonfattening meals, my husband often asks me, "Why wouldn't everyone want to eat this way?" "They don't know how yet," I reply. Read on and you will.

Chapter One

A Diet Is a Diet Is a Diet:
And You Don't Need One
to Get the Body You Want

DIET *n.* 1. food and drink considered in terms of qualities, composition, and effects on health: *Milk is a wholesome article of diet.* 2. a particular selection of food, especially as prescribed to improve physical condition or cure a disease: *a diet low in sugar.* 3. such a selection or a limitation on the amount a person eats for reducing weight: *No pie for me, I'm on a diet.* 4. the usual or regular food or foods a person eats most frequently: *He would be happy on a diet of meat and potatoes.*

The next time they do an update of Webster's dictionary, the source of the above, they should include a few new definitions of diet: 5. something used to get Americans to shell out a lot of money for false hope: *Buy this diet tea and you'll slim down in no time.* 6. a bogus product developed for false purposes: *Go on this diet (only $99.99!) and we guarantee you'll be a new person.*

In my mind the purpose of most diets is to get you to buy something, whether special meals or special supplements or just bad advice. The purpose of a diet is not to give you a real education on eating well. And let's define eating well: eating in a way that satisfies your mind and your heart, and suits your lifestyle and body type. To eat well you need to learn about food, not about dieting.

But why is it that so many intelligent people are susceptible to diet ruses, the snake oil of the modern age? Why is the speedy old five-pounds-in-five-days weight-loss scam so easy to sell when we all know that the fat comes back in no time flat? Why has the simple, natural task of feeding ourselves become a nightmare? In short, how did we end up so confused about how to eat happily and healthfully, and how can we get out of this big, *fat* mess?

Before I begin to explain all of the above (and trust me, I can), let me tell you a little parable of what has happened in this country over the last fifty years. It's a simple explanation, taken from nature because, really, we are animals, human animals.

Visualize a herd of beautiful long-legged giraffes, roaming the plains of Africa, going from tree to tree, eating leaves. Giraffes don't need personal trainers or gyms to meet their ideal weight because they move all day long. The leaves they eat (designed by Mother Nature) provide all the nutrients the giraffes need to be strong, lean, and healthy. The giraffes don't complain about not being able to add some ketchup, mustard, or special sauce to the leaves, nor do they sample the monkeys' bananas or try to grab a little raw meat from a lion's feast. They manage to grow strong, long, and elegant on a diet of foliage.

Imagine, though, if you decided to take the giraffes and herd them into a small corral—a corral that prevented them from roaming around all day long. Or put them on a little island (Manhattan, perhaps) covered with cement. There wouldn't be enough trees to keep them all fed, so you'd have to import some leaves. Since it's cheaper to make faux leaves than to go back to Africa and get the real thing, you'd manufacture them, probably adding some chemical preservatives, colorings, and flavorings to the formula. You'd want the giraffes to be healthy, so you'd supplement the leaves with chemical versions of vitamins and other nutrients, too. Since you'd want the animals to find them appealing, you'd also add some bright green coloring, some leaf flavoring, and package them all very nicely. *Voilà.* You now have instant leaves.

Then, let's say you keep them on that island for four to five decades.

It doesn't take long to figure out that the giraffes would start to gain weight from lack of roaming and that the endless barrage of chemicals would probably affect their systems, causing their bodies to operate improperly. The giraffes would probably become obese and develop heart disease, cancer, and a variety of other diseases. They would, of course, have baby giraffes and these baby giraffes would also live sedentary, chemical-filled lives. And the babies would have babies and they'd all grow up on giraffe junk food until they became an island of giraffes with a nationwide problem: fat. They'd have thick legs, large necks, big bellies. In other words, they'd be nothing like the species they were supposed to be and not at all happy about it.

Okay, so it's a little bit of an exaggeration, but doesn't it sound familiar? Doesn't it sound a little bit like what has happened in this country? We were never meant to move so little and eat so much, particularly the refined, polluted food we consume today. We have been consuming chemically processed, nutritionally void food for forty to fifty years. What an experiment!

How, then, do we get out of this mess? Not by diet programs—whether they promise two-pounds-a-week weight loss or not. Go on any *diet*—I don't care if it's called Zoneland, Scarsdale, Fit for It, Diet with Jesus, the Richard Simmons program, or the Buy-a-Tiny-Meal-a-Day weight loss plan—and if you stick to the rules you will lose weight, probably at a rate that isn't comfortable for your body. As a result, you'll feel the great need to kick the diet, eat what you want; you'll gain back the weight and then kick yourself. It's a vicious circle and we're all tired of it.

To some people, the greatest mystery in the world is how to lose weight and keep it off *without* dieting. Without, that is, sticking to some regimented program that inhibits your personality and prohibits all your fun. But it's no mystery at all. The way I teach it, you can like your body *and* be able to enjoy food again. What a concept!

It all revolves around what I call T & C—time and consistency.

When a client calls me for a consultation and I hear something like "I've got two months until a wedding [reunion, party, convention, you name it] and I have to lose twenty to thirty pounds by then," I say, "Wrong number." I don't hang up, though. Instead I explain that I simply don't work that way; I only offer long-term weight loss, something that takes time and consistency. In fact, depending on how much weight a person has to lose, I may work with them for three-month, six-month, or even year-long increments. But the work we do is the key to lasting success: incorporating real food into their real lives, and designing a personal roadmap to healthy, low-fat choices (that still allows for some fun fattening foods) for each of them. This approach takes longer to get the weight off than any of those quick-fix diets, but it also lasts longer—it lasts forever.

Your body is designed to adapt to changes over a certain period of time. It will respond to a change you ask it to make (such as living on fewer calories) by accepting the assignment, living with it for a little while (what's known as the diet plateau), then, if directed to make another change, adapting once again. But you can't rush your body into accepting changes too quickly. Remember, you're fighting Mother Nature herself when you keep attempting to drop weight fast. And guess what? Mother Nature will win time and time again—causing you to rebound to your old weight and then some—if you don't play by her rules.

And it's not just your body that will rebel. You need time to adjust psychologically to a change in your weight. For a lot of people, quickly dropping thirty, forty, fifty pounds is shocking. Friends and family notice—almost too much, and so much attention, even if it's positive attention, can be disarming. You must give yourself time. Aim for consistency over the long run.

There you have it: the foundation of my philosophy on losing weight.

What comes next are the specifics, guidelines for you to follow so that you don't have to enter another futile diet zone or rip-off weight center or have to take another side trip from your life in order to get leaner and healthier.

Fifteen Keys to Food Happiness

People get so much information every day that they've
lost their common sense.

—Gertrude Stein

1. Count your diets. Count how many times you have restricted your eating. If you have been on more than four diets in your life and not achieved a lasting goal, you are not getting to the crux of the matter. Don't buy the idea that you're a "fat slob by nature." That's the kind of self-hating propaganda that undermines anyone's efforts. Battering your body with quick-fix "diets" will never work—you will always end up back where you started. Resolve right now to lose weight the right way, with a lifetime plan for healthy eating.

2. Consider the *kinds* of foods you're eating. Are they highly processed and laden with preservatives? If so, it's no wonder that your body is not taking kindly to them. You need *real* food: fresh fruits and vegetables, whole grains, legumes, nonfat dairy—food that satisfies your system and keeps it in good working order.

3. Get your facts straight—don't buy the sales pitch. Your body does not get fed the sales pitch on the front of a box, it gets fed the ingredients! The bottom line: Don't read what's on the front of the package, read the ingredients list on the back.

4. Find out what works for you. One week we are bombarded with nutrition news; the next week, everything has changed. What I can say with assurance, though, is that certain foods have been billed as evil and that's just dead wrong. It's true that some people have problems with sugar, salt, alcohol, and chocolate. But what's happened is that the message has gotten out that these foods are bad for *everybody*. You need to find out what foods work for you and which don't. Then decide what you're going to eat.

5. Make your own rules. Get rid of all the old diet "shoulds." All the rules like, "never eat after 6 P.M.," "always eat breakfast," and so on. Chances are, these rules have never worked for you and they probably never will. You need to make your own guidelines, ones that work for your personality. And don't be afraid to live by them. No one cares what your "thing" is with food. People will respect you for trying to eat well.

6. You eat it, you burn it. Learn to burn off what you eat. If you have partied the night before don't get depressed and defeatist. Let your body burn off the extra fuel you've given it. I can't stress enough how important it is to move. Exercise is the *only* way you're going to stay slim and healthy.

Throughout the past decade, experts have stated that you need at least thirty minutes of continual aerobic/cardiovascular exercise, three times a week, to stay fit and keep diseases like arteriosclerosis and even cancer at bay. Thankfully, experts from the Centers for Disease Control and Prevention and the American College of Sports Medicine have begun to revise their exercise recommendations. It's now believed that you can lower your risk of disease as much as 50 percent by accumulating thirty minutes of exercise throughout the day. That is, you don't have to put aside a whole half hour to go for a walk or to work out on a StairMaster; you can break it up, do it piecemeal, a little exercise here, a little there. There are many ways you can get in these thirty minutes—and all without breaking a sweat. What's most important is that *you* fit exercise into *your* daily routine in some fashion so that you get your blood circulating and your heart working.

Don't sit at your desk at lunch, put on your sneakers and take a walk. I especially recommend the stairs—it is kind of like doing a step aerobics class.

7. Don't go too low. Unless you are under a doctor's supervision and following your doctor's orders, never, ever go on any program that limits you to under 1,200 calories per day. Anything less than that is too restrictive and requires control that you probably don't have the time and energy to invest. You need and deserve a respectable amount of calories, if you're going to be happy, satisfied and plan to stick with the plan (exactly how many depends on how much you burn—see #6).

8. Never overhaul your life. Most diets try to get you to make huge changes in your lifestyle. No wonder they never work! What needs to change is not your lifestyle but the food in your world and your understanding of it. Making the small—but right—daily choices is what will make a long-lasting difference in your life. Those choices will add up.

9. Don't be perfect. Not only is it impossible to be perfect, it's boring! Food and joy are synonymous. If you try to be perfect by being "good" at parties or in other social situations, you'll only wind up unhappy. Plus, if you aim for perfection, chances are you'll fail, wind up miserable, and feel as though you're no good. Obviously, this doesn't mean you should stuff your face four nights a week. But do pay attention to the rhythm of your life so that you'll know when significant eating times are going to come up. Then plan for them. Eat well the rest of the time and enjoy the moment.

10. Embrace your plateaus. No one wants to have her weight loss interrupted by a plateau, that point where the pounds won't seem to budge. It can be discouraging, a real diet killer. But we are so inundated with the "lose two pounds a week" pitch that we can't stand it when the body does what it is naturally meant to do.

My advice is to accept your plateaus. Celebrate them even, don't become frustrated or depressed. It's your body's way of telling you that it has accepted this new set point for a week, month, maybe even two months. When it's time to move on and lose the next round, it will let you know. Just keep eating well; don't go back on the promises you made yourself.

11. Consider food your responsibility. If you don't take responsibility for the food in your life, you'll never be lean and healthy. Too many people have taken the attitude, "I'm too stressed to think about food. I don't have the time to cook a good meal. I'll just pick something up on the way home." Don't be a victim of America's fast food mentality. It's up to each of us to bring back good, low-fat, healthy food into our lives.

12. Be an activist consumer. This is where you can really exercise your ability to take responsibility. Make yourself aware and open to the surge of new and worthwhile products the health food industry has to offer. And, by the same token, don't buy foods that are produced without any regard to your health. All food industry advertising is targeted at women. They listen when we want something, so use your dollars to cast your vote. Stop buying junk cereals, breads, crackers, cookies, and soups and the industry will provide us with better ones. The health food industry responded when we said we didn't like our food brown and tasteless. Now let's get the mainstream food industry to start listening up. See Chapter 5 for more on wise ways to spend your hard-earned dollars.

13. Give up "diet foods"—they're junk. Don't try living on diet junk food, what I call fat-free flubber foods. They may help you get pounds off initially, but have you ever looked at the labels? Junk! Chemicals! And this is supposed to better your health? These foods never give the body what it really needs and craves. Live on them and you're just going to end up going back to real food, and probably eating too much of it to make up for lost time. Then, of course, you gain the weight back.

14. Be consistent. I'll say it again. Your body is a machine that understands—and craves—habit. It responds enthusiastically to receiving the same information at regular intervals.

Your appetite is also a function of habit, and what's so bad about that? You've got to retrain your body so that it gets used to different, healthier habits. To do so, you've simply got to be consistent about the new diet you're introducing your body to. Once it gets used to it, your body will crave those good foods. Perhaps you have already tried this in miniature by going from whole milk to low-fat. Remember how bad it tasted at first? Now it probably tastes fine. Your body adapted.

It's for this reason that jumping from diet to diet never works. It confuses the body. You never get a chance to get on track and settle in. Consistency is the best gift you can give your body, and it will give back by becoming efficient and healthy. It works.

15. Take your time. Last, but not at all least, take your time when you are losing weight. Give yourself a year to learn to eat healthy, low-fat foods and to incorporate some regular activity into your life. Stop chasing the great diet machine and you will have a better chance of finding your dream: a good body, good food, and a great life.

Chapter Two

Give Me a Reason:
Why Should I Choose Healthy, Natural Foods?

There is something I want you to ask yourself every time you contemplate consuming a food: *What's in it for me?* Will that food hurt you? Just as important, will it help you or is it just plain detrimental? *What's in it—or not in it—for me?*

Let's face some cold, hard facts about healthful, moderate eating and dieting: Most people don't like it. People all over the world, but especially Americans, prefer to eat junk food. They love fattening food, and they love to eat as much as they want. Ask anyone why and the answer is the same nine times out of ten: It tastes good. And they have a point: junk food and excessively fatty foods taste better than healthy, low-fat foods, especially when junk and fat are all your palate knows. Real cheese tastes better than fat-free cheese; a Big Mac is more inviting than a veggie burger; Coke has a lot more punch than flavored mineral water; and Ben & Jerry's Cherry Garcia ice cream is just insanely better than a fruit-flavored pop. Bummer.

There are distinct lines dividing the many different types of eaters. In one group are those people who eat healthfully—they actually *like* fruits and vegetables and go out of their way to consume them. Then there are those people who scorn the healthy eaters and think that junk food is cute, funny, or "real" food. Last are the people hooked on the latest *diet* junk foods, sold on the notion that eating these foods will transport them to the golden land called Thin. "Here's the ticket," they think, "these foods are satisfying in taste and since they don't have fat or are low in calories they won't make me look bad or ruin my health either." But relying on those foods has backfired for many people.

When I wrote *Food Cop* in 1991, I felt it was my job to educate readers about the excess fats in the foods many of them were eating on a daily basis. At that time most people were still into calorie counting; fat was still a mystery. Now, though, everybody knows a tremendous amount about fat and calories; they know so much, in fact, that some people focus on them to the exclusion of looking at other elements that affect a food's quality. But fat and calories are not the only criteria you should use to choose a food. It's critical to look at what *kinds* of fat grams and what *kinds* of calories you're consuming.

When you choose an apple rather than a candy bar, you get plenty of important nutrients; that, by now, should be pretty obvious. It's common sense. But I also want you to understand why you should reach for something like a natural fat-free cookie from a manufacturer like Jammers or Health Valley over a highly processed fat-free cookie from a company like Snackwell's. It has something to do with nutrients—an important word to think about. These two types of products may both be fat free—and come in chocolate flavor—but they're completely different products.

What's in them for you? I'll tell you. In the natural cookie there are whole grain oats with fiber and B vitamins to keep your body in peak form. There are also dried fruits with iron to help keep your energy level up and complex carbohydrates to satisfy your appetite. The Snackwell's offers you a sugar rush and some empty calories. In other words, not much.

Compare two foods that are seemingly the same and you'll find that they're actually incredibly different. This goes not only for low-calorie foods but for higher-calories ones too—some foods simply offer you more bang for the buck. Take, for example, the much-maligned egg. So many people on diets avoid eggs because of their dietary fat and cholesterol. If you are trying to lower your cholesterol then you are right to limit your intake of eggs, but if you are watching your weight an egg is an excellent choice. Yes, really, and I'll tell you why. For only 5 grams of fat you are getting vitamins A, D, E, protein, zinc, iron, and selenium (nutrients you'll learn about later in this chapter).

These 5 grams of fat are well spent. Five grams of fat from a doughnut, which comes with virtually nothing else of worth, are not 5 grams well spent. See the difference? So as you begin to look at your calories and fat grams, ask how will my body best benefit from this food? What's its value? How are those calories benefiting my body? What does that food do for my hair, skin, heart, nails, energy level, and immune system? It's time that we started to look at these questions as we make our food choices. Science can now give us answers about what Mother Nature has known for centuries: there are reasons we're meant to eat the natural, wholesome foods put on this planet. And when you comprehend those reasons it's far easier to make the right dietary choices.

For many people food has become so confusing that they just give up and eat whatever crosses their path. Clearing up food confusion is a large part of my practice in California. Everyone needs to learn to find a balance between eating mostly healthy, nonfattening foods and the occasional fattening, non-nutritious foods.

The recipes in this book aim to help you find that balance, and there are also lots of great products you can buy in the market that will help you accomplish the task. I'll get to those in the next chapter, but before I do, let's talk about what will help you make the right choices in the first place: *motivation.* I believe that motivation is the major key to adapting or changing anything in your life. So let's talk about what drives you to drink and eat in the manner that you do.

For Vanity's Sake

In our modern age, there are generally two forces that goad people into eating healthy foods. One is the message we receive from the medical front telling us that good food will ensure our good health. The other message comes from the media and diet industry, which play into our sense of vanity by pitching us—at high velocity—the idea that thin is beautiful. "Go on this diet" the message goes, "and you'll look good."

For better or for worse, it's the vanity message that captures most people's attention. Certainly, a minority of people eat healthfully out of good old common sense; they're the group that has kept health food stores alive all these years. Unfortunately, health concerns don't motivate the majority of people unless they themselves have been confronted with a bad health issue, or someone close to them has.

Okay, since vanity is the stronger of the two forces, let's talk about that first. Vanity is the number one reason most people switch over to a healthy diet. Because it's true: if you consistently maintain a low-fat diet of natural, nutritious foods, you will look better. I see it with every client I work with. Within two weeks of changing their diets their faces begin to look younger. The puffiness begins to diminish and their hair and skin glow.

Notice I said that their hair and skin glow and puffiness diminishes. I didn't emphasize the fact that they lost weight—although they did that too. But the point I'm trying to make is that if you're going to eat for vanity, don't just think about your body weight. Any old chemical-filled, nutrient-empty, fat-free diet food can help you slim down, but it's not going to do anything for the rest of you. Looking luminous doesn't come from eating diet junk food.

Plus, it's important to keep weight loss in perspective. Obviously, this book is geared toward helping you lose weight and maintain it. But weight loss and "thinness" are two different things. The one thing I could repeat until I plotz, is to stop shooting for thin. Thin is just not what the Big One ordered when He designed the entire human race. I hope that you will begin to accept your personal body style and natural weight and aim to be the best that *you* can be. Everything in the following chapters and recipes is designed to arm you with what you need to make low-fat choices so that you can achieve this natural set weight. Once you begin to accept that weight you'll end your battle with food and constant dieting. Life is too long to have food be a negative, constant problem. And food is too good to have a hateful relationship with it.

I'd also like to drive home the point that while shooting for a body as taut and lean as a model's or actor's might seem like a reasonable goal, when you're not getting paid for it, or aren't constantly rewarded in any way, you're not likely to stick with a rigid diet. Believe me, I've worked with many celebrities who are successful, rewarded on a regular basis, and highly paid, and even some of them have a hard time sticking with it. Remember that all the great bodies we see in magazines, television, and films are motivated by career maintenance. If that's not what motivates you, this type of vanity may prove to be only a temporary inspirational force.

Accept your given body type and size, eat well, exercise, and enjoy your life. Women are much tougher on themselves than men, particularly when it comes to the "nude scenes" in their lives. The best dose of healthy vanity you can give yourself is to cop the same attitude that Frenchwomen have: "I am woman, therefore I am attractive." It's true.

For Health's Sake

Unfortunately, good health seems only to motivate many people to eat well if they are over thirty-five or forty. Sometimes I do get a client in the early twenties or thirties who is concerned about his or her health, but nine times out of ten it's because a parent or relative has suffered from an illness. Otherwise, health is not a huge concern for the bulk of the population under thirty-five.

But it should be. I wish health were a stronger concern, especially for our children's sake. We need to understand that we don't have to hand down the same physical patterns that made us or our parents suffer.

So many times I've heard it said that America is stuffed on junk and starved of nutrients. It's almost as if our intestines are packed with Styrofoam stuffing. But how do you convince someone that they are suffering nutritionally if they feel great? How do you get the idea across that a whole grain is so much more valuable to your system than one stripped of its bran, germ, and the rest of its nutritional value? That processed foods simply have most of the nutrients processed right out of them? Without being accused of lining up with the health-nut culture of juicers, joggers, macrobiotic munchers, super-vegetarians, wheat-grass weirdos, and Adelle Davis do-wells, how do you teach someone that it's really worth it to choose a natural cereal over Cocoa Puffs, turkey breast over salami, baked tortilla chips over the Chee•tos? Let *me* tell you.

When your concern is to eat for your health, you will automatically lower your fat, sugar, salt, and processed food intake. And yes, yes, yes, your palate and tastes will change and adapt to the healthier foods. Everyone who has made the transition will tell you that you can actually lose your cravings for things you thought you couldn't live without. One day you'll wake up and that Coke will taste way too sweet to you (really!), that burger will just look like a pound of grease, unappetizing, and although the Snackwell's cookie will still taste good, it won't be worth it. If you'll brave your way through healthy eating for about six weeks, what you'll find at the end of the road is a body that will satisfy your vanity, feel better, and more than likely even live longer, too.

The Vanity and Health Nutrients

No matter what motivates you to eat well, the more information you have about the nutrients you need to do so, the better off you'll be. Here I zero in on the vitamins and minerals that affect the way you look and feel the most. As it happens, the nutrients that cater to your vanity are often also the ones that keep you healthy, too. What's going on outside your body often mirrors what's going on inside: If your hair lacks luster and your skin is sallow, chances are your health is not at its peak either. So keep in mind that when you're eating for peaches-and-cream skin you'll also be eating to fight disease and prolong your life.

Here's Looking at You

Eat wholesome, natural foods and you'll have wholesome, natural, beautiful skin, hair, and nails. That's mostly because healthy foods contain the big vanity three: *vitamins A, C, and E.* You might think of them like the primary colors, yellow, red, and blue—just about everything that happens within your body is based on them. Without A, C, and E other nutrients can't do their work.

The big three are all also antioxidants, substances that deactivate free radicals, molecules that do damage to the cells—including skin cells. In fact, I like to think of the word "antioxidant" as "antirusting" because antioxidants are thought to reduce wrinkling caused by ultraviolet light.

The antioxidants affect your looks in a host of other ways. Vitamin C, for instance, beautifies the skin by aiding in the formation and preservation of collagen, a substance that provides elasticity and keeps the complexion looking young. Without ample C—and it can be depleted by things like stress as well as aspirin and certain over-the-counter medications—your hair can become lackluster, your teeth and gums may not stay healthy looking, and you can even get hangnails. (Try to have something with vitamin C at least three times throughout the day; more if you are under stress or taking medication.)

Besides its free-radical–quenching duties, that other hall-of-famer, vitamin E, helps oxygen travel through your bloodstream, ensuring that you have good color in your cheeks. In combination with the mineral *selenium*, another antioxidant, it also helps preserve the elasticity of your skin.

Vitamin A, which sometimes comes in the form of a substance you've undoubtedly heard a lot about, *beta carotene* (the body converts beta carotene into vitamin A), also has untold effects on your looks. It can, for instance, affect the rate of your nail growth (as can *calcium*). It, too, helps keep locks lustrous and, like C, helps keep your teeth and gums healthy.

Antioxidants, though, aren't the only vanity nutrients. *Zinc* and the *B vitamins* aid in the formation of the skin and are essential for healing wounds and burns—including sunburn. *Protein*, of course, is the major source of the building materials for almost the entire body, including the skin, hair, nails, and muscles.

Feel as Good as You Look

I'll bet you wish you had a penny for each time you've heard that over a million Americans die of heart disease every year. Then count how many times you've heard that it can be prevented, if not reversed, by changing your diet and exercising. Unlike other fatal diseases, heart disease responds almost immediately to diet improvements—a small price for a big pay-off: A healthy heart means a healthy circulatory system, which benefits all the organs, since many nutrients are carried through the bloodstream to various parts of the body. The circulatory system also carries the oxygen to the brain, helping to keep your nervous system operating properly.

If you are severely overweight (more than 45 or 50 pounds), it's a good bet that your heart and circulatory system are not functioning at their best. Have your doctor examine you and make sure to get your cholesterol levels checked. More than likely your doctor will tell you to exercise and change your diet. So as you do the latter—and even if you're not overweight and haven't received doctor's orders to alter your dietary habits—keep these nutrients in mind: *vitamin C, selenium,* and *zinc,* which are necessary for the maintenance of your arteries, helping to protect them against arteriosclerosis; *magnesium* to help regulate your heartbeat; and *soluble fiber,* a heart saver, which helps lower LDL (bad) cholesterol levels. (*Insoluble fiber* is important for another reason: prevention of colon and rectal cancer.)

For heart health, also stick to *monounsaturated and polyunsaturated fats,* the ones that don't raise cholesterol levels (see Chapter 4) and make sure to include *vitamin E* and *folic acid* in your diet in good supply. Recent studies have shown that these may be two of the most important vitamins for preventing heart disease.

When it comes to health, you'll also do well to protect yourself against the effects of stress. Stress is the word of the nineties, and rightly so: our crazy lives can really take a toll on our health. Stress, for instance, is thought to decrease the body's immune function, leaving you open to the next floating virus that sneezes through your door. When you are under stress your body releases more adrenaline than usual, which can play havoc with your metabolism, meanwhile depleting your system of essential nutrients like *vitamin C, potassium,* and *phosphorus.* Emotional stress, in particular, can set your system askew, so now is the time to really eat with your health in mind.

Calcium and *magnesium* are important antistress nutrients because they help the brain release the neurotransmitter serotonin, which gives the body a feeling of well-being. Magnesium also helps regulate the heartbeat, helping to keep you calmer.

Calcium, of course, also plays a role in keeping your bones strong. Strong bones may not be something you are currently thinking about, but it will be of major importance as you get older. According to the National Institutes of Health, osteoporosis is the fourth leading cause of death in women today. Most women can prevent this disease of brittle bones and hunched backs by getting a sufficient amount of calcium. Men should be wary too—they're not immune to the disease, although they are less susceptible.

Prevention is the key to maintaining bone density for everyone as they grow older. So I don't want you to take the issue of calcium lightly, or try and slip it in under the rug by just popping supplements. Keep in mind that women need a minimum of 1,000 milligrams calcium per day (the RDA for men is 800) and that calcium is best absorbed into your system when it comes hand-in-hand with *vitamin D*. The best sources of the two are milk products, so I encourage you to add more 1 percent and nonfat milk to your daily diet. One 8-ounce glass of skim or 1 percent milk gives you about 300 milligrams of calcium, so it's worth it. If I could ever give you a reason to drop the powdered coffee creamers and start to add milk to your coffee or tea, this is it.

The last nutrients I want to mention have to do with reproductive health. As a woman menstruates she loses *iron*, and often, as a result, energy too. Stock your diet with iron-rich foods to stave off fatigue, and keep up with your *B vitamins*—they help regulate hormone production and relieve some of the tension caused by PMS. Men need the Bs, too, in particular *folic acid*, which assists in the production of sperm. (Folic acid has also been linked to prevention of heart disease and cancer, so it's a particularly important B.) Selenium and zinc are also needed in good supply because a zinc deficiency can result in infertile sperm, and selenium, lost during ejaculation, needs to be replenished.

Getting the Nutrients You Need

Now that you know all that you need, how do you get it? How will you remember all those As, Bs, and Cs?

Don't worry. Packing all those nutrients mentioned in the preceding paragraphs is not as complicated as so many professionals make it seem. In fact, it's really very simple—and you don't need to pop all kinds of vitamins and mineral supplements to achieve nutritional nirvana either. If, that is, you don't go below 1,200 calories a day. I say so in the preceding chapter and this is one of the reasons: to get all the nutrients you need, you have to eat enough food.

Sure, supplements can be a great *addition* to a healthy diet, but they are there to enhance and assist the foods you eat; they do not make up for a diet of nutritionally empty junk food. The idea that to be healthy or thin you should take a pill has never worked and never will.

What follows are good *food* sources of all the vanity and health nutrients I've been telling you about. The best approach is to plump up your diet with as many of these nutrient-rich foods as possible. As you'll see in the next chapter—on how to eat by my (not the USDA's) pyramid plan—they all fit into a well-balanced diet.

Vitamin A Think orange-red and deep green, that's where you'll usually find beta carotene (which the body converts to vitamin A) hiding out. Sources: cantaloupes, mangoes, nectarines, papaya, tomatoes, sweet potatoes, red bell peppers, raw spinach, leafy greens, broccoli, green beans.

B Vitamins These vitamins, usually lumped together because they work together, include folic acid, thiamin, niacin, riboflavin, vitamin B6, and vitamin B12. Sources: green leafy vegetables, green beans, corn, alfalfa sprouts, bean sprouts, brewer's yeast, whole grain breads and cereals, eggs, lean meats, dairy products.

Vitamin C Try to have something with vitamin C at least three times a day, more if you're taking aspirin or medication or are under stress, all of which can deplete C. Sources: oranges, grapefruit, kiwi, strawberries, cantaloupe, watermelon, pineapple, tomatoes, red and green bell peppers, red cabbage, snow peas.

Calcium Dairy products are, of course, the prime source of calcium, but you can also get the mineral from other sources. Go for kale, spinach, dark leafy greens, canned salmon, sardines, and tofu processed with calcium sulfate.

Vitamin D Fortunately, the body manufactures this nutrient on its own after being exposed to sunlight. But all milk is also fortified with D (some cereals are, too), and you can get it by consuming fish and eggs.

Vitamin E Getting this nutrient is a little tricky for people watching their fat intake—it's usually found in fatty foods. Try to vary your intake with both nonfat and fat-containing foods. Sources: dark leafy greens, spinach, asparagus, egg yolks, wheat germ, all vegetable oils, nuts, and seeds.

Insoluble fiber All whole fruits and vegetables contain insoluble fiber, but bananas and apples are particularly good sources. Other sources: beans, whole grain (corn, wheat, rye, barley) breads, cereals, and anything made with whole grain flours.

Iron The kind of iron most readily absorbed by the body comes from animal foods. However, you can still rely on vegetarian sources; just make sure that you eat a lot of them. Where the iron is: eggs, fish and poultry, organ meats, molasses, green leafy vegetables, dried fruits, and cherry juice. To make an iron-rich hot "toddy," try adding a teaspoon of molasses and a teaspoon of honey to a glass of skim milk; microwave for a few seconds to warm.

Magnesium Magnesium deficiencies are rare, but it doesn't hurt to bone up on this mineral. Sources: seafood, whole grains, dark leafy greens, molasses, nuts. Try using a little molasses on your bagel, toast, or cereal in the morning (mix it with honey if you don't like the taste) or add a little to the batter when you're baking cookies and muffins.

Phosphorus Soft drinks are a source of phosphorus, but not one you want to depend on (drink too many and you'll get too much phosphorus, which can sap bone strength). Instead go for: lean meats, fish, poultry, whole grains, vegetables, beans, eggs.

Potassium This mineral can be found in oranges, bananas, dried fruits, lean meats, poultry, dairy products. The easiest way to make sure you get enough potassium is to keep bananas in your office or around the house at all times. You'll get the nutrient you need and be less likely to snack on junky sweets.

Protein Choose the leanest sources of protein you can find; e.g., white meat poultry without the skin, seafood, lean meats, egg whites, nonfat dairy products, beans. Grains also contain some protein. If you're a vegetarian who finds it hard to get enough protein in your diet, look for precooked beans and lentils in convenient healthy cup o' soups and in cans. Toss them into salads, or just mix with rice sprinkled with a little hot sauce for flavor.

Selenium This mineral is found in many vegetables, but there's no telling how much a vegetable contains because it depends on the soil it was grown in. Other sources: shrimp, tuna, herring, eggs, wheat germ, whole grains, sesame seeds. To sneak a little more selenium into your diet, toss chopped hard-boiled eggs into your salad.

Soluble fiber Most fruits contain soluble fiber, but especially good sources include apples, blackberries, and the white pith of citrus. Other sources: beans, oat bran, wheat bran, rice bran, raisins, whole grain (corn, wheat, rye, barley) breads, cereals, and anything made with whole grain flours.

Unsaturated and monounsaturated fats It's easy to get the moderate amounts of unsaturated fats you need in your diet: they're found in lean meats, poultry, seafood, nuts, seeds, and vegetable oils. You want to aim mostly, though, for monounsaturated fats, found in olive, canola, peanut, almond and avocado oils, olives and avocados. What you *don't* want are unhealthy saturated fats abundant in fatty meats, whole-milk dairy products, palm and coconut oils, and hydrogenated oils and margarines. (See Chapter 4 for a complete rundown on fats.)

Zinc Most people have (wisely) cut back on red meats, but unfortunately red meat is also an excellent source of zinc. It can, however, also be found in: wheat germ (sprinkle it on your cereal, add to your baking, and toss it into turkey burgers, chicken burgers, and turkey meatloaf for a nutty flavor), fish such as herring and tuna, oysters, shrimp, chicken, eggs, chickpeas, red kidney beans, pumpkin and sunflower seeds, mushrooms, soybeans. For a zinc-saturated meal, have some roasted oysters over a salad of baby greens.

Do yourself and your body a favor. Remember all the reasons that you should choose the most nutritious foods possible, even if it's a simple choice between whole grain and white bread. The payback for choosing natural, healthy low-fat products over junk is that you'll look and feel great. It's worth it.

Chapter Three

What to Eat and How Much: Refining the Pyramid Eating Plan

In the preceding chapters I've talked about some keys to slimming down and maintaining weight loss. I've talked about some foods that can help you look better and some that can help you stay healthy. Those are all *components* of a smart eating plan; now let's look at the big picture. How do you work the keys to living slim and the foods you need for good looks and good health into your daily diet?

One of the nicest things the government has done for us lately was to develop the pyramid eating plan. Thought up by the U.S. Department of Agriculture, the pyramid, pictured on the next page, is an at-a-glance guide to nutritious eating geared toward helping you get in heaping amounts of grains, fruits, and vegetables while moderating your intake of fat and protein.

One of the things I like about it is that it incorporates all kinds of foods. I've always been an advocate of eating all of the natural food groups. Frankly, I hate diets based on the idea that by eliminating a food group you have a guaranteed road to good health. The notion that leaving out all dairy, eliminating sugar, or never letting certain other foods cross your lips will cure you of all ills is simply someone's opinion, not fact, and has never been proven scientifically. I myself do not eat red meat, but that's my personal choice. That choice may not be right for everyone. Likewise, some people like to cook with fats—I don't advocate it, but that doesn't mean I expect you never to use them again. The USDA recognizes that there's a place for all natural foods and its pyramid helps make that clear.

That's the good news.

The so-so news is that, in my opinion, the USDA pyramid doesn't relate to our real eating habits. Now, it's certainly a vast improvement over the old four-food-groups structure that governed our eating habits for so long. (You remember the old box, which by virtue of its equal-size sections—one for fruits and vegetables; one for meat, poultry, and seafood; one for grain foods; and one for dairy products—indicated that we should eat the same amount of everything.) Yet the problem with the pyramid is that, just like so many other

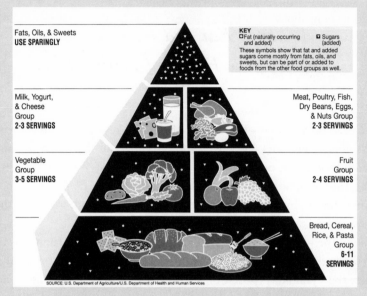

Food Guide Pyramid
A Guide to Daily Food Choices

Fats, Oils, & Sweets
USE SPARINGLY

KEY
□ Fat (naturally occurring and added)   ▨ Sugars (added)
These symbols show that fat and added sugars come mostly from fats, oils, and sweets, but can be part of or added to foods from the other food groups as well.

Milk, Yogurt, & Cheese Group
2-3 SERVINGS

Meat, Poultry, Fish, Dry Beans, Eggs, & Nuts Group
2-3 SERVINGS

Vegetable Group
3-5 SERVINGS

Fruit Group
2-4 SERVINGS

Bread, Cereal, Rice, & Pasta Group
6-11 SERVINGS

SOURCE: U.S. Department of Agriculture/U.S. Department of Health and Human Services

WHAT'S A SERVING ACCORDING TO THE USDA PYRAMID?

GRAIN FOODS: 6–11 PER DAY
1 slice of bread; 1/2 cup cooked rice, pasta, or cereal; 1 ounce cereal

VEGETABLES: 3–5 PER DAY
1/2 cup chopped raw or cooked vegetables; 1 cup leafy raw greens

FRUITS: 2–4 PER DAY
1 piece of fruit or melon wedge; 3/4 cup juice; 1/2 cup canned fruit; 1/4 cup dried fruit

DAIRY PRODUCTS: 2–3 SERVINGS
1 cup milk or yogurt; 1 1/2 to 2 ounces of cheese

PROTEIN FOODS: 2–3 PER DAY
2 1/2 to 3 ounces cooked lean meat, poultry, or fish; 1/2 cup cooked beans; 1 egg

FATS, OILS, SWEETS—USE SPARINGLY

eating strategies offered up by health professionals, it doesn't bridge the gap between an ideal nutritional world and the real world; it doesn't jibe with most people's real-life eating habits. As it stands, the pyramid gives you information only about the foods stocked on the perimeters of our supermarkets. True, those foods, mainly dairy, meats and poultry, and produce, are mostly healthy and natural. But it's the foods in the middle section of the market—processed foods—that fill most people's carts and the USDA pyramid gives you no idea what to do about those.

What I want to give you is an approach to eating that will be that "bridge over dietary waters." I've come up with my *own* pyramid plan, one that I believe is better suited to most people's lifestyles and is even healthier than the one suggested by the USDA.

Yolanda's Pyramid

The first tier: fruits and vegetables. The USDA has placed grain foods on its bottom tier; I believe the bottom should belong to fruits and vegetables. Of all foods, it's produce that we should be eating the most of, but right now it's the food group that's most neglected.

Fruits and vegetables taste good and are good for you. Five to six servings

junk food, processed food, diet sodas, sodas, foods with empty calories, **(1 per day if needed)**

fats, oils, sweets, nuts, seeds, **(sparingly)**

low-fat dairy **(2 servings)**

non-fat dairy or fat free **(2 servings)**

grains, cereals, rice, bread, **(3 times per day only and one serving at each meal)**

meats, poultry, fish, beans, **(2-3 servings but 6-8 oz., at two of your meals)**

fruits & vegetables- **(as much as you like, at least five times a day)** of fruits and vegetables, the amount the USDA recommends, is a nice number to ask for, but I say eat even more. Always top your cereal with a banana or berries. Cut up melon, put it in an airtight container, and bring it to work so you have a healthy snack and don't head for the vending machine. Eat big salads for lunch, fill sandwiches with grilled vegetables. When you order a sandwich at a restaurant and it comes with fruit on the side, eat the fruit first before you're too full. Make two vegetable side dishes for dinner, not just one. You really can't eat too many vegetables.

Luckily for vegetable haters and fruit snubbers, though, a serving size is smaller than you might think. One medium apple, ½ cup of cooked fruits or vegetables, or ¾ cup fruit juice all equal one serving. So having lettuce and sliced tomato on your sandwich counts. Topping your frozen yogurt with fruit counts. The banana on your cereal counts, as do the applesauce on your toast and onions on your burger—all these little additions count, so slip them in.

The second tier (left side): grains, breads, cereals, rice, pasta, potatoes. Many people are now finding that a fat-free diet hasn't helped them lose weight. What does that have to do with starchy carbohydrates like grain foods? Plenty. One of the main reasons Americans can't lose weight is because they are eating too much starch, coated with sugar and/or salt. You can't expect to eat tons of pasta or rice and lose weight, especially if you're *sedentary*. These foods may be nutritious and fat free, but they still contain calories. Thus, six to eleven servings a day is quite a bit, particularly since no one really measures a serving. Someone thinking her morning bagel is one serving of grain food may be surprised to learn that in fact it's equal to two servings. This sets the stage for overeating. I think three servings a day of grain foods is plenty.

The second tier (right side): meats, poultry, fish, beans, eggs. The USDA recommends that you eat two to three servings (2.5–3 ounces) of protein daily. I disagree. I've never been an advocate of a low-protein diet, and recommend that you eat two to three larger servings (6–8 ounces) of protein daily. If you stop to consider how important satiety is to losing and maintaining your weight, then limiting protein intake to small amounts is a mistake. I understand that by limiting your intake of animal foods you also limit your intake of saturated fat; however, if you make wise protein choices you can still eat more than the USDA suggests and stay well below the limit for saturated fat.

Let's be realistic here. As long as you are having lean protein and it doesn't take you over the calories and fat limit you've set for yourself, then have your protein. Because it's very satisfying it will help you stick with a healthy diet and dampen your desire to binge.

The third tier: low-fat and nonfat dairy products. I want to emphasize that milk and milk products are very healthy and satisfying, and recommend that you eat more dairy: Where the USDA says 1 ounce, I believe a more practical 3 ounces of a low-fat or nonfat milk product are in order. Tiny serving sizes of dairy seems unrealistic to me. I have yet to meet the person who consistently limits their portions to one slice of cheese, or ½ cup of cottage cheese.

The fourth tier: fats, oils, sweets, nuts, and seeds. I am in complete agreement with the USDA: Fats, oils, and sweets should be used sparingly (and I detail why in the following chapter). One thing to think about when you do spend your allotted fat grams—I believe 30 to 40 grams per day should be your maximum whether you're a man or a woman—spend them on fats that have some nutritional value, like the 5 grams of fat in an egg, or the 2.5 grams in a glass of 1 percent milk, both of which come with a bevy of nutrients. Even a teaspoon of olive oil has something to offer, by way of potentially lowering your cholesterol.

I have also added nuts and seeds to this category (the USDA lumps them with the protein foods) because, for little guys, they carry a lot of fat (3.5 ounces = about 40 to 50 fat grams) and it can really add up. They also provide nutrients like selenium, zinc, and vitamin E, so they're healthy, but do use them sparingly.

The fifth tier: junk food and highly processed foods. I've added a top tier to my pyramid because I think these foods should be in a category of their own. They, more than any other foods, should be limited in all diets. One serving a day is actually more than I want to see anyone consume, but it allows for the occasional piece of candy, cookie, or snack that you feel you just have to have. That serving size doesn't mean a whole bag of fries, or all the processed fat-free cookies you can eat. A reasonable serving size is generally about the size of your palm or, if the food comes in individual pieces, then no more than three.

Keep in mind . . .

Both my version of the pyramid and the USDA pyramid are general guidelines, not specifics. Make sure that you fulfill these guidelines with healthy foods and maintain a calorie and fat intake suited to your level of activity.

Chapter Four

We Love 'Em, We Hate 'Em: America's Fat, Sugar, and Alcohol Dilemma

There is nothing that Americans love more than fat, sugar, and alcohol. There is nothing that Americans struggle with more than fat, sugar, and alcohol. We want them, but we shouldn't have them. Or should we?

Inherently, none of the "big three" is so bad. The trouble is, too many people consume them in excessive amounts. But even if you don't have a tendency to go overboard, you've probably been overwhelmed by the flood of conflicting information; every diet expert seems to have a different idea about how much of each is healthy.

I've been listening to all of them, weighing opinions, reading studies, searching out the facts to come up with my own philosophy on the subject. But more than that, I've been paying close attention to my clients to see what happens to their bodies when they eat fat and sugar and drink alcohol. I like to listen to what people are really going to do, really going to eat, and how they live—the "let's get real" approach. So what I'm about to tell you regarding the big three comes from what I've witnessed and studied; it's not just theory.

Just the Fats, Ma'am

Some people say that fat-free foods, this whole "no-fat thing," is just another fad. I say it's not. A good deal of scientific evidence shows that excess consumption of fat may be linked to a number of chronic diseases, including obesity, diabetes, heart disease and certain kinds of cancer. What's more, studies suggest that reducing fat in the diet helps prevent some of these diseases. That makes it pretty clear that if you want to have a long, healthy life you have to get the fat out of your diet. The questions that lurk, though, are how much fat do you have to get rid of? How much should be saturated fat, monounsaturated fat, and polyunsaturated fat? Do you need to go completely fat free?

Lose All the *Added* Fat

The answer to the last question is a big NO. When I wrote my first book, *Food Cop*, I said that people who wanted to lose weight should eliminate all *added* oils and other fats from their diets, and I still feel the same way. But this doesn't mean that you have to go completely fat free. The truth is, there really is no such thing as a fat-free diet. Fish, poultry, lean meats, whole grains, legumes, and even vegetables have some fat, which is a good thing—the body needs it. Fat supplies essential fatty acids that the body can't make itself. These fatty acids help transport vitamins A, D, E, and K, which, among other things, help keep a woman's reproductive system working properly as well as our skin and hair glowing and healthy.

Yet, while you need fat, you don't need a lot of it. Some researchers believe that the body does fine with as little as 7 to 10 percent of calories devoted to fat. Nonetheless, studies have shown that the average American derives about 36 to 42 percent of his or her total daily calories from fat. The current dietary guidelines endorsed by groups like the American Heart Association recommend limiting fat intake to 30 percent of calories.

I don't, however, agree. Frankly, these groups feel that asking Americans to go below 30 percent is unrealistic. But with all the great new products available today, I think it's *very* realistic. The time has come for us to realize that this is the way of the future. In this sedentary world, we simply cannot afford to eat a lot of fat.

What is the bottom line? How much fat should you eat? If you want to lose weight you should barely eat any *added fats* at all; if you're trying to maintain your weight, you can eat a little bit more. By "added" fats, I mean oils or fats like butter and lard added to your cooking or mixed into products you buy. I'd say 10 to 20 percent of calories as fat is a good number to aim for, but I hesitantly make such a generalization. It really is an individual matter.

Consider, for example, the needs of a slim, young seventeen-year-old boy on the high school track team. His body is using both fat and carbohydrates to fuel his workouts; he's going to need more fat than someone who is slightly overweight and has a desk job. However, as he grows older and cuts back on intensive training (you know the story—gets a real job, settles down, gets stressed out), he too will probably need to cut back on his fat intake.

You have to be the judge of what's right for you. If you're holding on to body fat, you're probably eating too many calories, or at least consuming more than your body is burning. Obviously, you don't get all your calories

from fat, but fat is *calorie dense*—1 gram has 9 calories, while 1 gram of carbohydrate and protein have only 4 calories each. If you're eating too many
calories, you're probably eating too much fat.

What Kinds of Fat?

There is also the matter of what *kind* of fats you should eat. Most fatty foods
contain primarily three different kinds of fat: saturated fat, monounsaturated
fat, and polyunsaturated fat. But while saturated fat has been shown to promote heart disease and raise cholesterol—even more than dietary cholesterol—the latter two fats have been shown to *lower* overall cholesterol levels.

There are actually two kinds of cholesterol in the body that doctors worry
about: low-density lipoproteins (LDL), aka "bad" cholesterol because it's in-
dicative of the amount of plaque deposited on the arteries, and high-density
lipoproteins (HDL), aka "good" cholesterol because it *guards against* plaque.
You want to maintain a low overall blood cholesterol level (under 200 milligrams according to the National Cholesterol Education Program), but also
aim for low LDL levels (less than 130 milligrams) and *high* HDL levels (40
to 50 milligrams).

I know this may sound complicated, but understanding the various cholesterol levels may also help you understand why some fats are better than
others. Saturated fat raises overall cholesterol levels as well as LDL cholesterol levels. It coagulates in your arteries. Polyunsaturated fat lowers total
cholesterol levels, LDL levels *and* HDL levels (the ones you want to raise).
So while these fats are beneficial in some ways, they're far from perfect.
Monounsaturated fat seems to be the best of all because it lowers overall cholesterol levels and LDL levels without lowering the good HDL levels.

I'll reiterate that I'm the biggest proponent of using no added fats and
keeping consumption of natural fats to a minimum. That said, when you do
eat fat, do your utmost to make it something other than saturated fat. According to most health organizations, only 10 percent of the fat you eat
should be saturated fat. I believe maintaining that level of saturated fat in
your diet is fine if you're an athlete or growing child (an *active* growing child).
But if you're neither you should try to avoid saturated fats entirely just to be
on the safe side. This is particularly important if you're on a weight loss or
maintenance program.

Where does saturated fat lurk? Like dietary cholesterol (which is found
only in animal products), high percentages of saturated fat are contained in
meat, poultry, whole dairy products, and eggs. (See chart, on next page, for
other sources of saturated as well as polyunsaturated and monounsaturated

fats.) The truth is, you'd have to be a complete vegan to avoid saturated fat. Eat, say, a lean chicken breast, and you're going to get a little of it. But very little of it because you're choosing the least fatty version of an animal food. The fattier the type of animal food you choose—a big, thick, juicy steak, for example—the more saturated fat you're going to end up with in your diet.

WHERE THE FAT IS

SOURCES HIGH IN:

saturated fat	coconut and palm oils; beef, pork, lamb; eggs, butter, whole milk, cheese, ice cream; hydrogenated oils, margarine
polyunsaturated fat	corn, soybean, safflower, sunflower, and sesame oils; tuna, salmon, mackerel
monounsaturated fat	olive, canola, peanut, and almond oils; olives

---

The Butter Versus Margarine Debate

What about the most often cited sources of fat, butter and margarine? Butter is just plain old bad-for-you saturated fat; margarine, though, has always enjoyed a glossier reputation. Yet I must tell you that when I started counseling clients about their diets years ago, I was antimargarine. Today, it looks like my instincts were correct. Perhaps you've heard the words "trans fatty acids" being batted around. Trans fatty acids are the by-products of hydrogenation. The process of hydrogenation, which is how margarine is made, calls for adding hydrogen atoms to liquid oils in order to make them solid and less likely to go rancid. But hydrogenation also "saturates" fats so that even those derived from vegetables take on the LDL cholesterol-raising characteristics of animal-based saturated fat. At least that's what scientists suspect so far, and why take chances?

Rather than butter *or* margarine, I prefer to cook with vegetable oil sprays, which just barely glaze the pan. They give you just enough fat for flavor and preventing foods from sticking, but not so much as to add lots of calories or health hazards to a meal. I'll talk more about them in Chapter 5.

Let's Keep Olive Oil in Perspective

The healthier choice we've all been hearing about, of course, is olive oil. Virgin or not, it still has a great reputation. Olive oil, like canola and peanut oils, is high in monounsaturated fat, the kind that lowers overall cholesterol levels and bad LDL levels *without* lowering the good HDL levels. When you eat this type of fat it stays "liquid"—that is, it doesn't coagulate and become solid—which is why it can kind of Roto-Rooter through the LDL cholesterol, helping to clear your arteries.

Though olive oil and other monounsaturated fats might be considered good for you, they are still fat. They may be great for your arteries but not for your waist, hips, or thighs. If you are trying to get the padding off your body don't add oil, even olive oil, to your food. Use an olive-flavored vegetable spray for the flavor. And even if you're not trying to slim down, keep your oil intake to a minimum. Regardless of whether a fat is saturated, monounsaturated, or polyunsaturated, it has 9 calories per gram—9 calories that your body has no trouble converting into body fat, a task it finds much easier than to convert carbohydrates or protein. (Think about it, dietary fat is already much like body fat, while protein and carbohydrates have a very different chemical structure.)

Believe me, leaving these oils behind is easier than you think. Yes, it takes some adjustment. But I truly find it amazing that some people complain about giving up olive oil or butter, but think nothing of the alternative. Allow a plastic surgeon to insert a tube into their thighs and suck out the fat? Okay. Have their stomach stapled, jaws wired shut? Sure. Take all kinds of pills and have sheep's urine shot into their bloodstream (one of the more appalling Hollywood fat remedies)? No problem. Take diet pills with unknown side effects, diuretics, and laxatives? Absolutely. Starve themselves into bitchiness? Every other month. Play follow the leader with Oprah? Sounds good (until they realize what a personal chef costs). But give up oils and other fats? Don't think so, too hard.

Well, you've got me. It's been the easiest thing I've ever done. You'll be amazed at how quickly your body changes its habits. Trust me. After you try all the ways to prepare food without fat according to the recipes I include in this book, as well as trying some of the products I recommend, you'll see what I mean.

Flubber Foods—the Fats That Will Never Get You Thin

When I go into schools to give talks to students, I often bring a few props. To show the kids what fat substitutes are like I start by making yogurt from scratch. There are three basic ingredients: water, yogurt culture, and nonfat dry milk powder. Then I start to add the things that are in many of our yogurts today, like added starches and sugars. Next I add a big glop of hair gel to the yogurt. Their inevitable response is "Yuuuuck!" and who could blame them? "Yuuuuck" is just the way I feel about chemical fat substitutes or, if you will, flubber foods.

When the public demanded that fat be removed from products, the food industry went straight into their kitchens—oops! I mean straight into their laboratories—and came up with fat substitutes that they hoped would match the taste and texture of real fats. They don't. Most of them taste terrible and they're full of chemicals. Plus, because they don't have the qualities of real fat, the food producers have had to add more sugar and salt to products to cover up the lack of flavor in the fake fats. When you buy a flubber-laced food, you're usually getting a lot of junk, but you'll never know it unless you read the ingredients list.

For example, you probably think you're doing the right thing by pouring fat-free dressing on your salad. But take a look at the actual ingredients of a popular brand of fat-free Italian salad dressing: *Water, corn syrup, sugar, vinegar, modified food starch, natural flavor, salt, cellulose gel, xanthan gum, citric acid, artificial color, potassium sorbate, calcium disodium EDTA, lactic acid, egg whites, phosphoric acid, carrageenan, propylene glycol alginate, mustard, flour, spice.* Basically, you have water, lots of sugar, vinegar, starch, salt, the flubber, and some more additives and flavorings.

Now compare that to the ingredients of a fat-free salad dressing from a natural foods store: *Water, organic apple cider vinegar, organic grape juice concentrate, organic garlic, organic onions, sea salt, organic basil, organic oregano, herbs and spices, xanthan gum.*

The natural food is, well, more natural. Although both use xanthan gum, a natural fat substitute derived from the bacteria on cabbage leaves, the mass-market product also includes lots of ingredients that are laboratory formulated. Cellulose gels, for instance, are chemically altered substances. Not the kind of stuff you want to be putting into your body. Keep in mind that these products are created not by chefs but by "nutritional scientists," experts in the lab, not the kitchen.

There are some fat substitutes out there already that really aren't so bad;

you might even consider them a godsend. One of the newest is called Opta-Grade. It's made from cornstarch (hey, Grandma used it to thicken gravies, how bad could it be?) and maltodextrin. Maltodextrin sounds scary, but in fact it's an enzyme derived from corn, potato, wheat, or tapioca, and it's considered natural. OptaGrade is used in some sour creams, yogurts, cheeses, mayonnaise, salad dressings, and frozen desserts.

Many cooks and natural food companies are replacing fat in baked goods with powdered fruit fibers from apples, prunes, and figs, which provide moistness. As I will mention in many of my recipes there are now some great, natural fat substitutes for baking based on fruit purees. And, besides xanthan, there are other natural gums that I think are reasonable: guar, alginate, locust bean, and carrageenan (a seaweed derivative). When a food that normally contains fat is advertised as fat free, look for these kinds of substitutes and try to avoid the ones made by "mad scientists."

Sugar Is Sweet

It's common opinion that you shouldn't eat sugar if you're trying to lose weight and that you shouldn't have sugar, period. In my opinion, that's not true and somewhat unfair; "sugar" is an umbrella term used to describe a lot of different kinds of sweet stuff, but we've come to think of it as meaning only processed white granulated sugar.

Sugars are simple carbohydrates found in dozens of foods, including fruits and vegetables. In their pure form they are called such things as glucose (also known as dextrose), maltose, fructose, lactose, and sugar alcohols called sorbitol and xylitol. Of course, there are also honey, maple syrup, molasses, rice syrup, corn syrup, and fruit sugars like date sugar. Aside from a different molecular makeup, what differentiates these simple carbohydrates from complex carbohydrates (the kind found in such foods as pasta and potatoes) is that they don't usually come accompanied by any vitamins, minerals, or other essential nutrients. That's why sugar calories are known as "empty" calories.

Sugar, though, plays an important role in eating. We have taste buds especially designed for sweetness, and they like to be satisfied. What we *don't* need is sugar in everything we eat all day long, especially if we are trying to retrain our habits. Many of the fat-free products on the market now are packed with extra amounts of sugar to make up for the loss of fat. So pay attention to the ingredients—not the packaging! Sugar doesn't have a lot of calories—only 16 per teaspoon—however, if you eat enough of it, the calories add up. A product can have 0 grams fat but still be fattening if it has a lot of sugar.

Good examples of this are the fig and other dried fruit cookies on the market now. Their labels shout "fat free," not surprisingly, because dried fruit doesn't have any fat. Because it's moist, the cookie surrounding that dried fruit doesn't really need fat either. But dried fruit *is* high in concentrated fruit sugar. If you eat too many of these cookies you're not going to be free of any fat on your body. Treat your treats as they should be treated: something to eat once in a while.

What Kinds of Sugar

Okay, so you're going to eat sugar sometimes, and I use it in my dessert recipes. What kinds are okay? Is honey better than granulated cane sugar? Many people say that a sugar is a sugar is a sugar; your body can't really tell the difference. But years ago, they also said a calorie is a calorie, and now they tell us that the body is more likely to store fat calories than calories from other sources. So go figure. Personally, I think that natural sugars (like honey) are probably better for you than refined sugars. In my mind, anything heavily processed is just plain bad for you. And the only thing that processes honey is the bee; maple syrup is processed by trees.

The recipes in this book call for a variety of different sweeteners. I use honey sometimes; other times I use frozen apple juice concentrate or fruit sweeteners like FruitSource. I also like something called Florida Natural Crystals. Since this sugar is refined using only one step, it's not subjected to the same chemical agents as regular sugar, which is refined using a two-step process.

A note of caution: There's a lot of confusion about "fructose" these days. The word itself means *fruit sugar,* the natural sugar in our fruits and some vegetables. The fructose product sold in boxes, though, is crystallized fruit sugar, which is artificial and different from what is in a grape or an orange. Also, bear in mind that the ingredient "high-fructose corn syrup" is very much like Karo clear corn syrup. It's straight sugar—no nutrients.

What about Artificial Sweeteners?

I used to use a little NutraSweet in my morning coffee, but not anymore. My personal decision has been to stop using chemicals to replace what can be found in real food. I also distrust artificial sweeteners because I find that people get addicted to their heavy sweetness, which makes it hard to give up certain foods. Plus, we all know the person (we've all *been* the person) who orders

French fries and a diet Coke. Artificial sweeteners make you believe that you can take in calories elsewhere in your diet because you're being so "good." Switching from fake sugars to real ones may seem hard at first, but your taste buds will adapt quickly. Give it a try.

The Ongoing Debate about Alcohol and Weight

"I'm fat because I like to drink, and I like to drink because I'm fat!" This is how one of my more amusing clients started our first consultation. She was convinced that the relatively moderate affliction of oenophilia was responsible for her thick thighs and round behind. I had to remind her that French and Italian women are quite thin despite the fact that they don't think twice about a glass of vino. Believe me, wine, or even a couple of mixed drinks, never made anyone fat.

What does happen, though, is that drinking makes you relax—and relax your usual resolve not to eat certain foods. Down the hatch and cheers to the fettucine Alfredo and cheesecake. The alcohol itself is not the culprit.

Let me be clear about one thing: I'm talking about moderate drinking, not alcohol abuse. Many people take pleasure in a glass of fine wine, a refreshing beer, a delectable martini. And every culture around the world has an alcoholic drink attached to it—Russian vodka, Greek ouzo, French wine, Irish whiskey, Mexican tequila, Japanese sake. There is an old Russian proverb that says, "Drink a glass of wine after your soup and you steal a ruble from the doctor." In America it goes more like "An apple a day keeps the doctor away." Well, apples are wonderful for your health, but there is nothing like a nice glass of wine to end the day. And I've never toasted anyone with a Granny Smith. Drinking, kept in perspective, is a wonderful adjunct to eating well.

And the Russians are right: it may even be good for you. Many studies now show that there is a relationship between heart health and moderate drinking. Some research has shown that alcohol raises HDL (good) cholesterol levels; drinking red wine with a meal may counteract blood clotting and prevent the immediate risk of heart attack. Alcohol is also touted for aiding in digestion.

Still, many people are suspicious of alcohol. One day I was sitting in a newly opened restaurant in Los Angeles that serves only fat-free food. The chef, making his rounds, was sitting and chatting with a couple of women, one of whom asked him, "Does alcohol have fat?" Let me answer that. An emphatic no. Alcohol is basically fermented fruit juice or grain derivatives.

It's never had fat and probably never will. Of course, you can throw in some fat—the drink Kahlúa and *cream* comes to mind—but on its own alcohol doesn't contain fat. And it's not all that caloric. An average glass of wine has about 85 calories; a shot of whiskey (or other distilled spirit) has an average of 82 calories.

However, where alcohol really serves the weight- and health-conscious person well is in regards to cooking. I love to cook with wines, sherries, sake, and various liqueurs. They add flavor and body to many dishes, supplanting the need for oils and other fats. If you just want the taste but not the alcohol, rest assured that most of the alcohol cooks out. If you start a sauce with, say, wine, then gradually add the other ingredients and simmer them for a while, the alcohol will mostly evaporate. If you add the wine at the end of the recipe, though, your sauce will be more boozy. Either way, the flavor will be such that you probably won't miss the fat. I find that a dry white wine adds a salty flavor to food, so it's a great choice if you're trying to cut back on sodium.

Chapter Five

Put Your Money Where Your Mouth Is: A Guide to Good-for-You Shopping

They're listening to you. Who's listening? The food industry. Manufacturers are watching every dollar and cent you spend. They do surveys and studies on what you like and how you buy. Purchase a lot of bacon and they'll provide more of it. Spend your cash on a lot of foods laden with fats, sugar, and salt and they'll make more of them. They're not concerned with your medical bills or your dress size. They're concerned with selling what you will buy. Most companies truly don't have much of a conscience. They want you to be happy—being healthy is your problem. But you have more power than you think. If you buy natural, nutritious foods, manufacturers will get the message that those foods make you happy. And they'll make more of them.

Likewise, if you search out the companies that do care—care about both your happiness and your health—those companies will stay in business and other food manufacturers will try to emulate them. Everybody wins. And there *are* many wonderful companies out there that do have a conscience and care about making foods that will satisfy your taste buds, time schedule, and wallet. Health Valley, Hain, Barbara's, Westbrae, Auburn Farms, Fantastic Foods, and Imagine Foods are just a few, and I could list many, many more. If you want to be lean and healthy, put your money where your mouth is, and watch your body respond.

Finding the Right Foods: The Map to the Maze

Some of the brands mentioned above are commonly available in health food stores. But in every aisle of an ordinary supermarket, you'll find products that promote health and fitness. How to find them? What follows is a map to the supermarket maze. Under each category I list what to look for in a general sense so that you can learn to judge a healthy product from one that's not worth your while (let alone your hard-earned dollars).

Thankfully, the new nutrition labels make it much easier to figure out just what you're putting into your body. Yet label lingo can still be confusing, so it helps to know a thing or two about how those who make the rules, the (U.S.) Food and Drug Administration (FDA) and the United States Department of Agriculture (USDA), define the buzzwords stamped on a product. Do keep in mind, however, that the food industry still manipulates these buzzwords to its advantage.

Sometimes their tactics are so blatant that even a kid can see through them. I was giving a lecture to a group of sixth graders last year when a boy raised his hand and said, "I know what they do to the Healthy Choice raisin bran; they soak the raisins in sugar so they don't have to frost the cereal." This kid got a deputy badge from the Food Cop. If he can figure it out, you can too. And once you do, you'll feel as though you really understand food. It's a kind of freedom because you realize how many great products are sitting on the shelf right next to the junky ones.

What Does the Label Really Say on the Front?

It's important to distinguish the terms on the front from those on the back. Those on the front are a selling pitch, the back is hard copy.

"Fat free" To call itself fat free, a food must have 1 gram fat or less per serving. Warning: the serving size may be unrealistically small. Also, there are many products that don't contain any fat, but have so much sugar and/or salt to cover up their lack of flavor that they are detrimental to your health anyway.

"Percent fat free" (as in "98 percent fat free") *Warning: this is a reflection of the food's weight, not the amount of fat from calories.* If a serving of food weighs 100 grams and 2 of those grams come from fat, it can be labeled "98 percent fat free." *But that is not the same as 98 percent fat free in terms of calories!* One hot dog, advertised as 80 percent fat free, weighs 2 ounces, or 57 grams. That 20 percent fat by weight translates into 11 grams of fat. So no matter what the label screams out, always check the amount of fat calories as well as the ingredients list to see just what's in there.

"Light" This term means that the calories in a food have been reduced by at least a third of what they were in the regular product, or that the fat has been reduced by at least half. It can mean, too, that the sodium content has been reduced by half. Finally, "light" can also be used on labels to refer to the texture and/or color of a food—as long as the manufacturer makes clear what it's talking about.

"No cholesterol" This term has been splashed all over the supermarket in ways that mean almost nothing. Many products that *never had* cholesterol in the first place have it on their labels. Worse, so do many products that contain high amounts of fat. The fact is, products high in saturated fats have the potential to be even harder on the heart than cholesterol. Saturated fats, which include hydrogenated and partially hydrogenated oils, raise the body's LDL (bad) cholesterol levels. A product that rightfully advertises itself as cholesterol free is one that usually has no animal products in its ingredients. (Cholesterol is found only in meat, poultry, eggs, and dairy products.)

"Natural" By ruling of the USDA, which is in charge of the labeling of meat and poultry products, this means no artificial flavors, colors, preservatives, or synthetic ingredients. The animal-based product must also be minimally processed. Keep in mind, though, that fat, chicken skin, and other animal by-products may be natural but not necessarily good for your health. The FDA, which regulates the term on processed food products, has not set an official definition for it. So when you see the word "natural" on snacks like chips and cookies, it doesn't necessarily mean healthy.

"No sugar added" This phrase is different from "sugar free" or "sugarless." A product that sports the words "no sugar added" on the label may contain sugar substitutes such as sorbitol, NutraSweet, saccharine, etc. It can also contain naturally occurring sugars like fructose. In other words, it can still be a junk food. If you are trying to cut sugar from your diet, read the ingredients list.

"Low" It can mean various things, depending on what ingredient it refers to:
"Low fat"—3 grams or fewer per serving
"Low sodium"—fewer than 140 milligrams per serving
"Low saturated fat"—no more than 1 gram per serving
"Very low sodium"—fewer than 35 milligrams per serving
"Low cholesterol"—fewer than 20 milligrams per serving
"Low calorie"—40 calories or fewer per serving; for frozen dinners or
    meals, 120 or fewer per 3.5 ounces

What Does the Label Really Say on the Back?

It's always been my contention that the truth lies on the back of the label. By all means, start by reading the front, but then work your way around to the back, where the ingredients and nutritional information will allow you to determine the product's actual worth. Remember, your body digests the ingredients, not the flashy promises on the front.

"Serving size" Although the serving size is standardized for similar products (that is, the serving size for Wheat Thins crackers is likely to be the same as for Triscuits), and a lot more realistic now than in the past, it still may not relate to how much you are actually going to eat. This is especially true for products like salad dressings, chips, cereals, and soups, on whose labels the manufacturers indicate a super-small serving size in order to make it appear as though the product has very little fat or calories. I often see labels that state that a product has "0" fat grams—but from the ingredients list I can see that the product contains oil! Anything below a gram of fat does not have to be accounted for on the label and if the serving size is small enough, there *will* be under a gram of fat, allowing a manufacturer to call a food "fat free" whether it truly is or not. However, if you eat four servings, that fat will add up. I find the deception unacceptable. You have a right to fat-free foods that are truly fat free.

"Percent daily value" This tells you how much of a day's worth of fat, sodium, vitamins, minerals, and other nutrients the food provides. It's calculated using the RDAs (recommended daily allowances). As a rule, if a food has 20 percent or more of the daily value for a nutrient, it's high in that nutrient. If it has no more than 5 percent of a nutrient, it's low in that nutrient.

"Calories from fat" How much of a food is made up of fat? This term lets you know. For instance, if a food has 100 calories per serving, and 75 of them come from fat, you know that it's high. A product label should also tell you how many total fat grams a food has, another way you can tell if it's fattening or not.

Unfamiliar Words You Don't Have to Worry About

Believe it or not, there are some mysterious-sounding ingredients on food labels that are innocuous and sometimes even good for you. As food science expands, researchers are finding natural ways to enhance food (usually with thickening and emulsifying agents) and to extend their shelf life (with stabi-

1. A food's ingredients are listed in descending order according to how much of each ingredient is used. The ingredients listed in the beginning of the paragraph are used in abundance; those listed at the end are used in lesser amounts.

2. Above all, the first words you read on a label should be food words—like whole wheat flour or skim milk or tomatoes—not chemical words.

3. If a food is wholesome, it won't have an extensive paragraph listing the ingredients. As a rule, the longer the paragraph, and the more daunting the scientific words it's made up of, the unhealthier the product.

4. Sugar, salt, and oil in large quantities should be avoided, but if the product does contain them, they should be at the end of the list.

5. Beware the various monikers of sugar and salt. Sugar can be listed as corn syrup, high-fructose corn syrup, dextrose, dextrin, fructose, glucose, levulose, maltodextrin, and malt syrup. Salt can be listed under a variety of names, most which begin with the word sodium.

6. Just because a manufacturer has highlighted the few good ingredients contained in its product doesn't mean the product is healthy. Read on. Many companies add junk ingredients—they just don't advertise them. Remember, the real story is on the back of the label.

7. Trans fats are saturated fats in disguise. Outside your body they have no cholesterol; on the inside they create cholesterol. Trans fats are found mostly in margarines and other foods made with partially hydrogenated oil and shortening, and they act like saturated fats. There are many studies, and strong evidence that they raise the LDL ("bad") cholesterol in your system. Labels are not required to list the trans fats—yet. So you have to do the old ingredients check for shortenings, margarine, and partially or fully hydrogenated oils.

lizers). I'm going to list just a few of the most common natural additives you needn't worry about when you see them on the label—to list every additive currently on the market would require a whole other book.

• *Acetic acid* Present naturally in vinegar, cheese, wine, apples, and tart fruits, it's a flavoring agent used to control the pH balance in many foods.

• *Algae* There are many varieties of seaweed that are used for thickening, stabilizing, and emulsifying (keeping ingredients from separating). The most common are *carrageenan, dulse, agar-agar,* and *kelp.* There is some controversy about whether or not these additives are safe; if the waters they come from are polluted, the seaweed probably is, too. Trust the health food industry manufacturers to utilize algae from the safest waters possible.

• *Amino acids* These organic compounds—*cysteine, glycine, lysine,* and *methionine,* among others—form the basic constituent of proteins and are needed by the body for the repair and replacement of tissue. They are used in various ways to enhance food texture and flavor.

• *Annatto* A natural yellow food coloring from the seeds of a tropical tree.

• *Bicarbonates and carbonates* These are found naturally in tissues and fluids in the body. In foods they are used as leavening agents and to neutralize acidity.

• *Carotenes* Yellow-orange pigments occurring naturally in fruits and vegetables; especially prevalent in carrots, spinach, and turnip and beet greens. Carotenes, which the body converts into Vitamin A, are thought to help guard against cancer.

• *Dextrose and glucose* Food sweeteners obtained from corn sugar.

• *Fructose* Fruit sugar.

• *Gelatin* An extract of collagen, it's a protein that helps make up the connective tissue in the body. The kind of gelatin used as an additive usually comes from pigs or cattle and is used to thicken and jell food.

• *Glycerin (glycerol)* This clear, thick, sweet liquid is an alcohol found in all fats. It's used in foods to maintain water content so they remain moist.

• *Guar gum* A complex sugar gum that is extracted from the seeds of the guar plant. It's used in food processing as a stabilizer, thickening agent, and texture modifier.

• *Lactose* This milk sugar is the main carbohydrate in dairy products. It's used to improve flavor, texture, color, and aroma.

• *Lecithin* Commonly occurring in plants and animals, it's usually extracted from soybeans and added to foods as an emulsifier and antioxidant (a rancidity retardant).

• *Pectin* Occurring naturally in most plants, pectin strengthens the cells' walls. Citrus peels and apples are high in pectin and are used by food producers to thicken, jell, and blend foods.

• *Xanthan* or *xanthan gum* From a natural bacterium found on cabbage leaves, this is used to thicken and stabilize foods.

Wise Buys: Healthy Eating Starts at the Supermarket

Sometimes we get so accustomed to buying the same foods over and over again that we don't look at what's right next to them on the shelf. The following guide to every section of the supermarket is designed to help you make the healthiest choices possible. This is how *I* shop.

One thing to remember: the healthy, natural foods are generally located on the perimeters of the supermarket. That's where you'll find the fruits and vegetables, milk and eggs, seafood, and poultry. Once you make your way into the aisles, choose especially carefully. Read labels, read labels, read labels!

Meat, Poultry, Eggs, Seafood

Beef Beef is a great source of protein but should be eaten in moderation (and if you have high cholesterol consider cutting it out of your diet completely). When you do buy it, make sure you go to a reputable butcher and ask for the leanest cuts—the words "choice" or "select" are a tip-off. Or just look for these cuts:

Eye of round	Porterhouse (steak)
Tip round	Sirloin (steak)
Top round	T-bone (steak)
Bottom round	Top loin
Tenderloin	Extra lean (hamburger)

Lamb Lamb is very fatty. Remove all the extra fat before cooking and prepare without oil. Choose:

Foreshank
Shank
Loin

Pork A lean 3-ounce pork chop gets 44 percent of its calories from fat, nearly 10 grams. That's not too terrible, but the same amount of skinless white meat chicken has only about 3 grams fat. Now, 3 ounces of pork spareribs get about 69 percent of their calories from fat, nearly *26* grams. Like beef, how fattening pork is depends on the cut you choose. In any case, make sure that the pork you get is from a good butcher. Remove all extra fat before cooking and prepare without oil. Choose:

Chop, lean	Ham, cured, lean
Loin, lean	Tenderloin, lean
Center loin	Top loin, lean

Poultry White meat without the skin is always optimal, whether you're watching your cholesterol or watching your weight. If you're buying ground turkey or chicken, make sure that it's derived from skinless white meat poultry—dark meat and skin are often added into the mix, making it a lot higher in fat. Ask the butcher to grind it specially for you if a lean version isn't already prepackaged. Even though there are lots of turkey and chicken frankfurters on the market now, most of them are fatty and unhealthy. I only recommend the brands Smart Dogs and Veggie Links, which are based on soy and don't actually contain any poultry at all.

Luncheon meats Although they've cleaned up their acts lately, most of the major brands are complete junk, and fattening to boot. There are new ones labeled "fat free," but they're loaded with fillers that can still be fattening or unhealthy. Some of the turkey slices are fine, but watch for the nitrates. Your best bet is to buy plain slices of roasted turkey, chicken, or roast beef from your butcher or the deli section of your supermarket. Most of the "rolled" or smoked versions are filled with nitrates and other additives. Also look for:

Healthy Choice turkey breast slices
Louis Rich sliced turkey breast
Trim Slice, Health Valley, and Shelton Farms soy-based luncheon meats, all of which are fat free (located in the freezer section)

Eggs The egg is an excellent source of protein, vitamins A, D, E, and B12, not to mention iron, zinc, and selenium. And just like fish, eggs are a great natural source of the natural fats we need. They are very satisfying, and healthy if eaten in moderation. One trick is when recipes call for eggs, use half the amount of whole eggs called for and egg whites for the rest. If you have a cholesterol problem you shouldn't be eating a lot of egg yolks. But eggs really aren't that fattening (they only have about 80 calories each)—it's cooking them in butter and oil that drives up the calorie count. There are many organic eggs on the market now, so keep an eye out for them. If you'd prefer to use a cholesterol-free egg substitute, look for Ener G egg replacer and Nulaid egg substitute.

Seafood I believe seafood is very good for your health. I wish it were more of a staple in the American diet. What little fat most fish contain is chock-full of omega-3, a polyunsaturated fatty acid thought to help protect the heart. These are natural fats that are also good for our skin and help transport necessary vitamins. There is still controversy about whether or not shrimp, which contains cholesterol, raises LDL cholesterol levels in the blood. Many studies have shown that shrimp contains enough omega-3 to counteract the cholesterol. Still, we don't know for sure, so if you have a cholesterol problem, eat shrimp only in moderation. Although fish isn't fattening, some canned fish—like tuna and sardines—are packed in oil. Look for the water-packed varieties. Eat more seafood!!!!

Dairy Products

Butter and butter substitutes I shouldn't have to tell you that butter is pure fat and high in cholesterol. Most butter substitutes are based on a minute amount of milk fat, and have added oils, gels, and gums to fill out a product that has barely any food value. Neither the real or faux thing is a winner if you're trying to eat healthfully. If you love the flavor, try a butter-flavored nonstick vegetable spray.

Cheese There are lots of fat-free cheeses on the market now, but some of them have either unnatural additives or added gums. You want to make sure that although your cheese is fat free or low in fat, it's still good food and not just a lot of chemicals. It is true that you lose most of the real cheese flavor when you lose all the fat, so you might think about combining half fat-free cheese and half low-fat cheese to get more flavor. Another option, especially if you don't eat dairy, is soy-based cheese, but you should know that, while they're natural, these cheeses usually have a lot of oil, which makes them high in fat. If you're watching your cholesterol, fine. If you're watching your weight, not so fine. There are some fat-free soy cheeses out today, but they barely resemble cheese in flavor or texture. Three of my favorite fat-free and low-fat cheese lines are:

Alpine Lace
Healthy Choice
Lifetime

Milk We all know that whole milk is high in fat, but milk is still a natural and healthy food rich in nine nutrients: calcium, vitamins B12 and D, riboflavin, phosphorus, magnesium, niacin, folic acid, and protein. Along with other health professionals, I recommend that children up to the age of two drink whole milk. After that age, 2 percent or 1 percent is fine for growing children. Milk (all milk) is a great source of calcium. Don't be afraid to add skim or 1 percent milk to your diet. Skim milk has 0 fat grams per 8-ounce glass, and 1 percent has a mere 2.5 fat grams. I wish all Americans would drop the powdered coffee creamers (powdered oil) and switch to real milk. Buttermilk is a great ingredient to add to salad dressings and other recipes; despite its name, it contains hardly any fat at all. You can use powdered milk, the nonfat kind, and evaporated skim milk to thicken sauces and gravies.

If you have high cholesterol, look for the soy milks—they now also come in light and fat-free versions. Be aware, though, that soy milk does not taste very good on its own, so it's usually sweetened.

More good news about milk has finally arrived. For many years, UHT milk in the box was sold in Europe and now it's on supermarket shelves over here. UHT means "Ultra High Temperature." The milk is flash heated at a temperature of 270° F. for a few seconds, which destroys the bacteria that makes milk sour but keeps all of milk's nutrients intact. The milk is then packaged in hermetically sealed cartons and is shelf-stable for up to 6 months. I am very excited about the arrival of this product. It should be stocked wherever those awful powdered creamers lurk.

Yogurt There are a lot of yogurts that contain NutraSweet on the market now, and though they are lower in calories than traditional yogurts, I wouldn't advise eating these chemical-laced versions very often. I especially don't advocate feeding them to children. Of course, I do recommend the nonfat or fat-free yogurts (low-fat is fine for growing children). Do, however, check the labels because some of the new fat-free yogurts have fillers (starches and gels) or contain a lot of sugar. If the yogurt has honey or sugar just make sure it's low on the list of ingredients. Note: Make sure your yogurt lists "Live or Active Cultures" on the label. It's the bacteria that gives yogurt its health benefits over a custard or pudding. Also, avoid all yogurts with added nuts, which just add calories and fat. If you have high cholesterol, you might try the new soy-based yogurts. Some of the better yogurt companies are:

Alta Dena	Stonyfield Farms
Continental	White Wave (soy)
Dannon	

Grain Foods

Pasta Pasta has really been put to the test in the last few years. When we finally realized that pasta was not high in fat after we took away the heavy, oily sauces, we were ecstatic. Then a few people started saying that pasta and other starches raise insulin levels, thus causing the body to store fat. This set off a whole anti-pasta scare last year, a typical example of how people in this country are quick to jump on the first bandwagon that comes along.

Nonetheless, when the pasta backlash took hold, many people dropped their high-carb diets like a hot potato and began opting for high-protein diets instead. Many of them lost weight, too. Do I think protein has some magic power and that starchy carbohydrates are evil incarnate? No. What I think is that given the option of eating foods like chicken breast and fish versus pasta, people simply ate fewer calories and so they lost weight. (Protein also causes the body to excrete a lot of water, so some of those pounds coming off are fluid.)

Eating fewer calories is a great idea if you want to slim down, but that doesn't mean you have to give up pasta. The real story behind pasta is that too much dough makes your body doughy! Any food, if you eat enough of it, will make you fat, and that's been the problem with pasta: many people just go overboard and eat too much of it. Add to that the fact that they eat nothing but bread, bagels, pretzels, and cereals the rest of the day and you see why they have a problem.

Eaten with discretion and topped with a light sauce, pasta is a very healthy, nonfattening food. A lot of pastas are made with bleached flour, but I don't consider them junk. Better, though, are pastas made from whole wheat flour, buckwheat (the main ingredient in Japanese soba noodles), or other grains, like kamut, amaranth, corn, and quinoa. Fresh pastas, while they cook up more quickly than dried, often have egg or oil in them to bind the ingredients. So take the time to cook dry pasta and cut the extra fat.

Bread There isn't a person in the world who hasn't felt guilty about eating bread. Even though we now know not to butter our bread and that breads made without added fats are not especially fattening, many people are still confused. Well, here's the very simple truth about bread: Bread calories, like those of pasta and any starchy carbohydrate, add up. Eat dough all day and, yes, you will put on weight. But you won't if you eat it wisely—and if you pick the right loaf: bread made from unbleached whole grain flour, free of added butter or oils, chemicals, preservatives, and flavorings.

The first thing you should look for on the label when selecting a bread is whole grain flour. White breads made with refined flour have hardly any fiber and that goes for (sorry) French and Italian breads, too. This isn't to say you should never bring home a baguette, just that you should opt for whole grain breads (the choices range from plain whole wheat to whole grain rye, pumpernickel, sourdough, and multigrains) whenever possible. If you're buying from a bakery, ask at the counter what the ingredients are. When buying packaged bread, check the ingredients list to make sure the first ingredient is whole wheat flour (or some other whole grain flour), not just "wheat"—that's just another name for white flour stripped of fiber and nutrients. The word "whole" is key.

Many of the natural-brand breads have added nuts, raisins, or dried fruits, which makes them healthy but fattening. They're great for growing children, but if you're watching your weight avoid the breads with seeds and nuts. Fortunately, most breads don't have added oils or, if oil is added in, it's usually just a smidgen. Again, check the ingredients list when you're buying a supermarket variety of bread or ask at the bakery counter. Focaccias, for instance, are almost always full of olive oil. The basic thing to remember about bread is that the list of ingredients need not be a paragraph long or contain any words that sound like they come out of a chemistry textbook—flour, yeast, water, and salt are all that's really needed to make a good bread. If a loaf feels like foam rubber, that's usually a good tip-off that a lot of other (usually unhealthy) stuff has been tossed in.

Cereal Cereal can be a wonderful food—or a horrible one. Those coated with sugar are horrible, and I think the companies that market these candies in disguise should be—well, let's just say shut down. No cereal should have more than 5 to 7 grams of sugar per serving, and it should be made from whole grains to provide you with fiber. Remember, kids' cereals are placed on the middle shelves at children's eye level. A walk down the aisle is like one long commercial to kids. So help yours look up to the higher and lower shelves for better choices.

There are many cereal companies that are making natural whole grain products with natural sweeteners—and all the cartoons your kids need on the box as well. Look for those with ingredients lists that read simply. Three good examples:

Kellogg's Nutri•Grain Nuggets: Whole wheat flour, malted barley flour, dates, salt, yeast
Barbara's Shredded Wheat: 100% whole wheat
Apple Stroodles: Organic whole wheat flour, organic corn flour, organic maple syrup, apple juice concentrate, dehydrated apple pieces, cinnamon. (A great kids' cereal with natural sweeteners and fun cartoons.)

Today, only a few cereals have added fat, but watch out for them; those that have added fruit and nuts aren't so bad, but it's probably a good idea to skip them if you're trying to drop weight. The health food industry is coming out with new fat-free cereals every day, and the taste keeps getting better and better. So if you haven't found one you like yet, keep trying.

Crackers and grain cakes Cracker trends seem to come and go, so what's available to you is always changing. My best advice is to beware of the major manufacturers and their fad cracker of the week, which often contains some new, fattening ingredient. Or the cracker that may be fat free, but is mostly bleached flour, sugar, salt, and flavorings. Not a lot of nutrients there. Like bread, the ingredients list on a box of crackers shouldn't be a paragraph long. A few simple items, such as whole wheat flour, water, and salt, identifiable as food, are all it takes to make a cracker, and many companies are making great whole grain fat-free crackers that are nutrient dense. Also, try branching out. Oriental rice snaps, for example, are delicious and very low in fat. Crispbreads are also excellent low-fat choices, as are matzos (except for egg matzos).

Most of the grain cake manufacturers offer a good variety of plain nonfat cakes, ranging from rice and millet to popcorn, sesame, and rye, both salted and unsalted. They have, however, caught on to the fact that by flavoring them with oils, sugars, and other extras, they have a bigger market, so always check the ingredients list.

Granola As you have probably heard already, most granolas are fattening, coated with oil, honey, coconut, and other sweeteners. But there are now many on the market that have no added oil. Make sure, though, that the package says "fat free," not "no added fats," which means they may still have lots of nuts and seeds, and so may still contain a fair amount of fat. The best kinds of granola can be found in local health food markets. One word of caution: even the fat-free granolas are relatively high in calories because they're usually dense with both grain and sugar.

Muffins The very word "muffin" sounds cozy and satisfying. Plus, muffins are easy to grab, a great breakfast food when you're on the run. But somewhere along the way, "muffin" and particularly "bran muffin" came to mean healthy and nonfattening, which is not always the case. Many muffins are made with a lot of fat, and those that are packed with nuts, chocolate chips, coconut, or candy lost their "healthy" status long ago. Some of these can have as many as 40 grams of fat! Note, too, that while muffins loaded with dried fruit may still be healthy, they are also more caloric.

Fortunately, there are now many small bakeries that are making wonderful fat-free muffins. Usually they moisten the muffins by adding yogurt, applesauce, fruit-based purees, and/or dried fruit. Don't, however, count on these healthy fat substitutes to be in every muffin that bills itself as low fat. Always find out what goes into the batter. If your local deli, coffee shop, or bakery isn't willing to give you an ingredients list, pass on it. There are too many good muffins out there now to settle for those that are unhealthy and fattening. Look for muffins that have oil very low on the ingredients list. And, as with bread, look for muffins made with whole grains rather than white flour. If your good-muffin source is out of the way, buy a dozen when you go and freeze them.

The best option, of course, is to make fat-free muffins on your own. Check out the breakfast breads section beginning on page 89, or use a muffin mix. To make a mix fat free, use WonderSlim (see page 53 for explanation of WonderSlim) instead of oil. Some healthy brand-name mixes to look for:

Arrowhead Mills	Hain
Fearn	Morgan Mills

Rice and rice mixes Always look for brown rice and natural grains instead of white rice. Most white rice is bleached and has the bran removed, so it loses a lot of its vitamin and mineral content in the process. The exception to this rule is basmati rice, which is a light beige color.

As with any natural grain, rice benefits from having flavor added to it. Tossing in some herbs, spices, and other extras with rice—as in most ethnic cooking—can make rice taste so wonderful that you don't need to add any butter or oil. However, many companies that make rice mixes have managed to make a mess of it. Instead of just adding some herbs and spices and leaving it at that, most manufacturers load rice mixes with sugar, salt, MSG, and other additives.

But, once again, there's a healthy solution—several of them, actually: Arrowhead Mills, Casbah, Fantastic Foods, Hain, and Lundberg all make a variety of mixes in terrific flavors such as Spanish, Cajun, curry, and mixed pilaf. Whatever kind of rice mix you're making, keep in mind that you don't have to follow the directions when they tell you to add oil or salt. Just eliminate them, and replace the oil with a cooking wine, vegetable oil spray, or defatted chicken broth. Also, avoid the mixes with almonds or other nuts, which add fat and calories to the dish.

Other grains Yes, the world is getting smaller and we have access to more than just rice. To get more grains into your diet, don't just limit yourself to rice, wheat, and pasta. There are many different kinds of grain mixes available in stores, and the grain bins in your local health food store are chock-full of wild rice, kasha, couscous, quinoa, millet, barley, and other delicious varieties. As with rice, you can add defatted chicken broth to the cooking water instead of oil.

Fruits and Vegetables

Canned and frozen fruit Fresh fruit is always best, but frozen is the next best. Because they are flash frozen right after being picked, frozen fruits maintain more of their vitamin and mineral content than canned— sometimes even more than "fresh" produce that has been sitting around at the grocery store a long time. If you do buy canned fruit, watch out for added sugars and syrups, which make an otherwise low-calorie food fattening. Small cans or plastic containers of fruit are great for packing in sack lunches.

Dried fruit You might wonder why I often tell people to skip the dried fruit. It's not that it's so bad; as a matter of fact, it's very nutritious. But dried fruit is higher in sugar, and thus calories, than fresh fruit. Plus, most dried fruits have sulfites added. To find them without this preservative, you usually have to look in your local health food markets. If you give your kids dried fruit leathers, buy ones without added sugar—the fruit is sweet enough on its own.

Fruit juice Fruit juice is wonderful; fruit drinks, fruit-flavored drinks, and fruit cocktail drinks are not. They're all loaded with sugar and artificial additives. Look for plain fruit juice or fruit juice concentrate that has been mixed with water. One word of warning: If you are buying a juice or juice spritzer that contains a mix of juices, make sure that grape juice concentrate or grape juice is not high on the list. White grape juice concentrate is basically just a sweetener with little nutrient value, as is fructose, or high-fructose corn syrup. Manufacturers fool with these ingredients until they basically become sugar water. The plainer your juice, the better. Also, check for the vitamin C content on the label, and opt for the ones with the highest amount.

Jam, jelly, fruit syrup Just about every jam and jelly manufacturer is now making a jam or line of jams without sugar. Jam and jelly don't need sugar to taste sweet. Nor do they need artificial sweetener. Just look for the no-sugar varieties. There are also many fruit syrups on the market like Robbie's, Knudsen, and Wax Orchards that are made from fruit and fruit juice concentrates only.

Canned and frozen vegetables Once again, fresh is best; frozen without any added sauces, next best; canned and jarred vegetables come in third. Avoid all frozen vegetables with sauces, added sugar, salt, and flavorings. Likewise canned. Otherwise eat vegetables to your heart's content. I generally try to stick with fresh or frozen, but three canned vegetables I like to keep on hand are water-packed artichoke hearts, hearts of palm, and water chestnuts. They're all great quick snacks, particularly if you're trying to lose weight.

Pickles and relish Pickling in and of itself is a natural method of preserving food, so I don't see why some companies add chemical preservatives. Or colorings for that matter—avoid any pickles with yellow dye, as some food colorings have been linked to cancer. While pickles are not fattening, they are generally very salty. You can, however, buy unsalted pickles. Relishes are more likely to have added sugar, syrups, and chemical additives. Look for those without the extra goop.

Olives Some people sit in front of an hors d'oeuvre tray and toss back one olive after another, never bothering to consider that olives are what olive oil comes from. Olives contain fat. They are fine in moderation, and look for ones that are canned without preservatives.

Prepared Foods

Frozen Dinners Frozen dinners represent the worst of the industrialization of food. In order to make frozen dinners edible once they've been thawed and cooked, the manufacturers have added a lot of conditioners, fats, chemicals, artificial flavorings, salt, and sugar. There are very few that I can recommend. Even the new ones labeled "healthy" or "no cholesterol" or even "fat free" tend to be loaded with nasty ingredients. Ninety-eight percent of these dinners, especially those with diet labels, are loaded with junk. Even if the entree accurately reports its fat and calories, and the ingredients read just fine, you are getting a portion so small that you'll end up hungry later. Many of them boast that they're under or around 300 calories per entree. Well, a good dinner should supply no less than 500 calories, in order for you to be satisfied. I suggest that you make your own foods in bulk and freeze them at home, and many of the recipes in this book allow you to do so.

Soup There are endless varieties and choices of soup on the market. So when you can have something laden with vegetables and/or grains, why opt for one of those creamy soups packed with salt and preservatives? But even buying a vegetable soup can be confusing. You may look at a label, see all the vegetables, and think a soup is natural. Yet the presence of vegetables in a soup doesn't mean the manufacturer hasn't added artificial ingredients. Sometimes major manufacturers also add oil to soups that don't need them, so keep an eye on the fat content, too. If you find that some of the new fat-free soups taste a little bland, sprinkle in a little salt, garlic powder, or other seasoning. You usually can't go wrong with these soup makers:

Baxter's	Pritikin (any)
Hain (fat-free)	Shelton Farms (fat-free)
Health Valley (fat-free)	Westbrae Fat-Free Soups of the World
Legume	

Soup mixes in a cup are another thing altogether. Most dry soup mixes are loaded with chemicals and fats, but because they're dry and just require that you add water, they seem harmless. In fact, some ramen soups (Top Ramen, for instance) are loaded with fats. The good news is that there are now wonderful instant cup o' soups and ramens available, most of which are low in fat, if not entirely fat free (if they do have fat, it's usually on account of beans, which have some natural fat). I recommend them highly.

Look for:

Fantastic Noodles (all varieties)   San-J miso cup o' soups
Instant Cup Miso   Soken fat-free ramen noodle soups
Just Delicious (varieties prepared   Taste Adventure Instant (all varieties)
   without oil)   Westbrae Natural (all varieties)
Nile Spice cup o' soups

Fats, Dressings, Condiments

Cooking sprays Years ago the best chefs and nutritionists turned their noses up at cooking sprays, and with good reason: they were mostly chemicals. You'd never catch my mother the gourmet chef harboring a can of Pam in her cupboards. But today cooking sprays are different and even top cooks use them to cut down on fat.

Just what exactly is in those cans and which ones should you buy? Typically, the ingredients are some kind of oil, lecithin (a natural thickener), alcohol, a propellant, and sometimes a flavor like butter, garlic, or olive. Most of the propellants now used in cooking sprays are a combination of carbon and hydrogen, substitutes for the chlorofluorocarbons of the past (chlorofluorocarbons, as you might recall, were banned because they contribute to the destruction of the ozone layer). Propellants are generally used in minimal amounts.

Consequently, you can't really go wrong with the cooking sprays on the market today. You can, however, go wrong when using them. Remember that you're still spraying fat onto your cooking surface, so don't be heavy-handed. If you've sprayed so much that the oil runs in rivulets when you move the pan around, then you may as well have poured oil from a bottle. The idea is to spray so that the oil lightly coats the pan.

If you still don't like the idea of using a spray, use a basting brush instead and lightly brush a little oil across your cooking surface.

Margarine Despite what some TV commercials like to suggest, there is no way that margarine can be considered a nonfattening product: it's nothing but vegetable oil, water, and additives, processed to look like butter. Although I went over this in Chapter 4, I want to talk about it again. The process that margarines go through is called hydrogenation, which involves adding hydrogen molecules to the fatty acid chains in the liquid oil, which then converts them to solids. *Voilà*, you've got oil in stick form, resembling butter. Margarine in the tub is "partially hydrogenated," sort of halfway to solid form. The hydrogenation process creates something called trans fatty acids, which scientists suspect may raise LDL (bad) levels of cholesterol. Thus, margarine may be no better than butter in terms of your health.

My best advice is to use neither butter nor margarine; there are lots of other products you can use to give food flavor. But if you must use them, it's really a matter of taste. And if you're going to opt for margarine, consider these facts before buying:

1. The fewer fat calories a margarine has, the fewer trans fats it will have. (Some margarines are pumped up with air or solids to make them less caloric.)

2. Among those with equal fat content, the softer the spread, the fewer trans fats.

3. If you must use margarine, choose one made with soybean oil.

Mayonnaise This is a product I believe you should learn to live without unless you are consistently underweight, have no cholesterol problems, and exercise vigorously. Even then it should be used in moderation. The new so-called "fat-free" versions are so loaded with sugars, gums, and chemicals that I cannot recommend them either. The good news is that you will see many great alternatives for mayo in Chapter 8, "Let's Do Lunch—and Do It Right." Check out the mayo replacement on page 62, too.

Oils As you should know by now, all oils, no matter how healthy they are purported to be, are fattening. There are some oils that may reduce blood cholesterol levels (olive oil, primarily). And all vegetable oils are free of dietary cholesterol. *But*—and this is important—just because an oil has "no cholesterol" on the label does not mean that it's one of the oils that are good for your blood cholesterol! Some oils, like palm and coconut, are full of saturated fat, which raises blood cholesterol. The healthiest oils you can choose are olive oil and canola oil, because they are high in monounsaturates (peanut, avocado, and almond oils are too, although not quite as high). Corn, soybean, safflower, sunflower, and sesame oils are also fairly innocuous. But, I repeat, all oils are still fattening and an *excess* of any kind of fat in the diet is not healthy.

Salad dressings Today you'll find many dressings with "fat free" on the label, but these are the most mislabeled products on grocery store shelves. Keep in mind that when you eliminate oil from a dressing you need to add something to give it enough body to cling to the lettuce and vegetables. Some manufacturers add gums like carrageenan and xanthan, which are natural and okay in my book. But many other manufacturers of fat-free dressings load them up with sugar, salt, starches, and gels. These aren't okay. Plus, watch out for those dressings that claim to be fat free but have oil in their ingredients list anyway. Look for the term "oil free" and always check the ingredients on the back; no matter what the claim on the front says, many still contain partially hydrogenated oils.

If you sample some of the healthy no-oil dressings on the market, I think you'll find one or more that you like. But if they seem too bland, add apple cider vinegar, rice vinegar, or some Dijon mustard to give them more flavor. (If you don't like the no-oil dressings and can afford the extra calories, buy a regular dressing made with olive or canola oil.) Another good tip to add more flavor to your fat-free dressing is to cut it in half with a low-fat dressing. Also, consider that no-oil and fat-free salad dressings are not just for salads. They can be used as marinades and sautéing liquids. Some healthy, good-flavored ones to try:

Ayla's	Pritikin
Cook's Classics	S & W
Good Seasons oil-free mixes	Très Classique Grand Garlic and
Hain no-oil mixes	Caesar
Herb Magic	Uncle Henry's Mustard Tarragon
Paula's	Walden Farms

See Chapter 10, "Slimming Sides, Salads, Soups, and Sauces," for more information and recipes.

WonderSlim and Just Like Shortening You will see these two products mentioned throughout the book. Both are all-natural fruit purees that can be used to replace the oil and other fats in baking. They really work, making cakes, muffins, and other baked goods come out very moist. If you can't find them, refer to the tips on page 96 for how to use applesauce, plum purees, and other fat substitutes.

Sauces and Gravies

Pasta sauce As with any prepared condiment or food, you've got to watch out for preservatives and other additives in pasta sauces. Watch out for olive oil on the ingredients list, too, since most commercial pasta sauces contain a fair amount. There are, however, many small companies and even some larger ones that put out very simple sauces without oil or additives. You can make your own (see pages 169–179), or look for:

Ci'Bella	Millina's
Enrico's	Muir Glen
Healthy Choice (has sugar)	Pritikin

Salsa Fresh salsa is healthier, but bottled salsa is fine (check for preservatives). Think of salsa not just as a dip but as a topping for baked potatoes and other vegetables; a sauce for meat, poultry, and fish; a spicy pasta sauce. It goes well on anything and everything (okay, not ice cream, but everything else). And there are many variations today. Salsas don't need oil, so check the ingredients list because some salsa makers add it anyway. Some brands to look for:

Enrico's	Newman's Own
Guiltless Gourmet	Pace
Jardine	

Gravy Most canned, bottled, or prepared gravies are fattening and junk. The only one I can recommend is the Hain packaged dry mix, which is all natural. Also, see Yolanda's Famous Gravy, see page 272.

Snack Foods and Beverages

Nuts, chips, pretzels, and other snacks Nuts are high in fat and should be avoided by anybody who's watching his or her weight. And even if you're not watching your weight, consider that a handful of peanuts (about 3½ ounces) has 585 calories and 50 grams of fat. Ouch. The same goes for all nut butters and spreads. Peanut butter, for instance, is not an unhealthy food when it's pure, made without salt or sugar. But it's really meant for growing children, not as a main staple in an adult's diet. Defatted peanuts are available, so check the brand for calories and fat content. The exception to the rule of the nut world is chestnuts. Chestnuts are the only nut with vitamin C—$3\frac{1}{2}$ ounces provide 43 percent of the RDA, and have only 2 grams of fat and 245 calories.

All seeds also contain fat, which is why oils come from them: sunflower, sesame, canola. A $3\frac{1}{2}$-ounce serving of sunflower seeds has 570 calories and 50 fat grams. No wonder birds can survive on them! Once again, they are healthy but fattening, and to be avoided when you're trying to shed pounds, and eaten in moderation any other time. (For an alternative, see Marinated Water Chestnuts, see page 133.)

It's common knowledge that potato and tortilla chips and cheese puffs are fattening. Some of the new "baked-not-fried" kinds are better, although you should still check the ingredients list to see that no oil has been added. Check the list for pretzels, too, which are easily made without fat though some manufacturers persist in adding hydrogenated oils.

Also check the ingredients list when you buy popcorn. Air-popped popcorn is a perfect example of food trickery. The "air-popped" on the label leads you to believe that the popcorn is oil free, but in fact the manufacturer adds oil after the popping to get the salt to stick.

If you make air-popped popcorn at home, you can spray it with a little butter-flavored cooking spray, then sprinkle it with salt or salt-free popcorn seasoning. Most of the microwavable and instant-pop varieties of popcorn on the market are junk. However, they are changing every day, so look for natural ones.

Dips Many of the commercial cheese spreads and canned dips are junk, but there are so many healthy fat-free alternatives now that you'll never miss them. Look for fat-free bean dips, fat-free cheese dips, fat-free guacamole and salsas, both fresh and bottled.

Soda Most commercial brands of soda have little if any food value and most of them, particularly diet sodas, contain a lot of chemicals. Although I honestly couldn't tell you the scientific reason, and I don't think any studies have been conducted, I swear that sodas are addictive. It's obvious that those that have caffeine will make people develop a habit, but many are caffeine free and people are still fanatic about drinking their six-pack per day. Be careful of this habit as there is some evidence that the phosphorus in colas and root beers (although not citrus sodas), diet or regular, depletes bone density, setting you up for osteoporosis.

The following is a list of the natural-drink manufacturers that make just fruit juice and mineral water sodas, which are good for your health and your weight since they're not too caloric.

After the Fall	Mott
Calistoga	Knudsen
Crystal Geyser	Sundance
L & A	Tree Top
Martinelli	

Desserts and Sweets

Cake mixes Dry cake mixes are notorious for their chemical content; however, the natural food industry has come out with a few healthy contenders. And even when you use those, I recommend that you replace all the oil, butter, or margarine that's called for in the directions with WonderSlim, the natural fat substitute. Cake mixes to look for:

Amaranth	Hain
Arrowhead Mills	Mixed Company
Fearn	Morgan Mills

Cookies, cakes, pies, and pastries Let's face it, dessert is dessert, and most of the time that means fattening (though not always—see Chapter 13). Dessert is also a treat—and should be treated that way. The main words of caution here are *Don't overdo it!* Even many of the new "fat-free" versions of traditional desserts aren't much lower in calories than the regular kinds. All the sugar, gums, added starches, and flour used to compensate for fat add up. Also, don't assume that just because a sweet is made by a health food company that it's low in calories. Many of the health food cakes and cookies may not have processed sugar or saturated fats, but they are often still made with oil, nuts, and dried fruit, making them highly caloric. Your best choices are fat-free versions of health food sweets, such as Health Valley or Barbara's cookie nibbles. Another great choice is angel food cake, since it is a dessert that's naturally low in fat, but still sweet and satisfying. Have a little sugar, a little sin, and keep desserts down to a minimum.

Fudge sauces I just had to make this a category of its own. For someone who started dieting in 1969, like me, a healthy fudge sauce is heaven sent. There are now two companies that make delicious, natural sauces—butterscotch, fudge, and a variety of flavors like amaretto fudge and orange fudge. The fudge sauces are based on natural fruit juice concentrates and cocoa, and they're delicious! Several of the dessert recipes in this book call for the sauces, but you can just drizzle them over frozen desserts or use them instead of frosting to dress up cakes. Look for Wax Orchards and Newmarket, the two best brands, in your local gourmet or health food store.

Frozen fruit bars Most frozen fruit bars have sugar added to them, but they still make a great nonfat snack. Avoid the ones mixed with cream or frozen yogurt, which can drive up the fat and calorie count.

Ice cream, frozen yogurt, sorbet Ice cream, of course, is loaded with fat, especially the premium kinds like Häagen-Dazs and Ben & Jerry's. Frozen yogurts, despite sounding healthy, can often have a large number of calories. Sorbet is the least fattening of the three because it's made without cream. If you love ice cream, you should treat yourself once in a while. There is a large variety of diet and light ice creams—essentially ice milk, which is less fatty by definition—on the market now. However, be aware that most of the so-called fat-free or diet ice creams are loaded with gums and chemicals, coated over with tons of sugar, and can actually be a lot worse for you than the real thing.

If you are buying frozen yogurt at the market, check the label to see where it stands in the fat department—they vary tremendously. I know you are tired of my repeating this but you have to read the ingredients, especially in this category. This is a bad news–good news category, and you really have to be your own detective. The bad news is that, like other desserts, there are no freebies here—even the alternatives still have calories. The good news is that many of them have many fewer calories and lots less fat than traditional desserts. But, again, check out the details.

If you're buying from an independent yogurt shop, insist on knowing the ingredients and fat content. Even then you can't always be sure of what you're getting. Often, yogurt shops add what they please to their mix, but still claim that what you're getting is nonfat or fat free. They may be fat free all right, but only when the serving size is minuscule and unrealistic. For example, the sign may say 1 gram fat per 4 ounces, but a regular small serving may have 11 to 12 ounces, which can add up to more than 1 gram fat. None of these shops are subject to FDA label laws and they get away with murder (murdering your thighs, that is). Some of the better commercial brands to look for:

Häagen-Dazs (fat-free sorbets)
Living Lightly (line of ice creams)
Sweet Nothings (line of nondairy ice creams)

Pudding, custard, and gelatin I consider most commercial brands of these—including the sugar-free ones—complete junk food and suggest that you and your children avoid them. Hain, however, does make a few natural gelatin and pudding mixes that are healthy, and Imagine Foods' fat-free pudding in the cup is respectable. If you must eat the diet junk food kind made with sugar substitutes, the Sans Sucre mousse is your best pick.

Chapter Six

Things You Oughta Know:
All the Tips, Ideas, and Tricks Inside My Head
(Or, as I Say to My Clients, Pick My Brain)

I have designed the recipes in this book for everyone who wants to have meals and snacks with four basic attributes: they're easy, low in fat, healthy, and delicious. And they work for everyone, from young people just starting out on their own, to working parents trying to put together a meal after a long day, to older people who are tired of cooking but want to eat well. These recipes and eating ideas are for everyone who wants to get food into their lives and eat happily ever after.

But it's not just recipes that you'll find on the upcoming pages. I'll be giving you every idea, tip, and trick that I have in my head and teaching you the skills I've developed preparing fabulous healthy food. I'm dedicated to helping you cook without added fats. The only fats you'll find here are the natural fats contained in poultry, seafood, grains, and other foods. Most low-fat recipes found in cookbooks today have some olive or canola oil added to them, but I've left it out, just as I do when I make food for my home delivery service. The delivery service meals are designed for clients who want to lose weight healthfully—and not gain it back. That's just what I believe these recipes can help you do, too.

At the end of almost every recipe in this book, you'll find a breakdown of the dish's nutritional makeup per serving. These figures come from running the recipe through one, sometimes even two (for verification) computer programs. The programs work by tallying up the ingredients' combined amounts of calories, fat, protein, and carbohydrate grams, and milligrams of cholesterol and sodium.

I've got to tell you, though, that these programs are not perfect. I feel confident in saying that the nutritional information provided here is as close as you can get to absolute accuracy, but just be aware that there is still a small margin of error. Not so much of a margin that you'll be seeing the numbers on your scale suddenly rise or your cholesterol level jump, but a margin of error nonetheless.

Also be conscious of the fact that, although I often advise adding a dollop of this or a sprinkling of that to garnish a dish, unless they're in the list of a recipe's ingredients, dollops and sprinklings are not counted in the per-serving breakdown. But just so you have an idea of what you're adding to a dish, here are the fat and calorie counts of some common garnishes you'll find suggested throughout the book:

1 tablespoon nonfat sour cream: 35 to 40 calories; 0 grams fat
2 tablespoons maple syrup: 100 calories; 0 grams fat
1 tablespoon fat-free salsa: 5 calories; 0 grams fat
$1/2$ cup brown rice: 90 calories; 1 gram fat
1 tablespoon grated Parmesan: 25 calories; 2 grams fat
2 tablespoons grated fat-free cheese: 40 calories; 0 grams fat

Most of all, I believe that what you'll be reading on the upcoming pages will help you begin to understand the principles of healthy cooking so you can apply them all the time. Anybody can open up a cookbook and follow a recipe, but that's really only half of what's involved in healthful cooking. The other half is knowing how to pare the fat from *any* dish, whether it be the meatloaf recipe that's been in your family for ages, the pasta you've served to guests for years, or your best friend's chicken entree. You need skills that make it possible always to have low-fat and nonfat food in your repertoire. You need some basic no-brainer tricks before you become a really talented no-brainer cook. So before you even get to the recipes, read through the following "Yolanda-isms" for cooking ideas.

Taking the Fat out of Frying

Frying, as you're well aware, involves heating oil or butter in a pan and tossing in your food to cook. The combination of fat and heat turns the food crispy on the outside and, usually, fairly juicy on the inside, with just enough grease to send the mouth into orbit. The truth is, the soles of your shoes would taste good fried in oil and salted.

Here's another truth and one you'll learn to love: You can get the same effect by using one of the following "nonfrying" techniques. Because different foods have different textures and water content, you'll need to use a different method for each kind of dish.

Nonfried chicken The trick here is in the coating. Use very cold *skinless* white-meat chicken, just out of the refrigerator or soaked in a bowl of ice.

Dip the parts in beaten egg white (or whole egg if you prefer a little fat), let the coating drip off, then roll chicken in flour or bread crumbs. Place in a pan sprayed with nonstick vegetable spray and bake for about 20 to 25 minutes at 350°.

Nonfried potatoes Cut potatoes (leave skin on) into thick slices, placing the slices on a paper towel to allow them to drain as you go. Spray a cookie sheet with nonstick vegetable spray and place the potatoes on the pan. Spritz the potatoes with nonstick vegetable spray, turning to coat them evenly. Sprinkle with salt and pepper. Place in a 400° oven and cook for 10 minutes on one side, or until browned. Turn and cook until browned all over.

Nonfried tortilla chips Have a spray bottle of water ready (it's the water that toasts the tortilla chips). Slice oil-free corn tortillas into quarters. Spritz a cookie sheet with nonstick vegetable spray. Place the tortilla chips on the pan and spray with water, then place the pan in a 450° oven. As the tortillas brown, turn them and spray again. When they're crisp on both sides, remove from the oven. Sprinkle with your favorite seasoning (I like popcorn seasoning) and allow to cool.

Nonfried stir-fry Instead of using a lot of oil to cook a stir-fry dish as is the tradition, use one of the many new delicious fat-free Asian sauces on the market today. They come in ginger, tamari, garlic, and Szechuan flavors and are thickened with natural gums so they add the body you need when stir-frying. If you are using a deep sauté pan rather than a wok, make sure it's a nonstick pan. If you're using a wok, spritz it lightly with nonstick vegetable spray before cooking.

Making Nonfat Yogurt Go 101 Ways

There's a very inexpensive tool available in most kitchenware and health food stores that I find indispensable: a yogurt strainer. It looks like the plastic cone from a coffeemaker (in fact, a coffeemaker cone with filter inside can double as a yogurt strainer) and is used to drain the liquidy part (whey) out of the yogurt. Strained yogurt is thicker and creamier than the kind that comes straight from the carton. You can add flavorings and use it as a replacement for mayonnaise, sour cream, cream cheese, and even cake icing. I'm thrilled with my yogurt strainer and think you'll love having one, too.

When you strain yogurt, it's best to use nonfat varieties with no gelatin added. Place the strained yogurt in an airtight container and it will keep for up to two weeks refrigerated. The following suggestions combine to make great creamy spreads and toppings (I call them Mayo-nots, the mayonnaise replacers).

Drain one pint of nonfat plain yogurt overnight in the yogurt strainer. Transfer to a bowl and combine with one teaspoon of any of the following seasonings:

Chef Paul Prudhomme's vegetable seasoning and 1 tablespoon maple
    syrup
Dijon mustard and 1 teaspoon minced onions
Lemon pepper
Minced fresh garlic and 1/2 teaspoon chopped chives
Mr. Spice
Parsley Patch Garlic Saltless Seasoning
Spice Islands Blends
Spike
Any one of your favorite spice blends

Miscellaneous Tips and Ideas for Low-Fat and Nonfat Cooking

• Cook fish, turkey, and chicken in the oven on top of aluminum foil, bending the foil so that the sauce you're cooking it in nearly covers the poultry or seafood. This "foil boat" helps the sauce's flavor seep in during the cooking. Reserve any leftover sauce to pour over your vegetables.
• When grilling foods without oil (say you've used a fat-free dressing or sauce instead), return them to their marinade after removing them from the grill—they'll soak up even more of it and be incredibly juicy. First, though, place the marinade in a saucepan and bring it to a boil on the stove (you can do this while the food is grilling). This will kill any bacteria that might have been on the raw poultry or seafood.
• Instead of butter or oil, use any of these other nonstick liquids for sautéing: nonstick vegetable oil sprays (plain, olive-flavored, butter-flavored, and garlic-flavored); wine; defatted chicken, beef, and vegetable broths; any flavor vinegar; sake; oil-free vinaigrettes; lemon juice; flat beer; frozen fruit juice concentrate.

• Leftover chicken or turkey can be used in an entirely new dish. Just rinse the leftovers under hot water for a few seconds so that they lose most of last night's flavor, then incorporate them into tonight's recipe.

• Boneless, skinless poultry is more expensive than the uncut kind. If you want to save money, buy your poultry with the skin on and bone intact, then remove them yourself at home.

• To enhance the flavoring process, poke holes in poultry and seafood with a fork before marinating.

• When you're steaming vegetables, make plenty of extras so you have left-overs in the fridge for snacks the next day. Or, use the leftovers the next night: Place them in the pan around the fish or chicken where they'll soak up the juices; serve as a side dish.

• Instead of using butter on corn on the cob, slather it with hot pepper jelly before cooking on the grill or microwaving. (If you're boiling the corn, spread on the cob after cooking.)

• I believe that fresh onions, bell peppers, garlic, and herbs add a great deal of flavor to food. But on many nights, I simply don't have the time or energy even to think of the word "chop." On those nights I use prechopped frozen onions and peppers and prechopped garlic. Lots of times I'll use frozen chopped vegetables, too (many markets also now carry fresh prechopped veg-gies). There's almost no difference in taste but the difference in time and en-ergy saved is tangible.

• True gourmets buy dried beans, soak them overnight, and cook them the next day with onion, celery, carrots, and herbs. If I had the time to plan that far ahead, well, so would I. Since I usually don't (and you probably don't ei-ther), I often depend on beans in jars or cans or dried bean flakes. Dried flakes, a relatively new product that comes in cartons, are similar to mashed potato flakes—the flaking process hastens the cooking process so they're ex-tremely convenient. You just add boiling water. If you're buying whole beans, look for those that are not packaged with added fats or sugar.

• Remember that when you cook without oil or added fat you have to replace it with extra liquid. Don't be afraid to add more wine, broth, or whatever liq-uid a recipe calls for during the cooking time; it will cook down so that your dish doesn't end up soggy.

• Most oil-free salad dressings are dull in taste, but I find that adding a little apple cider vinegar, Dijon mustard, or rice vinegar gives them some pizzazz.

• If you are watching your cholesterol, use egg whites instead of whole eggs in recipes that call for them. Use two egg whites to replace one whole egg, three egg whites to replace two whole eggs.

- Use frozen juice concentrates instead of sugar to sweeten your recipes.
- Rather than using bleached white flour, cream, or processed bread crumbs to thicken a dish, use pureed or finely grated vegetables, farina, oat bran, wheat germ, or stale whole wheat bread (run it through a blender to turn it into crumbs).
- Squeeze fresh lemon juice into an ice cube tray and freeze. That way you'll always have fresh lemon juice on hand even if you don't have fresh lemons. Each cube equals about 1 ounce or 2 tablespoons of juice.
- Do the same with leftover defatted chicken broth so that you don't have to open a whole can for every recipe.

Ethnic Food Made Easy

One of the biggest misconceptions about cooking without fat is that the food will have no flavor if it doesn't have any fat. One easy remedy is the liberal use of herbs and spices, which make your mouth sit up and pay attention. Just consider ethnic cuisine, with its myriad of flavors. One reason that ethnic food is often healthier than American food (and American versions of ethnic food) is that cooks in other cultures rely on flavorings instead of fat to give a dish pizzazz. Ethnic food is also traditionally made with fresh foods—ours is the only country in the world with miles of supermarket aisles laden with processed foods. Protein portions are generally smaller, too, while whole grains are given much greater play than in stateside cuisine.

I use a lot of spices, spice mixes, and herbs in my cooking, and I can understand how they can be confusing. What goes with what? When one of my clients, Robin Riker, an actress on the television show *Thunder Alley*, asked me to clear up the mystery of which spices and herbs go together, I decided to create a guide to cuisine from other countries. The following is a list of various ethnic foods and the quintessential flavors that give them their unique characteristics. They also happen to be the flavors that will give your dishes so much oomph, they won't need added fat. One caution, while the following spice blends contain no fat and are extremely low in calories, some, particularly those with salt and garlic and onion powder, are higher in sodium. If you are watching your sodium intake, simply adjust the amount added of the ingredients.

Keep some (if not all) of these flavorings on hand, and don't just stay wedded to this guide. Experiment! The best way to learn your way around a spice is to use it—and abuse it. Make mistakes, then try again. Keep an open mind about all of the spice mixes I have listed, and look for new ones of your own.

Ethnic Flavorings

Italian

Olive oil is the base of most Italian cooking, but it is very high in fat (13.5 fat grams per tablespoon). I prefer to use a little olive-flavored nonstick vegetable oil spray (one good spritz is less than a gram of fat), and sauté with wines instead. Plus, you can get just as much good Italian flavor in food by using garlic, fresh or dried basil, oregano, rosemary, and parsley. Many stores now have prechopped fresh garlic, a real time-saver, or try crushed, powdered, or granulated garlic. You can also simply buy Italian seasoning, a mix of most of the above herbs, or, if you can't find Italian seasoning, then you can blend your own:

Italian Herb Blend

2	tablespoons basil
2	tablespoons marjoram
1	tablespoon granulated garlic
1	tablespoon oregano
1/2	tablespoon thyme
1/2	tablespoon rosemary
1/2	tablespoon crushed red pepper flakes

Place ingredients in a bowl and combine thoroughly. Store in a glass jar (baby food jars are great for this).

Greek

Red wine vinegar, garlic, cinnamon, bay leaves, dried dill, marjoram, rosemary, olives, olive-flavored nonstick vegetable oil spray. Feta cheese, of course, is a staple of Greek food, but it's high in fat—1 ounce has an average of 75 calories and about 6 grams of fat.

Greek Herb Blend

2	tablespoons garlic powder
1	tablespoon grated lemon peel
1	tablespoon oregano
1/2	tablespoon ground black pepper

Place ingredients in a bowl and combine thoroughly. Store in a glass jar.

Indian

Look for the different kinds of curry blends in the spice section of your market, and try: fruit chutneys, tamarind paste, curry powder, garam masala, ground turmeric, coriander, cumin, yellow and black mustard seeds, ground and whole cardamom, ground cloves, saffron, crushed red chilies, red chili powder, curry pastes, ground ginger, tandoori spice mixes, raisins, and plain yogurt. Ghee, which is used in many traditional Indian dishes, is clarified butter—butter with all but the fat removed. Don't even think about it.

Chinese

Tamari, mirin (rice wine), plum sauce, Chinese chili sauce, fish sauce, oyster sauce, hoisin sauce, rice vinegar, Chinese hot mustard, curry powder, five-spice powder, red sweet ginger, star anise, Szechuan peppercorns, tofu. Many Chinese sauces are laced with oil and sugar, but some don't have either in the ingredients. If ordering Chinese take-out, always ask for the sauce on the side and cut it with low-sodium soy sauce and rice vinegar to reduce the fat.

Japanese

Pickled ginger, pickled cucumber, light soy sauce, miso, ginger, garlic, wasabi, pickled daikon, teriyaki sauce, sake, rice vinegar, plum paste, ponzu sauce, plum sauce, tofu. Premier Japan makes ginger, garlic and regular tamari sauces, and both Premier Japan and San-J make many great fat-free sauces for stir-frying. They can be rather powerful, but you can cut them with defatted chicken broth, sake, or water to lighten them up.

Thai

Tamari, curry pastes, dried lemon grass, chili-garlic sauce, dried ginger, crushed red chilies, curry powder, tofu. Tommy Tang's Thai sauces are excellent. Also look for low-fat and no-oil Thai sauces.

Mexican

Chili powder, a variety of dried chilies (ancho, tepin, pepin), crushed red chilies, fresh cilantro, dried cilantro, garlic, crushed garlic, cumin, mole sauce, Mexican oregano, green chilies, jalapeños, cayenne pepper, taco seasoning or chili seasoning, chili sauce, red and yellow onions. Cheddar cheese (use the low-fat or fat-free). Make sure you use plain corn tortillas (corn, lime, and water), and look for the new fat-free whole wheat tortillas on the market. There are many Mexican spice blends that I like to add to rice or beans. Or make your own:

Mexican Blend

1½   tablespoons cumin
1   tablespoon onion powder
1   tablespoon garlic powder
½   tablespoon ground ginger
½   tablespoon paprika
½   tablespoon oregano
½   tablespoon dry mustard
½   tablespoon cayenne pepper
½   tablespoon parsley flakes

Place ingredients in a bowl and combine thoroughly. Store in a glass jar.

French

Tarragon, rosemary, thyme, sage, parsley, herbes de Provence, garlic, shallots, red and white wines, olive- and butter-flavored nonstick vegetable oil spray, mushrooms, yogurt, nutmeg, cloves, and a variety of liqueurs like cognac, brandy, and anisette. The French do a lot of sautéing in butter and oil; simply replace them with wine or liqueur. Try this herb mix to give your food a French accent, too:

Herb Salt

2   tablespoons onion powder
1   tablespoon garlic powder
1   tablespoon parsley flakes
1   tablespoon marjoram
1   tablespoon salt
½   tablespoon basil
½   tablespoon tarragon

Place ingredients in a bowl and combine thoroughly. Store in a glass jar.

More Herb Blends . . .

Poultry Blend

2   tablespoons marjoram
1   tablespoon basil
1   tablespoon parsley

1 tablespoon dill weed
1 tablespoon paprika

Fish Blend

4 tablespoons parsley flakes
2 tablespoons chopped chives
2 tablespoons dill weed
2 tablespoons oregano
1 tablespoon rosemary
1 tablespoon thyme

Cajun Blend

2 tablespoons cayenne pepper
2 tablespoons paprika
1¹/₂ tablespoons onion powder
1 tablespoon freshly ground black pepper
1 tablespoon freshly ground white pepper
1 tablespoon garlic powder
2 teaspoons dried basil
1 teaspoon chili powder
¹/₄ teaspoon dried thyme
¹/₄ teaspoon mustard powder
¹/₈ teaspoon ground cloves
pinch crushed red pepper flakes

For each blend, place ingredients in a bowl and combine thoroughly. Store in a glass jar.

Basic Recipes You Should Have in Your Repertoire

No lean-thinking cook should be without the following easy additions to his or her fat-free act. They're so easy, make them one time and you'll remember them forever.

Aromatic Poaching Liquid

MAKES 2¹/₂ CUPS

Poached fish and chicken are so healthy—and so utterly boring. Unless, that is, you cook them in something like this aromatic liquid that will infuse them with a wonderful peppery-herb flavor. Add more fresh herbs to the mixture, if you like.

2¹/₂   cups water
1   medium carrot, sliced
1   medium onion, sliced thin
10   peppercorns, crushed
3   sprigs thyme

Place the ingredients in a saucepan and cook over high heat for 5–10 minutes. Do not allow to boil. Strain through a fine sieve. Use to poach fish or chicken.

Frozen Flavored Bouillon Cubes

EACH RECIPE MAKES 12 CUBES

These cubes are great to have on hand for flavoring soups, or anything you sauté. In particular, they all make a wonderful replacement for butter or oil in a vegetable sauté. Make an ice cube tray full of each variety, then place the cubes in a large freezer bag, and mark so you can tell which is which.

VARIATION #1

Mild and aromatic; use this for French meals, soups, chicken, vegetable, and bean dishes.

2   13-ounce cans defatted chicken broth
¹/₂   cup white wine
2   shallots, chopped
1   teaspoon dried thyme
1   teaspoon poultry seasoning

VARIATION #2

Rich and pungent; this is the perfect liquid for making an Asian stir-fry dish or to serve with fish.

2   13-ounce cans defatted chicken broth
$^1/_2$ cup sake
2   garlic cloves, chopped
1   teaspoon minced ginger root
$^1/_4$ teaspoon lemon juice
$^1/_2$ cup low-sodium soy sauce

VARIATION #3

Subtle and saltier than the other variations; try this in chicken soups, with fish, and in bean dishes.

2   13-ounce cans defatted chicken broth
$^1/_2$ cup vermouth
1   teaspoon celery seed
1   teaspoon minced onion
1   teaspoon freeze-dried parsley or chopped fresh parsley

Combine all ingredients in a 1-quart saucepan. Simmer for 20 minutes, or until reduced to about 1$^1/_2$ cups. Remove and let cool. Fill an ice cube tray with bouillon and freeze. When frozen, remove from the tray and place in freezer bags.

Roasted Garlic

MAKES 1 SERVING

Roasted garlic is all the rage these days and for good reason. The roasting brings out the mellow aromatic flavor of the garlic and softens it for spreading or cooking. Look for the little ceramic garlic roasters sold everywhere today; they make roasting even easier.

1   bulb garlic, papery skin removed
2   teaspoons water

Preheat oven to 400°. Slice about $^1/_2$ inch off the top of the garlic head. Place the garlic on a square of aluminum foil or in a ceramic roaster. Sprinkle 2 teaspoons water over the bulb. If using foil, pinch the edges together to make a package. Roast for 40–45 minutes, or until the cloves are very soft. Unwrap and let cool slightly.

Superquick cooking variation: Place the bulb on a plate in a microwave oven. Cook on high for 1 minute; turn the bulb, then cook for 1 minute more.

Use in sauces, dressings, and mashed potatoes, or cut in half and serve as a garnish or as a spread for bread.

Toaster Oven Roasted Onions

Roasting turns onions mellow and brings out their sweetness.

1   red or yellow onion, papery skin removed
olive-flavored nonstick vegetable oil spray

Preheat toaster oven to 350°. Spritz the onion with the vegetable oil spray and wrap it in foil. Place the onion in the toaster oven and bake for 20 minutes, or until soft. Slice and serve as a side dish, in sandwiches, or tossed in a salad.

Whole-Wheat Flour Tortillas

MAKES 18 TORTILLAS

I'm the first one to take the easy way—like buying premade whole wheat tortillas. But I also love fresh, homemade tortillas. There's nothing like them. Make a batch of these, then freeze them four to a bag, so you can have fat-free tortillas whenever you want.

3   cups whole wheat flour
¹/₂   teaspoon baking powder
1¹/₂ tablespoons WonderSlim Fat & Egg Substitute
1¹/₂ cups boiling water
nonstick vegetable oil spray

Combine the flour and baking powder in a large bowl with a whisk. Heat the WonderSlim in the microwave for about 15 seconds *or* place in a saucepan and heat over low heat for 2 minutes or until just melted. Gradually add the WonderSlim and water to the flour mixture, blending as you go so that you have a soft, nonsticky ball. (Add more water or flour if necessary.) Divide dough into 18 little balls, and roll out the tortillas with a rolling pin, turning as you roll, until they are thin circles with a diameter of 8 to 10 inches. Spritz a nonstick skillet with vegetable oil spray and heat until medium hot. Drop the tortillas into the skillet and cook 15 to 30 seconds on each side. Let cool and store in the refrigerator or freezer. When reheating them to serve, it's best to either steam them, or put them on a plate covered with a damp towel and heat in the toaster oven.

Per tortilla: *69 calories; 0.4 g fat (4.6 percent calories from fat); 3 g protein; 15 g carbohydrate; 0 mg cholesterol; 12 mg sodium.*

Chapter Seven

Breakfast on the Run

"Breakfast," my father used to tell me, "means to break the fast. While you slept last night you were fasting." By putting it that way, he hoped my siblings and I would understand why he insisted that we eat breakfast before going to school each morning. It was logical, he theorized, that if your body did not receive any sustenance for eight to ten hours, you'd awake hungry and in need of food.

I believe that there is some degree of truth in my father's breakfast philosophy, especially for children. However, the reality for teens and adults is quite a different matter. When was the last time you tried to get a teenager to sit down to "break" his or her fast? How often have you yourself been out the door without even giving breakfast a thought?

If we all ate a healthy dinner between the hours of 5 and 7 P.M., and had one little snack before going to sleep, most of us probably would wake up hungry, our bodies crying out for fuel. But, judging from 80 percent of the clients I see, breakfast ain't happening! The real scenario goes something like this: You manage to get out of the office somewhere around six or seven o'clock, and whether you're making dinner for your family or eating out, you probably don't see the first forkful until somewhere around eight or nine. Then after dinner, you might relax with a bowl of popcorn or a dish of ice cream, munching your way to bedtime. The upshot is that you don't wake up hungry. Despite the logic behind my father's theory, most people don't want breakfast, or, if they do want it, they bury their desire because they simply don't have time to sit down and eat.

Is this bad? Not the way I see it. If you're not hungry or you're pressed for time, so be it. If you aren't into eating breakfast, then don't. I know that sounds like nutritional blasphemy, but there's solid reasoning behind my thinking. Remember, one of the keys to food happiness (see page 4) is "Make your own rules." I have always taught people to be themselves with food, and breakfast is a fine place to start.

I will, however, add one caveat. I believe that it's very important for growing children to have a good breakfast. Not only do their growing bodies need all the nutrients they can get, children expend a tremendous amount of energy during the day; they need the calories. Although adults feel like they expend a lot of energy, too, it's usually mental energy, not physical. And, obviously, adults don't need the extra calories to help them grow (unless, of course, they don't mind if their hips and belly keep growing).

Yet many of us still eat whether we're hungry or not. One of the main reasons people overeat is that they don't listen to their stomachs, their hunger, their appetites. One of the basic rules of healthy eating is, if you aren't hungry, then don't eat, whether it's breakfast time or any time.

Three Keys to Morning Food Happiness

I'll admit that telling you not to eat breakfast is an unusual way to preface a chapter of breakfast recipes. But let's be honest. Some of you are going to skip right through this chapter and never make a thing in the morning. Those who like breakfast, though, will find all the ideas they will ever need to add to their morning repertoire. And people who are on the borderline may decide that the options here are so easy and delicious that they will opt for breakfast after all. I was never a breakfast person till a cute little coffee and bagel shop opened within walking distance of my house. Now after I get the kids off to school I take about 20 minutes to sit and have a caffe latte and a bagel. I can't tell you how much I enjoy it, and it starts my day so much better.

But whichever category you fall into, keep these three tenets of A.M. eating in mind:

1. If you skip it, snack! So, you're not a breakfast eater. I repeat: Don't eat breakfast. But beware of one thing: By 10 or 11 A.M., you're probably going to be starving, so don't let it catch you off guard. The easiest thing to do—and the worst for your waist—is to grab from the box of office doughnuts or jump up at the honk of the roach coach or bell of the pastry cart. If you know you're going to get hungry, why not just plan ahead? This is when you need to have lean, healthy snack foods around. If you'll be at work, you need to bring in food that will satisfy you and prevent you from taking the easy (i.e., fattening, unhealthy) way out. Likewise, if you're at home, you've got to have something satiating in the cupboard.

Here's a tale that illustrates my point. I call it "Polly's Peril": Polly is a very successful stockbroker at PaineWebber in Los Angeles. Every morning she gets up about 4:30 A.M. so she can make it to the office by 6:00 and start phoning New York, where the stock market is just opening. Obviously she does not want to get up and wolf down breakfast at 5:00 A.M.; her body is barely awake! Instead she does what the average busy and stressed-out professional does: She rises, gets dressed, makeup on, drives to the office, inhales a cup of coffee (with powdered dairy creamer), and gets on that phone.

By about 10:00 A.M., when she can no longer simply run on adrenaline, hunger pangs hit. Then she and a few fellow employees head for the company kitchenette, which, as in so many offices, is stocked with junk. Once in a while you might be able to find a lone, miserable apple or orange someone brought in an attempt to diet or get healthy, but when your stomach is growling, and your nerves are jittery, who wants it? So Polly and her peers heat up the microwave popcorn, pull out some bran muffins or bagels with cream cheese, or just grab any old pastry and head back to their desks until lunch (the next diet disaster—but that's another chapter).

Now, a "good" nutritionist would tell Polly to have a protein shake or glass of juice in the morning before she leaves for work so that she wouldn't be starving by 10:00 A.M. And it's sound advice. Realistically, though? It's not going to happen. At least not for more than two mornings. Allowing Polly to be Polly is a better idea than trying to force food down her throat when she doesn't want it or asking her to abstain from the 10 A.M. break. Polly's solution lies not in breakfast but in stocking her office kitchenette with some lean and healthy foods.

Believe it or not, we figured out that what Polly would like best around 10 A.M. is a baked potato! Who's to say a baked potato is not a morning food? Having one in the A.M. is a great idea. A potato is high in fiber and complex carbohydrates, and it's as easily microwavable as—and much less fattening than—microwave popcorn. Polly's mission was to make sure that she stocked her office kitchenette with potatoes and great toppings like salsa and nonfat sour cream. Making this switch (and cutting out the fatty powdered creamer she was using in her coffee) helped her to lose weight.

2. **When you do eat breakfast, do it right.** Now that I've officially excused all you breakfast haters from cereal and toast duty, let's talk about those who really look forward to their morning meal. Breakfast is the meal that's the easiest to make lean and healthy. At this hour, you're not likely to be eating for emotional reasons. You feel fresh, the stress of the upcoming day hasn't landed on your shoulders yet, and you want to start the day right. To some people that may mean having fruit for breakfast, but it's rarely the sole at-

traction. Most people's favorites are starches like cereal, bagels, and crois-sants.

Many health experts recommend a breakfast high in protein, which for most people means eggs. Scrambled egg whites, egg-white omelettes, or egg substitutes are not a bad idea for the A.M. You can even have a few whole eggs a week if you don't have a cholesterol problem. But there are other protein foods to consider if you're not fond of eggs. Nonfat yogurt is one. A chunk of low-fat or fat-free cheese is another. Also check out the breakfast burritos with beans in Chapter 7.

What you should eat, though, really depends on what you'll be doing in the next few hours. If you're going to be exercising sometime soon after breakfast, it's a good idea to have a complex carbohydrate like oatmeal or a bran muffin. If you're going to be sitting all morning, then go a little lighter and opt for plain fruit or have a soft-boiled egg. There's also something else you should consider, which brings us to . . .

3. Plan ahead. The most important advice I can give you about selecting breakfast foods, especially if you are trying to lose weight, is know what you're having for lunch (and dinner for that matter) when you are deciding what to eat for breakfast. If you have a big luncheon to go to that day and you aren't going to get to the gym, then eat a light breakfast. Likewise, if you know that you are meeting your friend for a run at the track and will barely be able to grab lunch that day, then have something hearty. Know what you're eating and how you're going to burn it.

No-Brainer Breakfast Ideas and Recipes

Keep in mind that you don't have to think of breakfast as a square meal you have to sit down to each morning. However, if you have the time to make a lovely brunch, more power to you. What follows are recipes and eating ideas that will get you through the morning, no matter what your schedule and eating preferences are like.

Cereal: The Nitty-Gritty and Nutty-Flaky on What's Out There (Hint: Get the Marshmallows Out!)

Some cereals are healthy—but fattening. Others are healthy—but boring. Some are nonfattening—and healthy. And some are just junk! Many have sales pitches on the box that sound like they'll save your life.

The most important thing to remember about cereal is that it's not supposed to be dessert. In other words, it's not supposed to have as much sugar as a candy bar. As a matter of fact, a one-cup bowl of Alpha-Bits has about 5½ teaspoons of sugar—that's the same amount of sugar as in ten Hershey's Kisses! So look at the ingredients list to see what sugars have been added; there should be no more than one kind. Also, many cereals now will tell you exactly how much sugar they have, which makes it easy to compare and contrast brands. Here, too, are some tips for souping up your cereal in the morning.

• Make sure that your cereal has less than 5 grams of sugar and no more than 35 milligrams sodium per serving, that it's made from a *whole* grain or contains bran, and has at least 2½ grams of fiber. Also, take a look at the serving size the manufacturer gives on the side of the box. Most say ½ cup; some say 1 cup; it varies. If you're likely to eat double the serving size, judge its nutrients and calories accordingly.

• Choose a nonsweetened cereal, then sweeten the milk with a ¼ teaspoon vanilla or almond flavoring.

• Stir your favorite no-sugar jam or apple butter into hot cereal.

• Use ½ teaspoon of melted honey on cold cereal—it goes a lot farther than room temperature honey, which clumps, and the heat seems to expand its sweetness. To melt it, just pop it into the microwave for about 10 seconds, then add it to the milk.

• Rethink cereal itself. Use cooked Kashi, brown rice, wild rice, couscous, or a blend of grains as cereal. Add about ½ cup of skim milk, a teaspoon of honey, and a tablespoon of raisins to 1 cup cooked grains; microwave for about 1 minute.

• If you're out of fresh fruit—your best cereal-topping choice—drain a can of peaches (packed in natural juices) and top your cereal with them instead.

Grab and Go: How to Stock Your Briefcase, Desk, Car, and Even Your Moped with A.M. Eats

This is the stuff you need to have on hand at all times—if not for breakfast, when the hunger strikes. We really have to learn to tote along good foods the same way we do our daily calendars. We pack our papers, gym clothes,

RollerBlades, and hairbrush for the day; why not good food? It's a junk food jungle out there, and we have to be prepared! Breakfast tips and tricks galore:

1. Too rushed even to pour a bowl of good healthy oat cereal? Then pack a few healthy fat-free oatmeal cookies with you in your bag. At about 50 calories each and with 0 grams fat, they have the whole oats you need and are great dipped in your morning coffee.

2. Along the same lines, there are many healthy fat-free granola bars. Health Valley, Hain, and Barbara's are among the best brands because they're made with whole oats and contain no refined sugar. You might also try a few whole grain fat-free crackers, which are great to munch on during your morning commute. Some of the new flavored rice cakes travel well, too.

3. A few years ago, "Pop Tart" was just another way to say "candy bar." Now we have great jam-filled pastries made with whole wheat flour and no-sugar jam. For convenience, they're packed in sealed individual packets that fit into a suit coat pocket. Auburn Farms and Health Valley are the brands to look for.

4. If you love to pop into your local deli and grab a bran muffin, thinking that you're doing the right thing—beware! As we've already learned, the bran in the muffin may be buried in fat. If you don't have access to the ingredients list, then either change delis or change your choice. Look for a muffin that has 2 or fewer fat grams per muffin if not one that's fat free. If you can't find either, go for a toasted bagel with jam instead.

5. Always keep some dried apricots, dried apples, or raisins in your bag, car, desk, or moped. They may be high in concentrated fructose and calories, but eating a handful in the morning may give you the energy you need to get going. And since they're healthy and chewy, they're satisfying—just make sure you don't down a whole bag. Keep your serving to between $1/2$ and $3/4$ cup.

6. Keep a bag of bagels in the office and some low-fat or fat-free cheese in the fridge. Slice some of the cheese and place it on half a bagel; microwave for about 1 minute. The protein in the cheese will help get you through the morning.

7. There's nothing wrong with slicing off about 4 ounces of fat-free cheese on your way out the door. The calcium and protein cheese provides are a good way to start the day.

8. If you have a piece of leftover chicken, turkey, or some sliced turkey breast, grab that on your way out. Remember, breakfast doesn't have to be breakfast food.

9. Keep your desk drawer or briefcase stocked with a few envelopes of instant oatmeal (many come in great flavors) so that you can add some water and microwave at work. It's a great snack, too. One caveat: some instant oatmeals are like candy, with lots of added sugar and chemicals, so check the ingredients lists before you buy. I'm partial to Erewhon's maple and applesauce instant oatmeal.

10. Health Valley makes a wonderful assortment of fat-free breakfast bars called Apple Bakes, Raspberry Bakes, etc.; the company also now makes an assortment of fat-free scones and granola bars. By the time you get into your third bite of one of these, you won't even miss that glazed doughnut or cheese pastry. And neither will your thighs.

11. The oldest, but still best, trick in the book: Slice up some fresh fruit into a carton of plain nonfat yogurt. It's an easy breakfast you can't go wrong with.

No-Brainer Recipes

I developed a lot of these for my darling fifteen-year-old daughter, Nolina, who looks at me with disgust when I insist (much like my father before me) that she break her fast and eat something before she goes to school. The threat that it will make her brain work better falls on deaf ears (what a cliché, Mom!); she doesn't care. For a while I tried telling her that breakfast will bring the oxygen to her head, making her skin glow, and giving her naturally rosy cheeks. She only bought that one until she discovered makeup.

So now I just try to offer her simple alternatives that don't really even seem like breakfast. On the occasion that she does leave the house without food in her stomach, so be it; I pack a snack in her backpack as a backup. I'm sure she will survive the day even if her brain isn't working optimally and her glow comes courtesy of Revlon.

Toast It and Take It

MAKES 1 SERVING

Toast made from healthy, whole grain bread is the easiest, healthiest breakfast around, not to mention low in fat: 1 slice generally has 60 to 70 calories and less than 1 gram fat. But just spreading some jam on top every morning can get monotonous. Here are five ways to take a plain old piece of toast and make it better.

VARIATION #1

1   slice whole wheat bread
1   tablespoon applesauce
1   ounce fat-free cheddar cheese

VARIATION #2

1   slice pumpernickel bread
$^1\!/_2$ banana, sliced
1   teaspoon raisins
1   teaspoon honey

VARIATION #3

1   slice sourdough bread
1   tablespoon fat-free ricotta cheese
1   teaspoon sugar-free jam

VARIATION #4

1   slice rye bread
1   tablespoon fat-free cream cheese
1   teaspoon Fakin' Bacon Bits (soy-based fake bacon bits)

VARIATION #5

1   slice cinnamon raisin bread (I like Pritikin)
1   tablespoon apple butter
1   tablespoon fat-free cream cheese

Pop bread into the toaster. When golden brown, remove and top with remaining ingredients. You can also top toast with Vanilla Yogurt Cream with honey and cinnamon (see page 281).

Pancake Roll-Ups

MAKES 2 SERVINGS

These are super simple, because they're made with frozen pancakes. I love to roll these pancakes and hand them to my kids and husband as they walk out the door. My four-year-old son calls them doughnuts—little does he know that they're good for you. You can use any of the frozen pancakes in the market, but I like Van's because they are all natural and made with whole grains. They have 90 calories and less than 1 fat gram each. They're great to have on hand for desserts, too.

VARIATION #1

2   frozen pancakes
1   tablespoon fat-free sour cream
2   teaspoons sugar-free blueberry jam
1   teaspoon honey

VARIATION #2

2   frozen pancakes
2   tablespoons nonfat cottage cheese
1   can mixed fruit without syrup

VARIATION #3

2   frozen pancakes
1   tablespoon pumpkin puree
1   teaspoon maple syrup
dash of cinnamon

VARIATION #4

2   frozen pancakes
2   teaspoons sugar-free strawberry jam
1   tablespoon nonfat strawberry yogurt

Heat or thaw pancakes according to package directions. Combine the remaining ingredients and spread half the mixture on each pancake. Roll up and serve.

Waffle Sandwiches

MAKES 1 SERVING

Van's frozen waffles, just like their pancakes, are natural and made from whole grains. But you'll also find many other low-fat frozen waffles in your market. Van's are about 90 calories each and under 1 gram of fat. Besides these variations, try a waffle sandwich made with Vanilla Yogurt Cream (see page 281).

Variation #1

2   frozen waffles
1   teaspoon fat-free cream cheese
1   teaspoon sugar-free jam

Variation #2

2   frozen waffles
1   tablespoon nonfat cottage cheese
1   teaspoon honey

Variation #3

2   frozen waffles
1   egg, scrambled
1   teaspoon Fakin' Bacon Bits

Variation #4

2   frozen waffles
1   tablespoon fat-free sour cream
1   teaspoon honey

Heat or thaw waffles according to package directions. Combine the remaining ingredients and place on top of one waffle. Top with the other and serve.

Average per serving: 218 calories; 1.5 g fat (6.1 percent calories from fat); 3.3 g protein; 50.1 g carbohydrate; 27 mg cholesterol; 150 mg sodium.

Breakfast Baked Apples

MAKES 4 SERVINGS

Yes, I know that baked apples are normally for dessert, but that was when they were made with tons of sugar. You can make these on the weekend, then pop one in the microwave for breakfast. They also make great snacks. I had a client who used to make them in batches for her seventeen-year-old daughter so she'd have them when she got home from school. Use any flavor sugar-free jam you like and any juice without added sugar.

    4   green Pippin or Rome apples
    4   teaspoons sugar-free jam
    1   cup orange juice or juice of your choice
    1   teaspoon cinnamon

Core the apples about ³/₄ of the way through; leave some apple meat at the bottom to hold the jam in. Drop a teaspoon of jam into each apple, then sprinkle a little cinnamon on top. Place the apples in a shallow baking pan; pour the juice in the bottom of the pan. Cover with a foil tent and bake at 350° for 15 minutes; remove the foil and bake for another 10 minutes, or until the apples are soft. Do not overcook or you will have applesauce.

Per serving: 120 calories; 0.6 g fat (4 percent calories from fat); 1 g protein; 31 g carbohydrate; 0 mg cholesterol; 3 mg sodium.

Granola-Stuffed Baked Apples

MAKES 6 SERVINGS

This is a variation on the baked apple theme that not only tastes terrific but helps you get some more fiber into your A.M. meal. Also keep them around for late-night nibbles, topped with fat-free frozen yogurt.

    6   Granny Smith or Rome apples
    Juice of 1 lemon
    1   cup cranberry juice
    ¹/₂   cup apple juice
    1   pinch ginger powder
    ¹/₄   cup maple syrup
    ³/₄   teaspoon cinnamon
    1¹/₂ cups fat-free granola

Preheat oven to 375°. Core the apples about ³/₄ of the way through and scoop out half of the fruit. Place the lemon juice, cranberry juice, apple juice, ginger powder, maple syrup, and cinnamon in a small saucepan. Heat briefly until the maple syrup has melted. Add the granola and stir to coat it evenly.

Place the apples in a shallow baking dish and fill each with granola mixture. Pour any leftover granola mixture around the apples, and cover with a foil tent. Cook for 15 minutes, remove the foil, and cook for another 5–10 minutes, or until the apples are soft all the way through.

Per serving: 181 calories; 0.4 g fat (1.9 percent calories from fat); 2 g protein; 47 g carbohydrate; 0 mg cholesterol; 120 mg sodium.

Baked Bananas

MAKES 4 SERVINGS

Instead of letting brown bananas go to waste, try this sweet and spicy mélange. Serve on top of cereal or spread on an English muffin. (It makes a great dessert topping for frozen yogurt or reduced-fat ice cream, too.)

4	ripe bananas
2	tablespoons frozen apple juice concentrate
2	teaspoons honey
1/2	teaspoon cinnamon
1	pinch nutmeg
1	teaspoon dark brown sugar

Peel and slice the bananas in half lengthwise. Place the sliced bananas side by side like soldiers on a long piece of aluminum foil. Fold the foil ends together to form a "boat." Spread the apple juice concentrate evenly over the bananas, then sprinkle the rest of the ingredients on top. Close the foil at the top. Place in a toaster oven set at 350° and cook for 15–20 minutes, or until the bananas are browned and all of the juice and honey has melted. When cool enough to handle, cut the bananas into 1/2-inch slices.

Per serving: 134 calories; 0.6 g fat (3.7 percent calories from fat); 1 g protein; 34 g carbohydrate; 0 mg cholesterol; 4 mg sodium.

Frothy Orange-Banana Smoothie

MAKES 4 6-OUNCE SERVINGS

This quick morning shake can also be made into frozen pops. Pour into freezer pop containers for a Dreamsicle-like snack.

6   ounces frozen orange juice concentrate
2   cups skim or 1 percent milk
2   teaspoons honey
1   teaspoon vanilla extract
1   banana
5   ice cubes

Combine all the ingredients except the ice cubes in a blender. Blend until smooth. Uncover, and with the motor running, add the ice cubes one at a time. Blend until smooth and frothy.

Per serving: 149 calories; 0.4 g fat (2.6 percent calories from fat); 5 g protein; 32 g carbohydrate; 2 mg cholesterol; 66 mg sodium.

Breakfast Burritos

MAKES 4 SERVINGS

Burritos have become a regular part of my family's life, and not just for lunch or dinner. The nice thing about burritos is that they hold everything together, allowing the flavors of their fillings to blend. Make a large batch and put them in an airtight container, then just hand them to your kids in the morning.

4   no-oil corn tortillas or no-oil whole wheat tortillas
nonstick vegetable oil spray
³/₄   cup salsa
¹/₂   cup chopped scallions
2   red potatoes, steamed until still firm and diced
1   tomato, seeded and diced
4   ounces canned green chilies, drained
salt and pepper, to taste
2   eggs
2   egg whites
1   pinch cayenne pepper
2   tablespoons fresh chopped cilantro
¹/₄   cup grated fat-free cheddar cheese

Heat the tortillas in a toaster oven on medium for about 2 minutes. Or you can put the tortillas directly on the burner (gas or electric) on medium heat for 10 seconds. Spritz a nonstick pan with vegetable oil spray and add half of the salsa. Add ⅓ of the scallions and the potatoes. Sauté over medium heat for 1 minute. Add the tomato and chilies and sauté until heated through, about 2 minutes. Season with salt and pepper (optional). Push the vegetable mixture to the sides of the skillet. In a small bowl beat the eggs, egg whites, and cayenne pepper with a fork. Pour the egg mixture into the center of the skillet and cook over medium heat, stirring the egg mixture with a wooden spoon, until some curds have formed but the mixture is still creamy, about 1–2 minutes. Sprinkle cilantro over the top, then stir the eggs and vegetables together. Adjust seasonings. Top each tortilla with the egg mixture. Fold two ends in first, then roll them into burritos. Top with the remaining salsa and scallions and cheese. If you are going to freeze the burritos, do not freeze the toppings. Just add them before you serve.

Per serving: 169 calories; 3 g fat (10.8 percent calories from fat); 12 g protein; 43 g carbohydrate; 106 mg cholesterol; 331 mg sodium.

Tomato and Hot Sauce Breakfast Burrito

MAKES 2 SERVINGS

This is for those who like their breakfasts hearty. You can make this as spicy as you like by adjusting the hot sauce. Serve with a fruit salad to cool your tongue.

2   **no-oil whole wheat flour tortillas**
1   **egg, beaten**
2   **egg whites**
nonstick vegetable oil spray
1   **tomato, chopped**
1   **ounce fat-free Jack cheese, grated**
¼   **cup shredded lettuce**
2   **teaspoons hot sauce, or to taste**

Heat the tortillas in a toaster oven for about 2 minutes, or go the traditional route and cook them on the stovetop: Place them directly on the burner (gas or electric) turned to medium heat for 10 seconds. In a small bowl, lightly beat the egg and egg whites together, then set aside. Heat a nonstick sauté pan and spritz with vegetable oil spray. Pour in the egg mixture and cook for about 1 minute until the eggs jell, then add the tomato and cheese and cook until done. Sprinkle lettuce on the tortillas, then top with the egg mixture and hot sauce. Fold two ends in first, then roll them into burritos.

Per serving: 133 calories; 2.7 g fat (12.1 percent calories from fat); 15 g protein; 29 g carbohydrate; 108 mg cholesterol; 440 mg sodium.

Honey Ricotta Breakfast Burritos

MAKES 4 SERVINGS

Who says burritos have to be spicy? These are sweet and creamy. They freeze well and are nice topped with sliced fresh fruit.

1/2	cup fat-free ricotta cheese
3	teaspoons honey
4	teaspoons sugar-free raspberry jam
4	no-oil whole wheat flour tortillas

Mix the ricotta, honey, and jam in a bowl. Spread the mixture onto the tortillas. Fold two ends in first, then roll them into burritos. Heat in the toaster oven for about 2 minutes, seam side down.

Per serving: 119 calories; 1.1 g fat (4.8 percent calories from fat); 12 g protein; 35 g carbohydrate; 3 mg cholesterol; 470 mg sodium.

Huevos Rancheros Burritos

MAKES 4 SERVINGS

This is a quick, high-protein breakfast. For variation, add any leftover vegetables (or diced chicken) to the eggs.

4	egg whites
2	eggs
	nonstick vegetable oil spray
4	ounces fat-free cheddar cheese, grated
1/4	cup chopped scallions
1/4	cup cooked corn
1/4	cup canned, drained pinto beans

4 tablespoons salsa
4 no-oil whole wheat flour tortillas
nonfat sour cream (optional)

In a small bowl, lightly beat the egg whites and eggs together. Heat a medium-size nonstick sauté pan spritzed with vegetable oil spray. Add the eggs and cook over medium heat until they just begin to jell, about 1–2 minutes. Spread the grated cheese, scallions, corn, and beans over half the eggs. When the eggs are solid on the bottom, fold the mixture in half (as if you were making an omelette). Let the eggs cook for another 2–3 minutes, or until firm. Take a spatula, slice the egg mixture into four pieces, and slide a piece onto each tortilla. Top each with one tablespoon salsa. Fold two ends in first, then roll them into burritos. Serve with a dollop of nonfat sour cream, if desired.

Per serving: 200 calories; 3.7 g fat (12.4 percent calories from fat); 21 g protein; 38 g carbohydrate; 109 mg cholesterol; 561 mg sodium.

Tomatillo Breakfast Burrito

MAKES 4 SERVINGS

Tomatillo salsa is not as strange as it sounds. Tomatillos taste like green, slightly tart tomatoes, and salsas made with them are sold in most salsa sections of the supermarket. It's a nice change from regular red salsa, but if you can't find the tomatillo kind, red salsa will work just as well.

4 no-oil whole wheat flour tortillas
4 eggs, lightly beaten
2 egg whites
1/2 teaspoon Cajun seasoning
salt and pepper (optional)
nonstick vegetable oil spray
1/2 cup grated fat-free cheddar cheese
4 tablespoons tomatillo salsa
nonfat sour cream (optional)

Heat the tortillas in a toaster oven for about 2 minutes, or go the traditional route and cook them on the stovetop: Place them directly on the burner (gas or electric) turned to medium heat for 10 seconds. In a small bowl, lightly beat together the eggs and egg whites. Add the Cajun seasoning, and, if desired, salt and pepper. Heat a nonstick sauté pan and spritz with vegetable oil spray. Add the eggs and scramble lightly with a wooden spoon. As the eggs begin to jell add the grated cheese, and continue to stir until cooked, about 3–5 minutes. Fill the tortillas with a portion of the cooked eggs and cheese, then top the eggs with salsa. Fold two ends of the tortillas in first, then roll them into burritos. Serve with a dollop of nonfat sour cream, if desired.

Per serving: 141 calories; 5.6 g fat (24.2 percent calories from fat); 13 g protein; 26 g carbohydrate; 213 mg cholesterol; 395 mg sodium.

Take the Time to Bake It . . . So You Can Make It Through the Day

If cooking meals has gone the way of the past, baking is almost extinct. I must admit that while I make dinner every night, baking had become something I only did around holiday time. But I finally got fed up with the so-called "fat-free" muffins I found at markets and bakeries. Most are either dry and tasteless and heavy, or not as fat free as advertised. So one Sunday I went into the kitchen, baked the whole day away, and came up with some great recipes for morning breads and muffins. I now freeze everything in separate serving-size plastic bags so that we have a choice of banana breads, muffins, and other goodies every morning. Since my husband drives a lot during his workday, I slip some into his briefcase for on-the-road snacks. I even slide one into my breakfast-hating daughter's backpack so she's ready when she feels like having a snack at school.

Behold the Fat-Free Biscuit

MAKES 18 BISCUITS

Biscuits conjure up thoughts of country mornings, the smell of a hearty breakfast on the stove, and memories of soaking, dunking, and dipping them into everything from fried eggs to gravy. Then there's the vision of the numbers moving up on the scale with each dunk. Well, switch to poached eggs, make the gravy on page 272, bake up a batch of these, and you'll be in country-morning heaven once again—without all the fat! These biscuits are light inside, crusty outside, and worth making an extra batch so you can freeze them.

1³/₄	**cups all-purpose unbleached flour**
2	**teaspoons baking powder**
¹/₄	**teaspoon salt**
2	**tablespoons grated Romano cheese**
1	**teaspoon grated Parmesan cheese**
1	**teaspoon popcorn seasoning**
¹/₄	**teaspoon ground red pepper**
2	**teaspoons WonderSlim Fat & Egg Substitute or 4 teaspoons applesauce or baby food prunes**
²/₃	**cup nonfat buttermilk**
	nonstick vegetable oil spray

Preheat the oven to 400°. Combine the flour, baking powder, salt, grated cheeses, popcorn seasoning, and red pepper in a medium-size bowl and stir well. In another bowl, combine the WonderSlim and buttermilk; add to the dry ingredients. Stir with a fork until the dry ingredients are moistened. Turn the dough out onto a lightly floured surface and knead lightly 3 or 4 times. Roll dough to ¹/₂-inch thickness; cut into about 18 2-inch rounds (use a cookie cutter if you have one or a drinking glass). Place the biscuits on a baking sheet spritzed with vegetable oil spray, then lightly spray the tops of the biscuits. Bake for 15 minutes or until tops are golden. Serve with maple syrup or sugar-free jam.

Per biscuit, not including maple syrup or jam: 53 calories; 0.4 g fat (7.6 percent calories from fat); 2 g protein; 10 g carbohydrate; 1 mg cholesterol; 91 mg sodium.

Cranberry Bread or Muffins

MAKES 12 SERVINGS

For the prune mixture in this recipe you can substitute prune butter, baby food prunes, or WonderSlim. I like to use a natural fruit sweetener when I can, and the FruitSource works well here. You can use sugar, however (if you must), or substitute grape juice concentrate, brown rice syrup, or maple syrup.

¹/₂	**cup pitted prunes**
2	**tablespoons water**

1⅓   cups all-purpose unbleached flour
1   cup rolled oats
¾   teaspoon baking powder
1   teaspoon baking soda
¼   teaspoon salt
¾   cup FruitSource or sugar
1   tablespoon honey
½   cup skim milk
1   teaspoon vanilla
2   egg whites, lightly beaten
½   cup cranberries
        nonstick vegetable oil spray

Preheat oven to 375°. Puree the prunes and water until smooth. Combine flour, oats, baking powder, baking soda, and salt in a medium-size bowl. In a separate bowl, mix together the prune puree, FruitSource, honey, milk, vanilla, egg whites, and cranberries. Pour the wet ingredients into the dry ingredients and stir until the dry ingredients are just moistened. Spritz a small loaf pan with vegetable oil spray or use a nonstick 12-cup muffin tin. Bake for 15–20 minutes, or until tops are golden brown.

Per serving: 96 calories; 0.6 g fat (5.7 percent calories from fat); 3 g protein; 19 g carbohydrate; 0 mg cholesterol; 187 mg sodium.

Meal in a Muffin

MAKES 12 MUFFINS

I have to admit that I'm one of those mothers who is thrilled when she sees her kids eat vegetables, so I try to serve them as creatively as possible—sometimes even in disguise. Incorporating wheat germ, apple, vegetables, and egg, these muffins are nutritional powerhouses.

1½   cups all-purpose unbleached flour
½   cup whole wheat flour
1   tablespoon cinnamon
1   teaspoon baking powder
1   teaspoon baking soda
½   teaspoon salt
2   cups grated carrots

1/2	cup grated zucchini
1	apple, peeled and chopped
1	cup raisins
1	egg, beaten lightly
2	egg whites, beaten lightly
1/2	cup apple butter
1/4	cup WonderSlim Fat & Egg Substitute or 1/2 cup applesauce or baby food prunes
1 1/4	cups FruitSource
1	teaspoon vanilla extract
	nonstick vegetable oil spray
2	tablespoons wheat germ

Preheat oven to 375°. In a large bowl, combine the flours, cinnamon, baking powder, baking soda, and salt. Stir in carrots, zucchini, apple, and raisins. In a medium-size bowl, whisk together egg, egg whites, apple butter, Wonder-Slim, FruitSource, and vanilla. Add to the dry ingredients and stir just until moistened. Spritz a 12-cup muffin tin with vegetable oil spray. Spoon the batter into the muffin cups until they're about 3/4 full. Sprinkle the wheat germ over the tops of the muffins and bake for about 15–20 minutes or until done.

Per muffin: 166 calories; 0.9 g fat (5 percent calories from fat); 4 g protein; 36 g carbohydrate; 18 mg cholesterol; 245 mg sodium.

Pumpkin Muffins

MAKES 12 MUFFINS

This is a great natural way to get beta carotene, a powerful anticancer, anti-aging antioxidant, into your diet without even knowing it! Eat these muffins for both the beauty of your skin and the good health of the rest of your body. This basic recipe can also be modified to make three different variations. See the next page.

1	cup unprocessed oat bran
2	tablespoons wheat germ
3/4	cup all-purpose unbleached flour
2	teaspoons baking powder
1	teaspoon pumpkin pie spice

1   teaspoon cinnamon
1/2   teaspoon nutmeg
1/4   teaspoon salt
1/2   cup molasses
1/4   cup honey
1   cup canned pumpkin puree
1/2   cup skim milk
2   egg whites, lightly beaten
2   tablespoons WonderSlim Fat & Egg Substitute or
     4 tablespoons applesauce or baby food prunes
nonstick vegetable oil spray

Preheat oven to 425°. Combine the oat bran, wheat germ, flour, baking powder, spices, and salt in a large bowl. In a medium-size bowl combine the molasses, honey, pumpkin puree, milk, egg whites, and Wonderslim; stir well.
Make a well in the center of the flour mixture and add the pumpkin mixture
slowly, blending well. Spritz a 12-cup muffin tin (or if you want to make a
bread, a small loaf pan) with vegetable oil spray, and spoon mixture into the
cups until 3/4 full. Bake for 20 minutes, or until done. Remove from the tin
and serve warm or at room temperature.

*Per muffin: 127 calories; 1.9 g fat (5.6 percent calories from fat); 4 g protein; 30 g car-
bohydrate; 0 mg cholesterol; 126 mg sodium.*

Muffin Variations

MAKES 12 MUFFINS

These are all spin-offs from the pumpkin muffin. Substitute the following
sets of ingredients for variation. With these healthy, natural ingredients, the
calories and fat grams stay roughly the same.

Banana Muffins

Use Pumpkin Muffin ingredients, but delete pumpkin puree and pumpkin
pie spice and substitute:

3/4   cup ripe mashed banana
1   teaspoon vanilla

Apple Muffins

Use Pumpkin Muffin ingredients, but delete pumpkin puree and pumpkin pie spice and substitute:

¹/₂ cup finely chopped apple
pinch allspice

Pear Cinnamon Muffins

Use Pumpkin Muffin ingredients, but delete pumpkin puree, pumpkin pie spice, and skim milk and substitute:

²/₃ cup nonfat plain yogurt
¹/₃ cup chopped pear

Follow Pumpkin Muffin recipe, substituting where necessary.

Corn Bread Muffins

MAKES 12 MUFFINS

These, of course, don't have to be for breakfast only. They're a great accompaniment to any Southwestern or Mexican dish.

nonstick vegetable oil spray
1   cup whole grain cornmeal, yellow or blue
¹/₂   cup all-purpose unbleached flour
¹/₂   cup whole wheat pastry flour
3¹/₄   teaspoons baking powder
¹/₄   teaspoon baking soda
¹/₂   teaspoon salt
1¹/₃   cups skim milk
1   large egg white, lightly beaten
¹/₃   cup maple syrup
3   tablespoons WonderSlim Fat & Egg Substitute or
          6 tablespoons applesauce or baby food prunes
1   teaspoon grated orange peel
¹/₂   cup roasted red bell peppers, finely chopped

Preheat oven to 400°. Spritz a 12-muffin tin or shallow baking pan with vegetable oil spray. Sift the cornmeal, flours, baking powder, baking soda, and salt together in a large bowl and set aside. In another large bowl, combine the milk, egg white, maple syrup, WonderSlim, and orange peel. Combine the two mixtures, add the peppers, and stir until the dry ingredients are moistened. Do not overmix. Pour batter evenly into the muffin tin or pan. Bake for 20–25 minutes, or until golden and springy.

Per muffin: 117 calories; 0.6 g fat (4.4 percent calories from fat); 4 g protein; 25 g carbohydrate; 0 mg cholesterol; 237 mg sodium.

No-Brainer Cajun Corn Bread

MAKES 10 SERVINGS

The preceding corn bread recipe doesn't exactly require nuclear physics to pull together, but this one is even easier and has a bit more spice and sweetness. This is the recipe I use for my corn bread stuffing and it's a perfect mix to experiment with. Instead of adding the ½ cup oil, butter, or margarine the package calls for, try the fat replacer WonderSlim, applesauce, or baby food prunes. If you can't find the corn bread mix called for here, use any mix that doesn't have added fats and sugars and, again, use substitutes for any fat called for on the package.

1   package Morgan Mills corn bread mix or other corn bread
      mix
¼   cup maple syrup
1   teaspoon Chef Paul Prudhomme's or other Cajun seasoning
      (see page 68 to make your own)

Prepare the corn bread mix according to package directions, but as you proceed, make these changes: substitute ¼ cup WonderSlim for every ½ cup oil, butter, or margarine. Or substitute equal amounts of applesauce or baby food prunes for the fat. As you prepare the wet ingredients, add the maple syrup and Cajun seasoning. Stir to combine and continue with package directions. Serve corn bread warm with a mild red salsa.

Per serving: 92 calories; 0.8 g fat (7.9 percent calories from fat); 3 g protein; 18 g carbohydrate; 22 mg cholesterol; 42 mg sodium.

Ten Ways to Make All Muffin Recipes
Healthier and Lower in Fat

- Replace every ½ cup of oil, butter, or margarine with ¼ cup WonderSlim.

- Substitute equal parts applesauce or baby food prunes for oil, butter, or margarine, or if WonderSlim is called for but unavailable, use double the amount of applesauce or baby food prunes.

- Substitute fat-free sour cream for the regular version. Regular sour cream has about 52 calories and 5 grams fat per 2 tablespoons, while the nonfat kinds have 20 calories and 0 grams of fat.

- Use nonfat vanilla yogurt instead of milk to give your muffins more body and flavor.

- For every whole egg called for, use two egg whites. One large egg has 79 calories and about 5½ grams fat. One egg white has 17 calories and 0 grams fat. Egg substitutes have about 25 to 40 calories (depending on the brand) and 0 grams fat per each ¼ cup.

- Fat carries flavor, so when you cut down on fat you'll need to add more flavor; i.e., cinnamon, vanilla, nutmeg, orange zest, or flavoring or extract of your choice.

- Another way to add more flavor: use frozen or fresh fruit juice as an alternative to any water or other liquid a recipe calls for.

- Replace at least one third of the all-purpose flour with whole wheat flour. Many stores carry apple fiber in the box, which you can also throw into the mix for added flavor.

- Substitute honey, FruitSource, molasses, maple syrup, or brown rice syrup for any refined sugar in a recipe.

- Mix diced dried fruit into the batter to add more minerals, texture, and flavor to your muffins.

Relax into Sunday Brunch

Okay. You finally have the time to give the morning meal some respect. Perhaps even share it with friends and savor the morning over good coffee, cappuccinos, maybe even mimosas. But you don't want to ruin everybody's day by filling them with enough fat grams to last a week. You want delicious and light—right? You've come to the right place.

Curried Sauce with Chopped Eggs

MAKES 4 SERVINGS

The sauce made from this recipe is delicious with or without the eggs. You can drizzle it over 1-inch chunks of tofu or pour it on a baked potato. Another variation: instead of eggs, stir pieces of cooked chicken, turkey, or shrimp into the sauce.

1¼	cups defatted chicken broth
1	onion, chopped
1	green bell pepper, diced
½	jalapeño, seeded and chopped
2	teaspoons finely chopped ginger root or powdered ginger
2	tablespoons flour
1	tablespoon curry powder
1	teaspoon ground cumin
¼	cup nonfat plain yogurt
2	tablespoons chopped fresh parsley
2	teaspoons lemon juice
2	hard-boiled eggs, cut into large chunks (optional)
2	hard-boiled egg whites, cut into large chunks (optional)

Heat ¼ cup of the broth in a nonstick saucepan over medium heat. Add the onion and green pepper and cook, stirring, until onion begins to color, about 5 minutes. Add the jalapeño and ginger; stir for 1 minute. Stir in the flour, curry powder, and cumin, and cook for 1 minute more. Gradually whisk in the remaining chicken broth until the mixture is smooth. Remove pan from the heat and whisk in the yogurt, 1½ tablespoons of the parsley, and lemon juice. If desired, gently stir in the chopped eggs and cover the pan to let the eggs warm for about 2 minutes. Top with the remaining parsley and serve over whole wheat toast.

Per serving: 100 calories; 3.1 g fat (27.1 percent calories from fat); 8 g protein; 11 g carbohydrate; 107 mg cholesterol; 218 mg sodium.

Eggs Milanese

MAKES 4 SERVINGS

You can add any leftover cooked vegetables to this egg dish. One quick way to cook the potatoes is to poke a few holes in them with a fork, place them in a plastic bag and put them in the microwave for 10 minutes. If they are baby new potatoes, cook for only about 5 to 7 minutes.

³/₄	cup defatted chicken broth
2	cups sliced mushrooms
1	medium onion, chopped
1	green bell pepper, chopped
¹/₂	teaspoon Italian seasoning
	dash crushed red pepper flakes
4	red potatoes, cooked and sliced
¹/₂	cup chopped frozen spinach, defrosted
3	eggs
3	egg whites
1	tablespoon Parmesan cheese
	fresh chopped tomatoes
	salt and pepper to taste

Heat ¹/₂ cup of the broth in a nonstick sauté pan until sizzling. Sauté the mushrooms and set aside. In the same pan, heat the remaining broth and sauté the onion and pepper until tender. Add the seasoning, potatoes, spinach, and mushrooms. Toss quickly. In a medium-size bowl, beat the eggs and egg whites together. Add the eggs and Parmesan to the vegetables, stirring until the eggs are set. Season to taste. Top with fresh chopped tomatoes and serve with garlic toast and fruit salad.

Per serving: 188 calories; 4.5 g fat (21.2 percent calories from fat); 12 g protein; 26 g carbohydrate; 160 mg cholesterol; 263 mg sodium.

Uno Omelette

This is really a primer in basic omelette making. You can add any filling you want to this simple recipe. Use your imagination.

1 egg
1 egg white
pinch salt (optional)
pinch pepper
nonstick vegetable oil spray

Suggested fillings

2 tablespoons salsa
1–2 ounces grated low-fat cheese
2 teaspoons sugar-free jam
1 teaspoon Fakin' Bacon Bits
1–2 tablespoons:
diced asparagus
diced artichoke hearts
diced carrots
chopped spinach
chopped tomatoes and basil
canned kidney beans
bean dip
diced onions or scallions
cooked rice pilaf
cooked lentils

Combine the first four ingredients in a small bowl and beat briskly with a fork. Heat a small nonstick frying pan over medium-high heat; remove and spritz with vegetable oil spray. Return the pan to the heat and pour in egg mixture. Stir until the bottom layer has set (about 10 seconds). Tilt the pan and, using the fork to lift the set edge of the omelet, allow the uncooked egg to flow underneath. Continue until the omelet is almost completely set, about 20 seconds. Spoon the filling(s) of your choice down the center. Use the fork to fold the omelette in half. Remove from pan and place on a plate.

Per serving (omelette without filling): 92 calories; 5 g fat (51.1 percent calories from fat); 10 g protein; 1 g carbohydrate; 212 mg cholesterol; 118 mg sodium.

Gingerbread Pancakes

MAKES 12 SERVINGS

Oh, these are worth the time to make! They're so heavenly you can even make them for dessert, topped with melted fat-free chocolate syrup, or a little liqueur, fruit, and Whip It Slim (see page 301). They also freeze well, so make a bunch.

1	cup hot water
3	tablespoons espresso or instant coffee
3	cups frozen apple juice concentrate
4	cups whole wheat flour
3	teaspoons baking soda
2	teaspoons powdered ginger
2	teaspoons cinnamon
1	teaspoon ground cloves
8	egg whites, lightly beaten
1/3	cup WonderSlim Fat & Egg substitute or 1/2 cup applesauce or baby food prunes
	nonstick vegetable oil spray

Combine the hot water and espresso or coffee in a large bowl. Add the apple juice concentrate and set aside. In another large bowl, combine the flour, baking soda, and spices. Combine the beaten egg whites and WonderSlim in a small bowl, then blend thoroughly with the coffee mixture. Add the liquid ingredients to the dry ingredients and mix just enough to moisten. The batter should be lumpy. For each pancake pour about 1/2 cup batter onto a medium-hot nonstick pan or griddle that has been spritzed with vegetable oil spray. When bubbles start to form in the pancakes, flip and brown them on the other side. Serve with maple syrup and Baked Pineapple (see page 104).

Per serving: 180 calories; 0.9 g fat (4.5 percent calories from fat); 8 g protein; 37 g carbohydrate; 0 mg cholesterol; 359 mg sodium.

Overnight Drenched French Toast with Cinnamon Syrup

MAKES 4 SERVINGS

This is a great brunch dish for kids, who consider it a special treat. I like to double the cinnamon syrup part of this recipe so I have some on hand later to use as a topping for toast, pancakes, and frozen yogurt.

1	egg
2	egg whites
3/4	cup skim milk
2	tablespoons FruitSource or sugar
1	teaspoon vanilla extract
1/4	teaspoon cinnamon
1/8	teaspoon baking powder
8	1/2-inch-thick slices Italian bread

butter-flavor nonstick vegetable oil spray

Cinnamon syrup

1/2	cup FruitSource or sugar
1/4	cup honey
1/4	teaspoon cinnamon
1/2	cup water
1/4	cup evaporated skim milk

To prepare the French toast: In a medium-size bowl, whisk together egg, egg whites, milk, FruitSource, vanilla, cinnamon, and baking powder until well blended. Take a fork and prick each slice of bread about three times on each side. Place the bread in a large, shallow baking dish and pour the mixture over the top; turn to coat evenly. Press a piece of wax paper directly on the bread to cover it, then cover the dish with plastic wrap. Refrigerate overnight. When you're ready to make the French toast, spritz a shallow nonstick sauté pan with vegetable oil spray and warm the pan over medium heat for about 10 seconds. Add the bread and cook until golden brown on both sides and no longer soggy in the middle, about 2–3 minutes per side. When all of the slices are cooked, serve with the syrup and Baked Bananas (see page 84).

To make the cinnamon syrup: In a small saucepan stir together Fruit-Source, honey, cinnamon, and water. Bring to a boil over medium heat, stirring constantly. Boil for 2 minutes, then remove from heat and stir in evaporated skim milk. Let cool and transfer to a small pitcher. Can be refrigerated for up to a week.

Per serving: 377 calories; 3.5 g fat (8.2 percent calories from fat); 11 g protein; 76 g carbohydrate; 54 mg cholesterol; 440 mg sodium.

The Wonder Waffle

MAKES 12 WAFFLES

There's no waffling on this one: Each waffle has less than 2 grams of fat—which is amazing! You can make these in large batches and freeze them (see page 81 for four ways to serve frozen waffles).

8   egg whites
4   cups skim milk
4   tablespoons WonderSlim Fat & Egg substitute or 8
      tablespoons applesauce or baby food prunes
2   cups oat bran
2   cups self-rising flour
1   tablespoon baking powder
1   teaspoon baking soda
nonstick vegetable oil spray

Beat the egg whites, milk, and WonderSlim together in a medium-size bowl until well mixed. In another bowl, mix together the oat bran, flour, baking powder, and baking soda. Slowly add the liquid ingredients to the dry ingredients, blending with a whisk as you go until smooth. Spritz a waffle iron with vegetable oil spray and heat well. Pour batter onto waffle iron—a four-waffle iron will take about one cup to fill. Cook for about 7 minutes, or until golden brown. Remove and respritz waffle iron before each batch. Top waffles with any of Knudsen's fruit syrups or maple syrup.

Per serving, not including syrup: 188 calories; 1.6 g fat (6.6 percent calories from fat); 11 g protein; 39 g carbohydrate; 1 mg cholesterol; 540 mg sodium.

Waffle Variations

Here are three ways to make the Wonder Waffle even better.

VARIATION #1—HONEY-APPLE WAFFLES

Ingredients for the Wonder Waffle, plus:

$1/2$	teaspoon cinnamon
1	tablespoon frozen apple juice concentrate
1	tablespoon honey

VARIATION #2—ORANGE VANILLA WAFFLES

Ingredients for the Wonder Waffle, plus:

1	tablespoon frozen orange juice concentrate
1	teaspoon vanilla
$1/2$	teaspoon cinnamon
1	tablespoon honey

VARIATION #3—BLUEBERRY WAFFLES

1	tablespoon blueberry syrup (I prefer Wax Orchards)
1	tablespoon honey

Follow directions for the Wonder Waffle. When all ingredients are combined, stir in the remaining variation ingredients. Pour batter onto the waffle iron spritzed with vegetable oil spray—a four-waffle iron will take about one cup to fill. Cook for about 7 minutes, or until golden brown. Remove and respritz waffle iron before each batch.

Average per serving: 259 calories; 2.2 g fat (7.6 percent calories from fat); 15 g protein; 54 g carbohydrate; 2 mg cholesterol; 743 mg sodium.

Hash Browns

Let these notoriously fatty potatoes see the "light." I like to use leftover potatoes, but if you don't have them on hand start from scratch and follow the instructions given here. Either way you'll have cut the fat to less than 1 little gram. And that 1 gram can be any flavor—use butter-, olive-, or garlic-flavored vegetable oil sprays for variation.

3   **medium potatoes, peeled and quartered**
olive-flavored nonstick vegetable oil spray
2¹/₂   **tablespoons defatted chicken broth**
1   **small onion, chopped**
¹/₂   **teaspoon salt**
¹/₄   **teaspoon pepper**
pinch paprika
1   **tablespoon chopped fresh parsley**

Place the potatoes in a medium saucepan and cover with cold, lightly salted water. Bring to a boil and cook 5–10 minutes, or until the potatoes are just tender. Drain and cool. Cut the potatoes into ¹/₂-inch cubes. Spray a large nonstick pan with nonstick vegetable spray. Add the broth and onion and sauté over medium heat until tender, about 5 minutes. Spray the top of the onion with vegetable oil, then add the potatoes. Allow them to brown, then spray again. Keep turning the potatoes as they brown, using the spray again as needed. Cook until brown all over, about 10–15 minutes. Season with salt, pepper, and paprika. Top with parsley and serve.

Per serving: *125 calories; 0.1 g fat (5 percent calories from fat); 7 g protein; 25 g carbohydrate; 0 mg cholesterol; 477 mg sodium.*

Baked Pineapple

MAKES 8 SERVINGS

Baking pineapple gives it a rich, syrupy taste, and serving this instead of just fresh pineapple makes a brunch feel like more of an occasion. You can serve a steaming slice in the A.M.—it's great with omelettes, biscuits, and jam—then chop the leftovers into cubes and use it to top chicken or fish later on.

1   **pineapple (about 3 pounds), peeled**
1   **teaspoon cinnamon**
1–2   **tablespoons light brown sugar (optional)**
nonstick vegetable oil spray

Preheat the oven to 350°. Cut off the top of the pineapple, then cut the pineapple in half. Sprinkle the cinnamon and brown sugar over the fruit. Spritz a baking sheet with vegetable oil spray and place the pineapple flat side down on the baking sheet. Bake for 45–60 minutes, or until soft and fragrant. Cut into slices.

Per serving: *97 calories; 0.8 g fat (7 percent calories from fat); 1 g protein; 24 g carbohydrate; 0 mg cholesterol; 2 mg sodium.*

Chapter Eight

Let's Do Lunch—and Do It Right

"Lunch" is a great word. Let's do lunch, meet for lunch, ladies who lunch, business lunch, the luncheon, lovers' lunch, power lunch, break for lunch, the lunch wagon, a picnic lunch, pack a lunch, and that long-awaited lunch whistle. But as wonderful as lunch is, it's most people's diet downfall—the meal that they find most difficult to make healthful and low-fat. Not coincidentally, lunch is also the meal that most fast food places make their living off of, taking advantage of the fact that very few people have lunch at home as a family meal (actually, I don't know *anyone* who does). Even full-time moms often find themselves either skipping lunch or grabbing it somewhere away from home while they're running around.

In my first book, *Food Cop*, I wrote a whole chapter on the best choices at restaurants and fast food joints. I'm happy to say that things have only improved since then. You can eat well at almost any eatery in America. And those where you can't? Avoid them. There's really no excuse for choosing restaurants that won't accommodate your needs when there are so many out there that will.

Granted, if you are in a business that requires you to "power lunch" frequently, you may often end up in restaurants that have so many delicious temptations, you'll want to throw low-fat eating right out the window. But remember: a business lunch is about business, not savoring every delight the restaurant has to offer. As I said to one client who was headed to a meeting at a fine restaurant in L.A., "If it's not your birthday and it's not a party, save your indulgences." Plus, if you're like most business lunchers, you probably frequent the same three or four restaurants, which gives you the perfect opportunity to make requests that only a regular customer can get away with.

Let the staff know that you don't like olive oil or butter all over your food. Let them know that you always like your baked potato dry with salsa, and your pasta with plain tomato, basil, and garlic. This will make it easier when you're ordering at a high-pressure lunch and don't want to feel uncomfortable making special requests.

Most of all, don't let low physical self-esteem be the price you pay for success. In other words, as you are climbing the ladder of success, don't bury the joy of being successful with a body you hate. That is not a sacrifice you have to make.

There are many businesswomen with loaded schedules who manage to maintain figures we all admire despite frequent power lunching. But even if business lunches aren't your thing—if the idea of sitting down to lunch at all is outrageous—there are still easy, no-hassle steps to a healthy lunch.

Moms like myself, who are usually eating on the run, in between dropping one kid off at day care and shuttling the other off to soccer practice, have to think ahead. Pack lean and healthy food. Moms learn to pack things along from the diaper-bag stage on. Why not good food? Don't just choose whatever crosses your path—especially if you've waited so long to eat that you're starving.

In the spring of 1995, I did a one-month stint on the *Mike & Maty* show. My task was to work with a group of women taking the show's "Change Your Life Challenge"—the show had challenged a group of working women and a group of moms to lose weight. One of the moms I was helping had a bad habit of diving into her kids' French fries. Keep a bag of fat-free crackers in your purse at all times, I told her, and you'll have the will to resist. When you are craving a fattening food, and eat a fat-free substitute (like the crackers) instead, you're likely to be satisfied by the third bite. After the month was up, she preferred the crackers to the fries! So it's worth it to have them with you. And if you're not going to pack food along, take the time to research the foods on your day's route. You would be surprised how many places around you have the food you need—and can fix it for you quickly.

To show you just how solvable lunch problems are, here are a couple of cases from my client file showing how we attacked lunch head-on.

Plan Your Route *or* Bring the Loot: Fran's Fulfillment

Fran is a full-time mom with two boys. She came to see me when her youngest was two and a half years old, and she was finally ready to tackle those last fifteen postpregnancy pounds. Fran complained of never being in the same place twice during lunchtime due to her kids' varied schedules. Yet when we looked closely at her days, we found there was in fact enough regularity to map out some strategies.

Most days, Fran would drop off her kids at their individual schools, then work out with a trainer. After exercising, she was generally famished, but only had about twenty minutes before she picked up her youngest son. A block away from the gym where she worked out was a little Italian restaurant, which she avoided, assuming it had only fattening foods. But when we called we found out that the restaurant makes a great chopped salad. Asking them to substitute chicken for the cheese and salami, then dress the salad with a little balsamic vinegar, Fran had her answer. She was getting a healthy dose of veggies and the protein she needed to satisfy her.

Next, we stocked her car. She never left the house without diapers and wipes; why not also include fat-free pretzels, lunch-size no-oil tortilla chips, and other munchies? That way, if she got stuck at Gymboree or at a soccer match she always had something healthful to eat.

Don't Be a Victim: Paula's Possibilities

Paula had an ordering-in lunch problem. Busy running her own production company, she was caught in the dangerous "somebody go get lunch" syndrome. Relegating lunch to someone else means that you also relegate responsibility for what you eat. Men are particularly susceptible to this—it's not in their nature to go over little menu details with their assistants, especially when they're busy. Many working women are now falling victim to the same problem, too.

Paula and I looked at about six menus from the restaurants she normally ordered from and discovered healthy, fat-free choices on all of them. It had been her habit just to let an assistant order the usual entrees instead of looking at the side dishes and appetizers, which are often lower in fat and can be pieced together to make a meal. I also pointed out that there was a huge supermarket within two blocks of Paula's office that had a great salad bar with oil-free dressings, and a deli with a number of healthy choices. Most people don't think of going to the market for lunch, but it's worth checking out.

Be a Leader: Sandra's Social Solutions

Sandra is a well-to-do woman involved in many committees, charities, and events. Her calendar is a social calendar, and lunch is always booked at fine restaurants. The problem was that Sandra was getting too fat for all of her designer clothes. I explained to her that although it is lovely to have the finest food put in front of you daily and have a lovely, gossipy lunch with friends, it is not lovely to have those lunches ruin your body and health.

I've always found it quite amazing that women around the table will talk about how they should lose weight, talk about their diets and exercise programs, complain about their bodies, but not spend any of that energy ordering lean food! That just seems crazy and ridiculous to me. The funny thing is, if one woman does get up the nerve to order healthfully, the rest usually follow suit.

So that's what I encouraged Sandra to do. Instead of going to some quack diet doctor and getting shots in her behind, the solution she had opted for previously, I asked her to be brave and take the lead. Lunch is a great time to have a salad, I told her. So have one—and have one with some grilled chicken, shrimp, or salmon, and a piece of bread, too, so that you'll be satisfied, not starving later. Elaborate salads are always a big lunch item at most restaurants and she could order it with oil-free dressing, pack along her own oil-free dressing, or ask for it served with salsa or balsamic vinegar. Ordering lean lunches made a huge difference in Sandra's overall diet.

No-Brainer Lunches

Some of the following recipes can be packed up and taken with you; some are for lunching at home. All are new takes on old favorites and make life easier, giving you time to use your brain for other, more important, matters.

Mini Pita Pizza

MAKES 1 SERVING

When most of us think about making pizza we think about mixing the dough, letting it rise, rolling out the crust, the brick oven, the paddle—the whole nine yards. That has its place (namely, in Chapter 11), but so does taking the easy way out: use a pita as your crust. And don't just limit yourself to these toppings. Use your imagination or steal some topping ideas from your local gourmet pizza eatery.

3   tablespoons Millina's or other fat-free brand pasta sauce
1   whole wheat pita

1   mushroom, sliced
3   slices green bell pepper
1   tablespoon grated Parmesan cheese

Spread the pasta sauce over the pita. Top with the mushroom and pepper slices. Sprinkle on the Parmesan and heat in a 350° oven or toaster oven for 3–5 minutes.

Per serving: 181 calories; 2.7 g fat (12.9 percent calories from fat); 9 g protein; 32 g carbohydrate; 4 mg cholesterol; 352 mg sodium.

Pita Ahorita

MAKES 1 SERVING

Everyone knows how to stuff a pita, but this gives you some idea of how to keep the fat out and flavor in. Instead of the yogurt you can use a low-fat cucumber-dill dressing. If you use a different type of tomato, take out the seeds or your pita will get soggy.

1   teaspoon lemon juice
1   tablespoon nonfat plain yogurt
1/2   teaspoon dill weed
1   whole wheat pita
1   Roma tomato, chopped
1/2   cucumber, chopped
1/2   can water-packed tuna, drained, or 1 mini pop-top can

In a small bowl, combine the lemon juice, yogurt, and dill. Fill the pita with the tomato, cucumber, and tuna. Top with the yogurt mixture.

Per serving: 145 calories; 1 g fat (8 percent calories from fat); 23 g protein; 11 g carbohydrate; 24 mg cholesterol; 293 mg sodium.

Open-Face Rice Cake Sandwiches

MAKES 1 SERVING

Rice cakes are typically thought of as snacks, but they're also put to good use at lunchtime. Here are three rice cake sandwiches that are a snap to make.

No-Brainer Lunch Tips

Pack it along. No one's asking you to stand at the counter for a half hour each morning making yourself a gourmet lunch. The following are all the great new, healthy, low-fat products and easy food ideas that you can toss into your briefcase, a brown bag, purse, gym bag, car, or desk.

- Mini 3.5-ounce pop-top cans of water-packed tuna or chicken breast
- Any of the natural cup o' soups and chilies (Health Valley, Fantastic Foods, Nile Spice, Westbrae; look for low-sodium varieties)
- Mini lunch-size bags of no-oil tortilla chips
- Mini lunch-size bags of caramel or popcorn cakes
- Small pop-top cans of fruits packed in their own juice or water
- Mini (yogurt-size) containers of nonfat cottage cheese
- Mini containers of applesauce and fruit applesauce
- Sandwich bags of flavored fat-free rice cakes
- Sandwich bags of fat-free crackers
- Sardines packed in water or mustard sauce
- Sandwich bags of fat-free pretzels
- Fat-free string cheese
- A potato or yam to microwave at work
- Fat-free granola bars
- Sandwich bags of fat-free cookies
- Mini lunch-size bags of fat-free potato chips
- Mini-size fat-free yogurt (4.4 ounces)
- Bags of precut veggies, or baby carrots
- Fat-free bagel chips
- Mini bags of dried apple snacks or carrot snacks
- Precooked soy hot dogs (low in fat and last longer than meat/turkey franks)
- Fruit, glorious fruit

The average rice cake is 50 calories and 0 grams of fat. Your topping calorie and fat counts will vary, but all of these are healthy and low-fat.

VARIATION #1

2   cheddar cheese-flavored rice cakes
1   slice fat-free cheese (your choice)
1   slice turkey breast

VARIATION #2

2   popcorn cakes
1   slice fat-free Monterey Jack cheese
1   Roma tomato, sliced

VARIATION #3

2   fat-free caramel corn cakes
1   slice part-skim Muenster cheese
1   tablespoon raisins

Top one of the rice cakes with the cheese. Place in a 350° oven or toaster oven and warm until cheese melts. Remove from the oven and divide the remaining ingredients between the two rice cakes. Serve open face.

Sardine Bites

MAKES 2 SERVINGS

The poor forgotten sardine. Here is a perfectly delicious and easy lunch—or snack—scorned by most Americans. Not only can you get low-fat, oil-free sardines packed in vinegar or mustard, they're also loaded with calcium. And we all know how important calcium is for bone strength. Truth be told, this was my favorite lunch (along with a few hard-boiled eggs) during my last pregnancy! Here's a two-minute way to prepare them. You can even pack the sardines and a box of crackers to work with you and make this meal in the kitchenette.

1   tablespoon Dijon mustard
1   tablespoon pickle relish
4   Wasa crackers or other fat-free whole wheat crackers
3   ounces fat-free Jack cheese, sliced
1   can sardines, packed in mustard

Spread the mustard and pickle relish on two of the crackers. Divide the cheese and sardines between the two dressed crackers, then top with the remaining crackers. If you prefer, use whole wheat bread instead of crackers.

Per serving: 118 calories; 2.6 g fat (22.8 percent calories from fat); 15 g protein; 5 g carbohydrate; 16 mg cholesterol; 582 mg sodium.

Tuna-Stuffed Baked Potato

MAKES 4 SERVINGS

This is just one way to stuff a baked potato—among hundreds. Other fillings include leftovers, fat-free sour cream, and chopped scallions. Also see Yam On, page 114, for more ideas.

4   large russet potatoes
1   can water-packed tuna, drained and separated with a fork
4   ounces fat-free cheddar cheese, grated
4   tablespoons salsa

Prick a few holes in the potatoes with a fork. Rinse with cold water and place the wet potatoes in a plastic bag. Microwave on high for 15 minutes, or until cooked through. If you're going to bake the potatoes, prick and wrap in foil. Place in a preheated 350° oven and bake for 1 hour. Remove the potatoes from the oven and slice them open. Divide filling ingredients evenly among potatoes.

Per serving: 182 calories; 1 g fat (5.3 percent calories from fat); 21 g protein; 21 g carbohydrate; 15 mg cholesterol; 376 mg sodium.

The Office Potato

MAKES 1 SERVING

This is a super-quick, satisfying lunch with a big carbohydrate and protein payoff to get you through the day. Always keep a jar of salsa in the office fridge. A can of black beans or one of the new fat-free bean dips will keep anywhere.

1   russet potato
3   tablespoons salsa

2   tablespoons canned black beans
1   teaspoon fat-free cheddar cheese (optional)

Poke a few holes in the potato with a fork. Rinse with cold water and place the wet potato in a plastic bag. Microwave on high for 8–15 minutes, depending on the size of the potato, or until cooked through. Remove the potato from the oven and slice it open. Top with salsa and beans. Sprinkle a little grated fat-free cheddar cheese on top if you like.

Per serving, not including cheese: 191 calories; 2.3 g fat (10.3 percent calories from fat); 8 g protein; 36 g carbohydrate; 0 mg cholesterol; 44 mg sodium.

Yam On: Five Variations on the Theme
MAKES 2 SERVINGS

The yam has become my new best friend. Not only is it satisfying, rich, and slightly sweet, it has all the beta carotene you need for one day. A medium yam has 150 calories and 0 fat grams. So don't wait for Thanksgiving to roll around. Stock up on some yams and try these variations.

VARIATION #1

2   yams
$1/2$ cup frozen corn, cooked
$1/2$ cup frozen peas, cooked
$1/2$ cup chopped red bell pepper
4   ounces fat-free Jack cheese, grated
pinch nutmeg
$1/2$ teaspoon cinnamon
1   tablespoon maple syrup

VARIATION #2

2   yams
1   banana, sliced
2   teaspoons honey

VARIATION #3

2   yams
2   tablespoons Guiltless Gourmet or other fat-free brand spicy
     black bean dip
4   ounces fat-free mild Mexican or cheddar cheese, grated
2   tablespoons salsa

VARIATION #4

2   yams
1/2 cup canned pumpkin
1   teaspoon pumpkin pie spice
1   teaspoon honey
1/4 teaspoon cinnamon
2   tablespoons nonfat vanilla yogurt

VARIATION #5

2   yams
1   teaspoon Cajun seasoning
1/2 cup frozen chopped onions, defrosted, or sautéed onions
1   teaspoon lemon juice
2   tablespoons canned black beans

Prick yams several times all over with a fork and rinse with water.

To cook in the microwave: Put the wet yams in a plastic bag and place in the microwave. Cook on high 10–15 minutes (depending on the size of the yams). Poke with a fork to see if they are soft all the way through.

To bake in the oven: Wrap the yams in aluminum foil and place in a preheated 350° oven. Bake for 15–20 minutes or until soft all the way through. When yams are done, slice down the middle and scoop out the flesh. In a medium-size bowl, mix with the remaining ingredients. Stuff the yam mixture back into the skin or transfer to a baking dish. Place back in the microwave for another 30 seconds, or in the oven for another 5 minutes.

Per serving: 132 calories; 1.2 g fat (7.5 percent calories from fat); 9.3 g protein; 22.7 g carbohydrate; 3 mg cholesterol; 227 mg sodium.

Tuna Salad with Tomatoes and Capers

MAKES 2 SERVINGS

I really think mayonnaise is passé. We can get along so well without it, and this recipe is proof. When I give my clients' fridges a makeover, the first thing I do is take out the mayonnaise, and they inevitably ask, "How will I make tuna salad?" Here's how (see the other tuna salads on following pages, too). And don't wrinkle your nose at the idea of tuna and cottage cheese combined. My mother recommended it to me when I was pregnant with my daughter, and I lived on it. It's a light, fresh mix, and a high-protein lunch.

1   6-ounce can water-packed tuna, drained
1   teaspoon red wine vinegar
1   cup fat-free cottage cheese
1   tomato, seeded and chopped
1   tablespoon capers
salt and pepper, to taste

In a medium-size bowl, separate the tuna with a fork. Sprinkle the vinegar over the tuna, then add the remaining ingredients. Mix thoroughly. Serve on Rye Krisp crackers.

Per serving: 188 calories; 0.9 g fat (4.7 percent calories from fat); 21 g protein; 19 g carbohydrate; 24 mg cholesterol; 420 mg sodium.

Mustard-Yogurt Tuna Salad

MAKES 2 SERVINGS

I like to use mini cans of water-packed tuna because you can pack them with you to the office or carry them in your purse. You can even open up the tuna, sprinkle on a little vinegar, and eat it right out of the can.

1/2   6-ounce can water-packed tuna, drained
1   tablespoon canned navy beans
2   tablespoons nonfat plain yogurt
1   teaspoon lemon juice
1   teaspoon Dijon mustard
1   teaspoon chopped scallions

In a medium-size bowl, mash the tuna with a fork. Add the remaining ingredients, toss to combine, and serve. Use to fill a sandwich or top fat-free cheddar rice cakes.

Per serving: 80 calories; 0.6 g fat (6.4 percent calories from fat); 13 g protein; 5 g carbohydrate; 12 mg cholesterol; 181 mg sodium.

Two Hearts Tuna Salad

MAKES 2 SERVINGS

Artichoke hearts and hearts of palm are vegetables we use far too infrequently. But perhaps the rarity of their appearance on the plate is what makes having this tuna and double heart salad seem like you're treating yourself to something special. If you want to spruce the salad up even more, toss in a few kidney beans or some grated Parmesan cheese.

1   14-ounce can water-packed hearts of palm, drained and sliced
      into $1/4$-inch rounds
1   14-ounce can water-packed artichoke hearts, drained and
      quartered
$1/2$ 6-ounce can water-packed tuna, drained
1   tomato, diced
2   tablespoons balsamic vinegar

Place the hearts of palm and artichoke hearts in a medium-size bowl. Add the tuna, flaking it with a fork as you combine it with the hearts. Add the tomato and drizzle the vinegar over the top. Toss and serve with whole grain crackers.

Per serving: 104 calories; 0.7 g fat (5.3 percent calories from fat); 14 g protein; 13 g carbohydrate; 12 mg cholesterol; 223 mg sodium.

Leisurely Lunches

On days when you do have the time to make a "real" lunch, these recipes allow you to have a gourmet meal without having to make a gourmet effort. It's always a good idea to make extra on these occasions so you have leftovers on hand for lunches the rest of the week.

Curried Chicken Salad

This is one of those dishes usually made with mayonnaise—delicious but fatty. Here I use nonfat yogurt to impart creaminess, then pour on the Indian spices to give it zing. If you don't have the pineapple-apricot jam called for, use apricot jam mixed with a couple of tablespoons of canned crushed pineapple. Also, if turmeric is not in your pantry, substitute mustard powder. This dish also makes a nice dinner entree; just add some cooked pasta like small shells or penne to make it heartier.

2	tablespoons maple syrup
2	cups nonfat plain yogurt
1	tablespoon curry powder (preferably Madras)
1	tablespoon pineapple-apricot jam
1	teaspoon turmeric
1/4	teaspoon cinnamon
pinch cayenne pepper	
4	6-ounce boneless skinless chicken breasts, cooked and cubed
1/2	cup raisins
1/2	cup sliced scallions
2	Golden Delicious apples, diced
1/2	cup diced celery
salt and pepper to taste	

In a medium-size bowl, blend the maple syrup, yogurt, curry powder, jam, turmeric, cinnamon, and cayenne pepper with a whisk. In a large bowl, combine the chicken, raisins, scallions, apples, and celery. Pour the yogurt mixture over the chicken mixture and toss to combine. Season with salt and pepper. Serve spooned onto plates or wrap salad in whole wheat chapatis, which is a type of unleavened bread. If you can't find chapatis, use fat-free flour tortillas.

Per serving: 243 calories; 2 g fat (7 percent calories from fat); 31 g protein; 28 g carbohydrate; 67 mg cholesterol; 148 mg sodium.

Thousand Island Chicken Salad

MAKES 5 SERVINGS

The dressing for this dish is also terrific over potato salad. If you can't find dry Thousand Island dressing mix, look for a fat-free bottled version.

Skinny Thousand Island Dressing

- ½ **cup tofu**
- ¼ **cup cider vinegar**
- ½ **cup ketchup**
- 1 **package dry Thousand Island salad dressing mix**

Chicken Salad

- 2 **4-ounce boneless skinless chicken breasts, cooked and cubed**
- 1 **tablespoon Fakin' Bacon Bits**
- 1 **tablespoon pickle relish**
- ½ **cup diced celery**
- ½ **cup sliced cherry tomatoes**
- 2 **ounces sliced black olives**

Combine the tofu, vinegar, ketchup, and dressing mix in a blender or food processor; process until smooth, about 1 minute. Place the chicken, bacon bits, relish, celery, tomatoes, and olives in a large bowl. Drizzle on the dressing; toss to combine.

Per serving: 115 calories; 3.1 g fat (23.1 percent calories from fat); 13 g protein; 10 g carbohydrate; 26 mg cholesterol; 428 mg sodium.

Broccoli and Wild Rice Salad

MAKES 4 SERVINGS

Rather than using wild rice in this dish, you can use leftover brown rice or any of the great rice mixes made by Arrowhead Mills or other natural food companies. Barley or cooked lentils are also great alternatives. This is one of the dishes I like to make a lot of so that I can have it for lunch during the week. If you don't have time to chop the vegetables, use a bag of frozen mixed vegetables. You can buy carrots already shredded in most produce sections, too.

2	cups wild rice, cooked
$^1/_2$	cup broccoli florets
$^1/_2$	cup peeled, sliced broccoli spears
1	cup oil-free Italian salad dressing
4	Roma tomatoes, seeded and diced
$^1/_4$	cup shredded carrot
2	tablespoons diced scallions
2	tablespoons diced green bell pepper
$^1/_2$	cup diced roasted red peppers, not marinated in oil

salt and pepper to taste

Cook the wild rice according to package directions. Drain and set aside to cool. Steam the broccoli florets and spears; set aside to cool. Toss all of the ingredients in a bowl; season with salt and pepper. Chill for at least one hour and serve.

Per serving: 130 calories; 1 g fat (6.5 percent calories from fat); 6 g protein; 28 g carbohydrate; 0 mg cholesterol; 28 mg sodium.

Burritos Supreme

MAKES 4 SERVINGS

Sandwiches are great because they allow you to get many of a day's recommended foods—vegetables, grains, protein—all in one shot. But let's face it, after a while, sandwiches get boring. That's where the lunchtime burrito comes in. It, too, is all-encompassing, but a nice change for the palate.

	nonstick vegetable oil spray
6	ounces ground turkey breast
2	teaspoons taco seasoning mix
4	no-oil whole wheat tortillas
6	ounces fat-free mild Mexican cheese or cheddar, grated
$^3/_4$	cup salsa
$^1/_2$	cup frozen corn, defrosted and cooked
4	tablespoons Guiltless Gourmet or other fat-free brand bean dip
$^1/_2$	cup shredded lettuce

nonfat sour cream and chopped scallions, for topping (optional)

Spritz a nonstick sauté pan with vegetable oil spray. Sauté the ground turkey and taco seasoning over medium heat, until the turkey is no longer pink. Transfer to a bowl. Briefly heat the tortillas in a toaster oven, then place on a plate. Place the remaining ingredients in separate bowls, arrange on a table, then let everyone assemble his or her own burrito. Or, lay the burritos flat, spoon some turkey mixture over each, then divide the remaining ingredients among each. Fold two ends of the tortillas in first, then roll the tortillas into burritos. Serve with some nonfat sour cream and chopped scallions, if desired.

Per serving, not including sour cream: 211 calories; 4.2 g fat (13.1 percent calories from fat); 28 g protein; 35 g carbohydrate; 30 mg cholesterol; 720 mg sodium.

Garden Burritos

MAKES 4 SERVINGS

Believe me when I tell you that this is one of the best-selling items from my home delivery service. I think the burrito is going to take the place of the sandwich in the future. This one, in particular, is chock-full of vegetables and, by extension, loaded with fiber, vitamins, and minerals. I make about six of these on Monday for the kids' lunches, or for an after-school snack. To spice it up even more, add 1/4 fresh jalapeño, diced, when cooking the vegetables.

1/4	cup defatted chicken broth
1	red bell pepper, seeded, cored, and chopped
1	cup frozen corn, defrosted
2	zucchini, diced
1/2	teaspoon oregano
4	tablespoons salsa
4	no-oil whole wheat tortillas
1	cup canned black beans, drained
4	ounces fat-free cheddar cheese, grated
1	cup shredded lettuce

nonfat sour cream and cilantro for toppings (optional)

In a medium-size nonstick saucepan, heat the broth over medium heat. Add the bell pepper, corn, zucchini, oregano, and salsa. Cook for 5–7 minutes over medium heat until the vegetables are just soft. Drain off any extra liquid. Take each tortilla and layer the drained beans, vegetable filling, and cheese (add extra fresh salsa if you choose). Fold two ends of the tortillas in first, then roll the tortillas into burritos. Serve on a bed of shredded lettuce topped with grated cheese and a dollop of salsa. You can also heat the burritos in a toaster oven and top with fresh chopped cilantro and nonfat sour cream.

Per serving, not including sour cream: 203 calories; 2.3 g fat (7.3 percent calories from fat); 18 g protein; 49 g carbohydrate; 3 mg cholesterol; 475 mg sodium.

Southwest Turkey Burritos

MAKES 4 SERVINGS

This burrito—my husband's favorite—isn't as spicy as the Burritos Supreme; however, it has a savory mix of spices that make the taste buds take notice.

¹/₂	red bell pepper, diced fine
1	tablespoon balsamic vinegar
2	tablespoons defatted chicken broth
¹/₂	pound ground turkey breast
2	teaspoons Chef Paul Prudhomme's Seafood Magic Cajun seasoning or other Cajun seasoning
4	no-oil whole wheat tortillas
4	ounces fat-free cheddar cheese, grated
4	teaspoons tomatillo salsa or green salsa

Place the red pepper in a small bowl and douse with the vinegar; set aside to marinate. Heat the chicken broth in a nonstick sauté pan. Add the ground turkey, then the Cajun seasoning as you stir. Continue cooking over medium heat until the turkey is no longer pink. Remove from heat and drain. Drain the pepper. Lay the tortillas flat and spoon the cooked turkey, grated cheese, pepper, and 1 teaspoon of the salsa onto each. Fold two ends of the tortillas in first, then roll them into burritos. Top with a dollop of fat-free sour cream, if desired. These store well in the fridge for up to three days.

Per serving, not including sour cream: 156 calories; 1.1 g fat (4.5 percent calories from fat); 25 g protein; 27 g carbohydrate; 37 mg cholesterol; 498 mg sodium.

Chicken Enchiladas

For those of you who don't live in a Mexican food haven as I do, the main difference between a taco, burrito, and enchilada is that the enchilada is baked and covered with sauce. The sauce is often fatty, but fat-free ones are also available now. This recipe is fairly basic and you can add your own touches. Toss some cooked corn, peas, or rice into the filling, for instance. Or use tomatillo salsa instead of red enchilada sauce. Let your creative juices flow.

4   4-ounce boneless skinless chicken breasts, cooked and
      shredded
1/2   cup chopped onion
2   tablespoons chopped cilantro
6   ounces fat-free mild Mexican or cheddar cheese, grated
1   teaspoon garlic powder
8   no-oil corn tortillas
2   cups fat-free enchilada sauce
2   teaspoons sliced black olives

Preheat oven to 350°. Combine the chicken, onion, cilantro (reserving some for garnish), grated cheese, and garlic powder in a large bowl. Place the enchilada sauce in a medium-size bowl and dip the tortillas into the sauce; place on a platter. Spoon a portion of the filling onto each tortilla, then roll them into tubes. Spoon some of the sauce in the bottom of a large, shallow baking dish. Lay the enchiladas in the pan so that they touch each other. Ladle the rest of the sauce on top and garnish with sliced olives and cilantro. Cover the dish with foil and bake for 10 minutes. Remove foil and bake another 10 minutes. Serve with Pinto Bean Fiesta salad, see page 146.

Per serving: 226 calories; 3.5 g fat (18.2 percent calories from fat); 27 g protein; 8 g carbohydrate; 47 mg cholesterol; 494 mg sodium.

Terrific Tacos

Tacos have come a long way, and not just from Mexico. What I mean is that this Latin alternative to the sandwich no longer has to be fat encased in a

Taco Tips

- To heat the tortillas, you can place them directly on a gas or electric burner turned to medium heat for about 10 seconds. Just be sure to turn them quickly before they burn. Lay them in a folded clean dish towel to keep warm.
- Use cooked ground turkey or chicken breast, turkey tenders, or cooked fish to fill your tacos. Sauté as you do the chicken in the above recipe.
- Some great fillers:
  Black olives
  Bean dips (spread on the tortilla)
  Chopped cilantro
  Cooked corn and peas
  Cooked brown (or any kind) rice
  Chopped tomatoes
  Chopped scallions
  Chopped onions
  Chopped celery
  Chopped cooked potatoes
  Scrambled eggs
  Chopped cabbage
  Grilled veggies
  Chopped red, yellow, or green bell peppers
  Cooked lentils

hand-held tortilla. The following is a basic taco recipe, but I'm also going to give you a list of the many items you can fill your tacos with so that they never get dull. Remember that a basic corn tortilla is just corn, lime, and water—it doesn't need fat, so watch out for the ones with added lard or preservatives.

¼	cup white wine
1	tablespoon taco seasoning mix
2	6-ounce boneless skinless chicken breasts, cooked and cut into strips
8	no-oil corn tortillas
1	cup chopped lettuce
4	ounces fat-free cheddar cheese, grated

³/₄ **cup canned pinto beans**
1 **cup salsa**
nonfat sour cream for garnish (optional)

Heat the white wine in a nonstick sauté pan. Add the taco seasoning, blend, and add the chicken. Sauté for 5 minutes. Heat the tortillas in the oven or on the stovetop (see Taco Tips, above). Hold one in the palm of your hand so that it forms a pocket. Spoon in chicken, lettuce, cheese, and a dollop of beans. Top with salsa and, if desired, a dollop of nonfat sour cream. Place assembled tacos on a plate or, if you prefer, serve the tacos unconstructed and allow everyone to assemble his or her own.

Per serving: 209 calories; 3.3 g fat (14.4 percent calories from fat); 22 g protein; 22 g carbohydrate; 35 mg cholesterol; 485 mg sodium.

Chicken-Apple Egg Rolls

MAKES 8 SERVINGS

Egg rolls are for take-out only, right? Wrong. They may seem complicated, but they're really as easy to make as sandwiches. This recipe calls for Chinese five-spice powder, which can be found in the spice section of your supermarket.

3 **4-ounce boneless skinless chicken breasts**
1¹/₂ **cups chopped Granny Smith apple**
1 **cup chopped cabbage**
³/₄ **cup grated fat-free Swiss cheese**
¹/₂ **cup chopped scallion**
2 **teaspoons Chinese five-spice powder**
¹/₄ **teaspoon salt**
8 **egg roll skins**
nonstick vegetable oil spray

Preheat oven to 400°. Place the chicken breasts in a saucepan and cover with water. Bring the water to a boil and poach the chicken until cooked through, about 8 minutes. Let cool. Remove the chicken breasts and slice into thin slivers. (If you like, you can use leftover cooked chicken, or canned chicken breast, drained, instead.) Combine the chicken and next 6 ingredients in a large bowl; toss well. Separate the egg roll skins. Spoon about 2 heaping tablespoons of the chicken mixture onto one wrapper and fold the lower right corner over the mixture. Then fold the lower left and top right corners over chicken mixture. Moisten top left corner with the spray and roll up. Line a pan with aluminum foil. Spritz the foil with the spray. Coat the rolls with the nonstick spray and place them seam side down in the pan. Bake for 15 minutes or until golden brown. Serve with plum dip or Marmalade Chutney (see recipe, page 172).

Per serving: *119 calories; 0.9 g fat (7.3 percent calories from fat); 17 g protein; 9 g carbohydrate; 28 mg cholesterol; 316 mg sodium.*

Chapter Nine

When It's Not a Meal, What Is It?
Snacks, Appetizers, and Starters

One of the first things I do when clients come to see me is talk schedule. Or, I should say, lack of schedule. It's already passé to talk about the fact that our lives are chaotic. But what people so often *don't* talk about is that the chaos in our lives disrupts our eating schedules. There is very little pattern to the way most people eat, or if there is a pattern it no longer resembles the ordered, three-meal-a-day plan of the past.

I like to call this "disordered eating"—eating that's out of order, in the sense that there's no logic to it. This isn't to suggest that there's no rhyme or reason to your eating habits, or that you have psychological problems. But you probably do have something in common with people who have true eating disorders: Your eating is out of control, though due to your lifestyle rather than to some deep-seated problem.

And it's frustrating. It's frustrating to feel that you can't get your food life in balance. You're undoubtedly already giving your all just to balance work, family, friends, and, don't forget, your fitness regimen. How much more can you be expected to juggle? Disordered eating makes you begin to feel as if food is just happening to you. You end up eating whatever crosses your path at whatever time that might be. And as a result, you don't eat healthfully. You rely on food that is convenient but junky; available but fattening.

A perfect example of someone who could very well have a disordered eating problem (if he didn't have a wife watching out for him) is my very own husband, Richard. He is a sales executive who spends a lot of time in his car, five days a week. He leaves the house at 7:45 A.M. and sometimes doesn't get home until 10:30 or 11:30 at night. When Richard started this job a year ago I was concerned that he would end up stopping off at fast food places, eating the worst junk possible and ruining his health. So before he began, we looked up all of the fast food places on his route, identified the best ones (or you might say the least bad), then looked for some other places he might stop, too. By doing so, we circumvented some of the bad meals he could have ended up having. Plus, no matter what he eats on the road, there's always good food waiting for him at home, even if he doesn't return until 11 P.M.

Some people might say, "Eating dinner at eleven, that's not healthy." But I disagree. As long as the food Richard is eating is lean and healthy, he will be too. The point is, you can eat well even if your eating pattern is disordered. If you're going to be eating at off hours, if you're not going to be eating meals at all—just snacking—if you're just trying to satisfy your cravings, whatever, you can still eat healthfully.

Which brings me to the reason that I have lumped snacks together with hors d'oeuvres and starters. Appetizers are rarely served at home, before the dinner hour, unless we are entertaining; we usually only eat them when we are dining out. There's no reason that certain kinds of foods should be reserved for specific occasions, especially if it makes sense to eat them anytime. A perfect example is Grilled Mushrooms (see page 130). I used to make them as a side dish, but would always grill them early, then set them aside until dinner. Well, grilled mushrooms are so succulent, soft, and chewy, that everybody just dove into them before dinner was even served. Now I just grill a bunch and serve them as appetizers or keep them around the house for snacks. They can be tossed into a salad to start off a meal or sliced and put in a sandwich.

Use your imagination with the following recipes. Anything here can be a mini meal, an appetizer, a snack, a craving satisfier. They fit right into even the most disordered eating schedule.

Brazilian Shrimp

MAKES 4 SERVINGS

It's probably easiest to serve plain steamed shrimp for an appetizer, but this simple mixture makes it memorable. Fresh shrimp are best, but here in nobrainer land we like our shortcuts. So look for frozen bags of shrimp.

olive-flavored nonstick vegetable oil spray
1/2   cup fresh lime juice
1   small onion, minced
2   teaspoons minced cilantro
1   clove garlic, minced
1/2   teaspoon salt

$^1/_4$ teaspoon pepper

$1^1/_4$ pounds medium shrimp, peeled, deveined, and thawed if frozen

Preheat the broiler and line a baking pan with aluminum foil. Spritz the pan with vegetable oil spray. In a medium bowl, combine the lime juice, onion, cilantro, garlic, salt, and pepper. Set aside. Place the shrimp on the baking sheet and spritz with the nonstick spray. Broil the shrimp 4 inches from the heat source for about $1^1/_2$ minutes on each side. Toss immediately with the lime juice mixture. Serve warm or cool with Papaya Salsa (see page 177).

Per serving: 168 calories; 2.5 g fat (13.6 percent calories from fat); 29 g protein; 6 g carbohydrate; 216 mg cholesterol; 615 mg sodium.

Tuna Pâté

MAKES 4 SERVINGS

Pâté is another one of those dishes you'd never expect to find in this book, but it just goes to show that very few foods can't somehow be slimmed down. This makes a great sandwich spread as well as a lovely appetizer. Make a large bowl on Sunday and have it for lunch or snacks all week long.

1   6-ounce can water-packed tuna, drained
4   ounces fat-free cream cheese
1   tablespoon nonfat sour cream
3   teaspoons lemon juice
$^1/_8$ teaspoon cayenne pepper
3   tablespoons capers, drained and chopped
2   tablespoons chopped fresh parsley
$^1/_2$ teaspoon dried thyme

Combine the tuna, cream cheese, sour cream, lemon juice, and cayenne in a food processor or blender. Process until smooth. Transfer to a small bowl and add the capers, parsley, and thyme. Stir to blend. Serve chilled with mini rye cocktail bread.

Per serving: 61 calories; 0.5 g fat (7.1 percent calories from fat); 11 g protein; 2 g carbohydrate; 13 mg cholesterol; 215 mg sodium.

Grilled Mushrooms

You can use any fat-free BBQ sauce, Asian sauce, or plain steak sauce to give these mushrooms some zing. When I'm in the mood for world travel (but am only able to go as far as my backyard), I doctor them with a fat-free curry sauce (like John Troy's), but you can use any of the fat-free sauces on pages 169–179. Serve these mushrooms as an appetizer or a side dish.

3/4   **cup Worcestershire sauce**
1/4   **cup steak sauce**
2   **tablespoons low-sodium soy sauce**
1   **pound large regular cap mushrooms*, stems removed**
nonstick vegetable oil spray

In a medium-size bowl, combine the three sauces. Add the mushrooms and coat them liberally. Heat the grill and spritz with vegetable oil spray. Place the mushrooms top side down on the grill. As the mushrooms start to sweat, turn and grill on the other side. Cook about 7 minutes, depending on the size of the mushrooms. After you take them off the grill, dip them back into the marinade to coat, and serve.

Per serving: 51 calories; 0.4 g fat (6 percent calories from fat); 2 g protein; 11 g carbohydrate; 0 mg cholesterol; 662 mg sodium.

Classic Quesadillas

This is a great example of a classic Mexican snack that's thought of as junk food, or if not junk, then just plain fattening. It doesn't have to be as you can see by the ingredients used here.

    nonstick vegetable oil spray
6   **whole no-oil, corn tortillas**
1   **cup grated fat-free mild Mexican or cheddar cheese**
1/2   **cup salsa**

*Substitute shiitake or portobello mushrooms if you like.

Spritz a nonstick medium sauté pan with vegetable oil spray and place over high heat. Place a tortilla in the pan and top with ¹/₃ of the cheese, leaving a half-inch border all the way around. Place another tortilla on top and cook until the bottom tortilla is lightly toasted, about 2 minutes. Turn and cook until the cheese has melted and the other tortilla is slightly brown. Transfer to a plate and cover with foil to keep warm. Repeat with the remaining tortillas and cheese. Cut into quarters, top with the salsa, and serve warm.

Per quarter quesadilla: 55 calories; 1.5 g fat (34 percent calories from fat); 6 g protein; 1 g carbohydrate; 2 mg cholesterol; 166 mg sodium.

Quesadilla Variations

These are a few variations of the Classic Quesadilla, all of which make wonderful appetizers, snacks, or quick lunch dishes. Follow the directions for the Classic Quesadillas, substituting toppings where necessary.

Nacho Quesadillas

A little spicier than the Classic Quesadilla, this variation is just as simple to make. Pepperoncinis or small marinated green peppers can also be used as toppings.

   nonstick vegetable oil spray
   6   **no-oil corn tortillas**
   1   **cup grated fat-free cheddar cheese**
   ¹/₂   **cup salsa**
   1   **can nacho rings (pickled chili slices sold in pickle sections)**

Per quarter quesadilla: 55 calories; 0.8 g fat (21.6 percent calories from fat); 6 g protein; 1 g carbohydrate; 2 mg cholesterol; 166 mg sodium.

Quesadillas Pinto Style

I'm fond of spicy pinto bean dip as a tortilla topper, but any fat-free bean dip will work fine in this recipe.

   nonstick vegetable oil spray
   6   **no-oil corn tortillas**

6	tablespoons fat-free spicy pinto bean dip
1	cup grated fat-free cheddar cheese
1/2	cup salsa

Per quarter quesadilla: 55 calories; 0.8 g fat (21.6 percent calories from fat); 6 g protein; 1 g carbohydrate; 2 mg cholesterol; 166 mg sodium.

Quesadillas Tomatillo

Tomatillo salsa has a fresh flavor and is milder than red salsa. It's available in jars and available in most supermarkets.

	nonstick vegetable oil spray
6	no-oil corn tortillas
1	cup grated fat-free Monterey Jack cheese
1/2	cup tomatillo salsa

Per serving: 50 calories; 0.4 g fat (12.6 percent calories from fat); 6 g protein; 1 g carbohydrate; 2 mg cholesterol; 158 mg sodium.

Crab Quesadillas

This quesadilla can also be made with bay shrimp or lobster meat. If you like, use both red salsa and tomatillo salsa to brighten the top of the dish.

6	ounces grated fat-free cheddar cheese
2	scallions, chopped
1/2	pound crabmeat, fresh or canned, shredded
6	no-oil whole wheat tortillas
1/2	cup salsa

Mix the cheese, scallions, and crab together in a bowl. Spoon equal amounts of the mixture onto three of the tortillas, leaving a half-inch border all the way around. Place another tortilla over the top of each and bake in the toaster oven for 5 minutes, or until cheese is melted. Cut into quarters, top with the salsa, and serve warm.

Per quarter quesadilla: 65 calories; 0.6 g fat (5.6 percent calories from fat); 10 g protein; 13 g carbohydrate; 16 mg cholesterol; 293 mg sodium.

Marinated Water Chestnuts

Like peanuts and popcorn, these have great crunch. And like peanuts and popcorn, they're great for zoned-out eating—you know, the kind where you bring your hand to your mouth over and over again without even thinking about it. But unlike peanuts or popcorn, these won't put a pound on you. Keep some in the fridge and munch on them anytime.

2 cans whole or sliced water chestnuts, drained
$1/2$ cup low-sodium soy sauce
1 teaspoon curry powder
$1/4$ teaspoon ginger
$1/8$ teaspoon salt
pinch red pepper flakes

In a medium-size bowl, toss the water chestnuts with the soy sauce and seasonings. Marinate for at least 20 minutes. Refrigerate for at least 15 minutes. Serve instead of nuts.

Per serving: 13 calories; 0 g fat (0 percent calories from fat); 1 g protein; 2 g carbohydrate; 0 mg cholesterol; 427 mg sodium.

Party Mix

This is a perfect example of how to take junk food and turn it into something lean and healthy. Add this mix to kids' lunches or tote it along on a hike instead of trail mix. I even gave sandwich bags of this for Halloween treats one year. You can use any of the cereals mentioned in Chapter 5 to make this mix, although make sure you use bite-size bits rather than flakes.

3 tablespoons honey
3 tablespoons light brown sugar
1 teaspoon cinnamon
$1^{1}/_{2}$ cups Barbara's Animal Crackers
$1^{1}/_{2}$ cups Health Valley Healthy O's
$1^{1}/_{2}$ cups Barbara's Spoonfuls (mini shredded wheats)
$1^{1}/_{2}$ cups puffed wheat cereal

1   **cup whole wheat pretzels**
raisins (optional)

Preheat oven to 350°. Place the honey and brown sugar in a small saucepan and cook over low heat, stirring, until melted and blended. Add the cinnamon and stir. Place the remaining ingredients in a 13 × 9 × 2-inch baking dish and drizzle the honey mixture on top. Toss to coat. Bake for 20 minutes, stirring occasionally. Cool and store.

Per serving: *99 calories; 1.1 g fat (9.3 percent calories from fat); 2 g protein; 22 g carbohydrate; 1 mg cholesterol; 62 mg sodium.*

Roasted Red-Pepper Ricotta Dip

MAKES 2¼ CUPS OR 12 SERVINGS

If you want to roast your own fresh red bell peppers, more power to you: Preheat the broiler. Cut the peppers in half and remove the seeds and membrane. Place skin side up on a foil-lined baking sheet. Flatten with the palm of your hand. Broil 3–4 inches from the heat for about 4 minutes, or until blackened. Transfer the peppers to a heavy zip-lock plastic bag and let sit for about 15 minutes. Remove from bag and peel the skins off. Otherwise, look for canned or jarred roasted red peppers, packed in *water,* not oil.

3   **cloves garlic, skin on**
1½ **cups roasted red peppers, fresh, or from water-packed jars,**
      drained
8   **ounces fat-free ricotta cheese**
2   **teaspoons balsamic vinegar**
pinch salt
¼   **teaspoon crushed red pepper flakes**

Preheat the broiler. Place the garlic cloves on a foil-lined baking sheet and broil about 2 minutes on one side, 2 minutes on the other. Remove and let cool. Peel the garlic and put in a food processor or blender with the red peppers; process until smooth. Add the cheese and process again until smooth. Transfer mixture to a medium-size bowl and add the remaining ingredients. Stir until thoroughly combined. Let chill before serving. Goes well with crudités.

Per serving: 19 calories; 0 g fat (1.4 percent calories from fat); 3 g protein; 2 g carbo-hydrate; 1 mg cholesterol; 37 mg sodium.

Ginger-Jalapeño Red Pepper Dip

MAKES 1 CUP OR 8 SERVINGS

This red pepper dip is spicier than the preceding one. I like to use it as a sauce for fish or chicken as well as a dip.

2	**whole roasted red peppers, fresh (see above for instructions), or 7 ounces from water-packed jars, drained**
1	**clove garlic, chopped**
1	**tablespoon gingerroot, peeled and chopped**
¹/₂	**jalapeño, seeded and chopped**
1	**scallion, chopped**
2	**teaspoons low-sodium soy sauce**
2	**teaspoons rice wine vinegar**
1	**teaspoon honey**
1	**tablespoon nonfat sour cream**
5	**tablespoons bread crumbs**

Place the peppers, garlic, and gingerroot in a food processor or blender. Process rapidly to blend thoroughly. Add the jalapeño, scallion, soy sauce, vinegar, honey, and sour cream. Blend again until smooth. Transfer the mixture to a medium-size bowl and add the bread crumbs. Blend with a fork or whisk. Chill for about 15 minutes before serving.

Per serving: 31 calories; 0.1 g fat (3.7 percent calories from fat); 1 g protein; 3 g car-bohydrate; 0 mg cholesterol; 77 mg sodium.

Roasted-Eggplant Garlic Dip

MAKES 1¹/₂ CUPS OR 6 SERVINGS

My mother used to roast an eggplant over the stove in the winter while we shared a glass of wine. I loved the smell of the roasting vegetable almost as much as I loved the taste of it after it had been mashed with garlic and we were dipping into it with our French bread. It's a classy dip to serve to guests and also makes a great sandwich spread.

1   large eggplant, skin on
3   cloves garlic, minced
$^1/_3$ cup lemon juice
     salt and pepper, to taste

Place the eggplant over a stovetop burner turned to low. As it starts to brown, turn it to the next side. Keep circulating the eggplant so it doesn't char on any one side. (Use an oven mitt!) You will notice that it gets softer as it cooks. When it's cooked on all sides, looks like a deflated balloon, and is soft all the way through, remove from the stove. Split it open and scoop the cooked eggplant into a small bowl. Add the minced garlic, lemon juice, and salt and pepper to taste. Mash with a fork to combine. Serve with fat-free crackers or sourdough bread.

Per serving: 25 calories; 0.1 g fat (4.4 percent calories from fat); 1 g protein; 6 g carbohydrate; 0 mg cholesterol; 3 mg sodium.

Use Your Bean

According to the newest nutritional guidelines, we're all supposed to be eating more legumes. But how to get them into our diets without just sitting down to a plate of rice and beans every night? One answer is right here: You can dip your way to good health.

The beans you can use for these dips come in various forms. You can puree canned beans, cook your own beans, or use the new bean flakes that come in cartons and are very easy to use. These bean dips can also double as sauces for fish, chicken, or rice dishes—just add a little defatted chicken broth to make them easier to ladle, and heat in the microwave or on the stove. I love to pour them over Cajun redfish, or even steamed spinach. Also think of them as sandwich spreads. With two slices of bread and a few vegetables scattered on top they are the best high-protein, low-fat lunches around. Store in jars in the refrigerator.

Homemade Black Bean Dip

MAKES 2 CUPS OR 10 SERVINGS

If you'd like to make this dip spicier, add some salsa, making certain to drain off most of the liquid first. You can also toss in some fat-free cheddar cheese if desired.

2 cups packaged black bean flakes
1 tablespoon chili powder
1/2 teaspoon cumin
2 tablespoons chopped red onion
1 clove garlic, minced
1 tablespoon fresh chopped cilantro

Prepare the bean flakes according to package directions. Add the spices, onion, and garlic and blend well. Top with fresh chopped cilantro and serve with oil-free tortilla chips.

Per serving: 136 calories; 0.7 g fat (4.5 percent calories from fat); 9 g protein; 25 g carbohydrate; 0 mg cholesterol; 10 mg sodium.

Monterey Navy Bean Dip

MAKES 2 CUPS OR 12 SERVINGS

White wine, Jack cheese, and Italian dressing give this dip its tangy flavor.

15 ounces canned navy beans, drained
1/2 cup white wine
1/2 onion, chopped
2 cloves garlic, minced
1/4 cup oil-free Italian salad dressing
1/4 teaspoon white pepper
4 ounces fat-free Monterey Jack cheese, shredded
pinch crushed red pepper flakes
1 teaspoon poultry seasoning

Place the beans in a food processor or blender and rapidly process until still chunky (don't overprocess). Pour the wine into a small sauté pan and sauté the onion and garlic over medium heat until just softened. Add the salad dressing and cook about 1 minute, stirring to blend. Pour the onion mixture into the food processor or blender with the beans. Add the remaining ingredients and process rapidly. Chill the dip in the refrigerator for about 15 minutes before serving. Serve spread on Quaker Oats mini white cheddar rice cakes.

Per serving: 138 calories; 0.5 g fat (3.2 percent calories from fat); 11 g protein; 22 g carbohydrate; 1 mg cholesterol; 102 mg sodium.

"Guacamole" Gets Thin

MAKES 2½ CUPS OR 12 SERVINGS

What's guacamole doing in this book? Well, it isn't really guacamole, but this spicy bean-based dip has a similar rich flavor.

15	ounces canned black beans, drained
½	cup white wine
½	onion, chopped
2	cloves garlic, minced
1	teaspoon garlic powder
½	cup diced tomato
⅓	cup picante sauce
½	teaspoon cumin
½	teaspoon chili powder
¼	cup shredded fat-free mild Mexican or cheddar cheese
¼	cup chopped fresh cilantro
1	tablespoon fresh lime juice

Place the drained beans in a bowl and mash slightly with a fork. Set aside. Heat the wine in a nonstick sauté pan. Add the onion, fresh garlic, and garlic powder and sauté over medium heat about 4 minutes, or until tender. Add the beans, tomato, picante sauce, cumin, and chili powder. Cook for 5 minutes, or until thickened. Remove from the heat and add the remaining ingredients, stirring until the cheese melts. Serve at room temperature.

Per serving: 76 calories; 1.2 g fat (14.7 percent calories from fat); 5 g protein; 11 g carbohydrate; 1 mg cholesterol; 79 mg sodium.

Garlic Watercress Dip

Here's a creamy green and white dip with a bit of bite to it. It makes a particularly good spread for a cucumber or tomato sandwich.

16   ounces canned navy beans, drained
1   tablespoon nonfat sour cream
1   tablespoon thyme
2   teaspoons lemon juice
1   clove garlic
1/4 cup chopped watercress
pinch salt
pinch pepper

Combine the beans, sour cream, thyme, lemon juice, and garlic in a food processor or blender. Process until smooth. Add the watercress, salt, and pepper. Stir to combine. Chill before serving.

Per serving: 45 calories; 0.2 g fat (3.7 percent calories from fat); 3 g protein; 8 g carbohydrate; 0 mg cholesterol; 182 mg sodium.

Chapter Ten

Slimming Sides, Salads, Soups, and Sauces

I know what you're thinking. You've just read the title to this chapter and you're picturing some of the things to follow. Just the word "slimming" evokes visions of dull, boring diet foods. Slimming sides? That must mean steamed broccoli and maybe some boiled potatoes. The salads must be lettuce with a little lemon juice, the soups some watery broths with a couple of sliced mushrooms floating on top. A slimming sauce? That must be pureed carrots or something along those lines. In other words, what's to come will be dull, dull, dull.

And why shouldn't you be under that impression? For years, those were the kind of offerings available to people who wanted to eat healthy and lean. Listen, I'm the first to admit that they're a turnoff. But side dishes, soups, salads, and sauces can also be the gorgeous jewelry that makes a simple dress stunning. They can really enhance your meals, not just accompany them. Our attitudes toward the makeup of the dinner plate have really changed, especially with the new food pyramid telling us to have more grains and legumes. Instead of seeing a huge piece of steak or half a chicken barely decorated by a few lowly side dishes, we now see grains and veggies playing an equal—and sometimes even bigger—part on the plate. And salad and soup shouldn't be something you have just to keep you busy while you wait for the real thing to come along. They are meals in themselves these days, and have expanded way beyond the wedge of iceberg lettuce clunked on a plate.

Let me reiterate, too, the importance of the vitamins and minerals that these sides, salads, and soups contain. By eating sides, salads, and soups, we get the "five servings a day" of produce that health watchdogs have posted in all of our supermarkets. So pile on the veggies and grains—and although plain veggies can taste great, why not have some fun?

Let's begin with side dishes. What follows is all you need to know to make accompaniments that you (and even your kids) will really love. Also note that all the sides here are great for packing in your lunch the next day, so make a lot.

No-Brainer Tips for Zipping Up Side Dishes

Vegetables

• Add chopped garlic to plain steamed veggies, especially spinach, while steaming.

• Squeeze some fresh lemon into the steaming water, then spritz some more on top of the vegetables before serving.

• Top steamed veggies with fat-free cheese or a little freshly grated Parmesan.

• Steam vegetables, then toss them into a sauté pan with some fat-free sour cream and a sprinkle of seasoning; cook until blended. This is a great way to jazz up leftover veggies, too.

• Poach vegetables in defatted chicken broth flavored with garlic and/or fresh or dried herbs.

• Roasted vegetables have a sweeter flavor than steamed or poached. To roast, cut veggies into 1-inch chunks, then spritz with an olive-flavored oil spray, sprinkle with salt and pepper, and bake about 8–10 minutes in a preheated 350° oven. Also, see the roasted vegetable recipes here, beginning on page 148.

• Grilling also gives vegetables a new personality, adding crunchiness and barbecue flavor. To grill, marinate veggies in oil-free salad dressing or sauce. Spray the grill with a nonstick spray, then cook until grill marks appear on both sides and vegetables are tender. After you grill the vegetables, put them back in the sauce or dressing so they soak it up and stay moist.

Grains and potatoes

• Even if the directions on the box call for fat, don't add any oil, butter, or margarine to your rice mixes. For moisture, replace half the water called for in a recipe with defatted chicken broth—it has a tiny bit of fat, which is enough to keep the grains from tasting dry.

- Add flavor to rice and grains by sprinkling poultry, Italian, or any other seasoning blend into the boiling water phase of cooking.

- Use one of the many flavored pastas on the market as a side dish. They have so much flavor you don't need to add any fat, let alone sauce—just rinse the pasta with defatted chicken broth after cooking to keep it moist and prevent sticking.

- Skip the sauce and serve cooked pasta tossed with either nonfat sour cream or grated Parmesan.

- Throw frozen vegetables into the boiling water as you cook rice or other grains—a great way to sneak more produce into your kids' (and your own) diet.

- Top baked potatoes with nonfat sour cream, Worcestershire sauce, hot sauce, ketchup, steak sauce, or light soy sauce.

- To make split-second mashed potatoes in the skin, slit baked potatoes down the middle, pour in $1/4$ cup skim or 1 percent milk, then mash in the skin with a fork. Season with salt and pepper.

- Peeling yams is a cinch if, immediately after cooking, you remove them from the pot and place them in a cold-water bath. The skins will slip right off.

Balsamic Onions

MAKES 4 SERVINGS

These go great with roast turkey, chicken, and cold sandwiches, and make a beautiful garnish.

    2   medium red onions, peeled and quartered
    1   cup balsamic vinegar

Preheat oven to 350°. Place the onions on a sheet of aluminum foil. Turn up the edges to form a "boat." Pour the balsamic vinegar over the onions, fold the foil at the top, and bake for 20 minutes, or until the onions are soft. If you want to serve the onions as a garnish, slice them in half, remove the center, and place "cup" side up in a baking dish. Pour the vinegar into the onion halves and bake for 20 minutes, or until soft.

Per serving: 39 calories; 0.1 g fat (2.5 percent calories from fat); 1 g protein; 10 g carbohydrate; 0 mg cholesterol; 3 mg sodium.

Grilled Veggies with Garlic Marinade

MAKES 4 SERVINGS

Don't just think of this as a side dish. Make a big batch and keep the vegetables in the refrigerator so you can grab them for a quick snack or toss them into a salad. After the vegetables are done grilling, dip them back into the marinade so the flavor really seeps in. Don't overgrill or you'll have charred veggies.

1	cup oil-free Italian salad dressing
1/4	cup lemon juice
1	tablespoon Dijon mustard
1/4	teaspoon cracked pepper
1	green bell pepper, cored, seeded, and sliced 1/4 inch thick
1	red bell pepper, cored, seeded, and sliced 1/4 inch thick
3	Japanese eggplants, sliced lengthwise
2	zucchini, sliced lengthwise
2	yellow squashes, sliced lengthwise
1	cup regular cap mushrooms, sliced 1/4 inch thick

Combine the first four ingredients in a medium-size bowl. Add the vegetables to the marinade and coat evenly. Place on a hot grill and cook until grill-marked on one side, then the other. As you remove the vegetables, place them back into the marinade.

To bake: Preheat oven to 400°. Place the vegetables in a baking dish and pour the marinade on top. Add 1/2 cup defatted chicken broth, cover, and bake for 20 minutes. To crisp the vegetables, place them under the broiler for 1 to 2 minutes.

Per serving: 40 calories; 0.5 g fat (8.9 percent calories from fat); 2 g protein; 9 g carbohydrate; 0 mg cholesterol; 51 mg sodium.

Nonfried Steak Fries

If you like your steak fries extra crispy, dip the raw potatoes in beaten egg white before baking. Serve with sugar-free ketchup.

4   large russet potatoes, cut into thick wedges
Nonstick vegetable oil spray
2   teaspoons garlic powder
2   teaspoons dried rosemary (optional)
1   teaspoon coarse black pepper
1   teaspoon salt

Preheat oven to 425°. Spray a baking sheet three times with vegetable oil. Spray the potatoes and place them in a gallon-size plastic bag. Sprinkle the garlic and rosemary in the bag and shake to coat the potatoes. Scatter the potatoes on the baking sheet, and sprinkle with pepper and salt. Place the baking sheet on the bottom shelf of the oven and bake potatoes for 45 minutes or until golden brown, turning every 10 to 15 minutes so they cook evenly.

Per serving: 88 calories; 0 g fat (1 percent calories from fat); 2 g protein; 20 g carbohydrate; 0 mg cholesterol; 273 mg sodium.

Herb-Baked Romano Tomatoes

Tomatoes are one of the best sources of vitamin C, but we hardly ever look beyond salads and pasta sauces as a way to eat them. Well, here's one way—a delicious way—to get more of them into your diet. If you're not fond of marjoram, use rosemary, thyme, or a garlic-spice blend.

1   pint plain nonfat yogurt, strained (see page 61)
1/2   teaspoon marjoram
1/4   teaspoon salt
1/4   teaspoon pepper
2   large tomatoes
nonstick vegetable oil spray
1/4   cup grated Romano cheese

Preheat oven to 400°. After straining the yogurt (2 hours to overnight), add the marjoram, salt, and pepper (or spice blend of your choice). Slice the tomatoes in half crosswise; remove the seeds and most of the pulp. Spritz a cooking sheet with vegetable oil spray. Place the tomatoes on the pan. Fill each half with the yogurt mixture and top with equal amounts of Romano. Bake for 30 minutes or until lightly browned.

Per serving: 104 calories; 2.3 g fat (19.6 percent calories from fat); 9 g protein; 12 g carbohydrate; 9 mg cholesterol; 310 mg sodium.

Creamy Mashed Potatoes (Without the Cream)

MAKES 10 SERVINGS

You will never miss the butter or cream in this slimmed-down but creamy mashed potato dish. The new nonfat sour creams are a wonderful replacement for their fatty counterparts. If you're not a sour cream fan, try using 1 percent or skim milk instead. Leave the peel on when you make these: the peel is the most nutritious part of the potato and it gives the dish a rustic, country look.

10	potatoes, peel on, cubed
1	cup nonfat sour cream
¹/₂	cup skim milk
1	teaspoon salt
1	teaspoon pepper

Cut the potatoes into cubes and place in a pot of boiling water deep enough to cover them completely. Cook until soft, about 5–7 minutes, and drain. Place the potatoes in a large bowl, add the sour cream and skim milk, and mash. Add the salt and pepper, and mash again until creamy.

Per serving: 94 calories; 0.1 g fat (1.3 percent calories from fat); 3 g protein; 21 g carbohydrate; 0 mg cholesterol; 227 mg sodium.

Asian Green Beans

These beans have a slightly sweet taste and are a lot more interesting than plain steamed beans. This recipe calls for frozen beans, but by all means use fresh if you have the time to shop and chop.

nonstick vegetable oil spray
1/4   cup chopped onion
1/2   teaspoon cornstarch
1/2   cup water
3   tablespoons rice vinegar
1   tablespoon frozen apple juice concentrate
1/8   teaspoon salt
pinch white pepper
2   whole cloves
1   bay leaf
1   9-ounce package frozen green beans, thawed

Spritz a large nonstick sauté pan with nonstick vegetable oil spray, and heat over a medium burner. Add the onion and sauté until tender. Combine the cornstarch with 1/4 cup water in a small bowl. Add to the onion. Cook 1 minute, stirring constantly. Add the vinegar, the other 1/4 cup water, and next 5 ingredients, stirring until blended and smooth. Add the beans, cover, and cook 6–8 minutes, or until the beans are tender. Remove the cloves and bay leaf and serve.

Per serving: 44 calories; 0.8 g fat (13.4 percent calories from fat); 1 g protein; 10 g carbohydrate; 0 mg cholesterol; 118 mg sodium.

Pinto Bean Fiesta

Every time I make this for a dinner party, it's the first thing to go. For variation, you can substitute chopped red, yellow, and green bell pepper for the corn and peas. This can also serve as a main dish, topped with grilled chicken, or spooned over brown rice. Beans are one of the best sources of protein and fiber—we could all stand to eat more of them.

2	cups canned pinto beans
2	cups corn kernels
2	cups frozen peas
3	Roma tomatoes, chopped
¹/₂	small red onion, diced
¹/₄	cup fresh lemon juice
¹/₄	cup fresh lime juice
1	teaspoon apple cider vinegar
2	tablespoons frozen apple juice concentrate
¹/₂	bunch cilantro, chopped
¹/₂	jalapeño, diced
	salt and pepper to taste

Rinse the pinto beans and set aside. Thaw the frozen corn and peas under hot water and drain. Mix all of the ingredients in a large bowl and toss until well blended. Let sit in the fridge for a half hour or more, but stir every 15 minutes. Serve on a bed of lettuce with baked tortilla chips.

Per serving: 149 calories; 0.9 g fat (4.9 percent calories from fat); 7 g protein; 31 g carbohydrate; 0 mg cholesterol; 49 mg sodium.

Wild Rice Bell Pepper Pilaf

MAKES 6 SERVINGS

This is a colorful side dish, and the leftovers can be eaten cold for lunch. If you can't find the Arrowhead Mills brand of wild rice mix, use 1 cup of cooked wild rice and 1 cup of cooked brown rice, mix with the poultry seasoning and bell peppers, then top with the Italian dressing.

1	box Arrowhead Mills wild rice mix
1	tablespoon poultry seasoning
¹/₄	cup white wine
1	red bell pepper, cored, seeded, and diced
1	yellow bell pepper, cored, seeded, and diced
³/₄	cup oil-free Italian salad dressing

Make the rice pilaf according to the package directions, but do not add any oil or margarine. Add the poultry seasoning when the water begins to boil, then continue cooking according to instructions. Heat the wine in a medium sauté pan. Cook the diced bell peppers until just soft, about 3–4 minutes. Add the Italian dressing. Stir and cook for one more minute. Remove from heat and add to the rice mix. Toss well to blend.

Per serving: 53 calories; 0.7 g fat (12.3 percent calories from fat); 1 g protein; 7 g carbohydrate; 0 mg cholesterol; 107 mg sodium.

Five Variations on Roasted Vegetables

Whenever anyone thinks about losing weight or trying to eat healthfully, they inevitably conjure up visions of endless piles of plain steamed vegetables—it's enough to send anyone into a pizza parlor. Roasted vegetables, however, are actually tempting, satisfying, even something to look forward to. During the roasting process they caramelize and take on a lovely sweetness. I like to make large amounts so that I have them as leftovers to munch on the next day, or to pack into a lunch.

Maple Roasted Acorn Squash

MAKES 4 SERVINGS

There's absolutely nothing more no-brainer than slicing up an acorn squash, doctoring it up, and roasting it. This is a great comfort food for winter nights and a wonderful source of beta carotene.

1   large acorn squash
olive-flavored nonstick vegetable oil spray
1   teaspoon cinnamon
2   tablespoons maple syrup
salt and pepper to taste

Preheat oven to 450°. Cut the acorn squash crosswise, remove the seeds, and slice into ¹/₂-inch-thick rings. Spritz with the vegetable oil spray and place in a roasting pan. In a small bowl, combine the cinnamon and maple syrup, then drizzle the mixture across the top of the squash. Season with salt and pepper. Roast for 15 minutes, or until tender.

Per serving: 70 calories; 0.1 g fat (1.7 percent calories from fat); 1 g protein; 18 g carbohydrate; 0 mg cholesterol; 4 mg sodium.

Roasted Tarragon Asparagus

MAKES 4 SERVINGS

I love the taste of plain steamed asparagus, but this is one more way to serve this spring veggie while it's in season.

1   pound asparagus, ends trimmed
olive-flavored nonstick vegetable oil spray
2   teaspoons minced onion
1   tablespoon freshly chopped tarragon
¼   cup white wine
salt and pepper to taste

Preheat oven to 450°. Line a shallow baking pan with aluminum foil, spritz the asparagus with the vegetable oil spray, and place in the foil-lined pan. Sprinkle the minced onion and tarragon on top, and pour the wine in the bottom of the pan. Season with salt and pepper, and roast for 10–15 minutes, or until tender.

Per serving: 38 calories; 0.3 g fat (6.4 percent calories from fat); 3 g protein; 6 g carbohydrate; 0 mg cholesterol; 9 mg sodium.

Orange Roasted Carrots and Parsnips

MAKES 6 SERVINGS

Parsnips are a vegetable lots of people don't like—only they've usually never tried them. This is a super introduction to the underused vegetable. If, of course, you are a confirmed parsnip hater, this recipe works just as well with carrots alone.

1   pound carrots
1   pound parsnips
olive-flavored nonstick vegetable oil spray
2   teaspoons frozen orange juice concentrate
1   teaspoon balsamic vinegar
salt and pepper to taste
1   teaspoon chopped parsley

Preheat oven to 450°. Peel the carrots and parsnips and cut into matchsticks. Spritz with the vegetable oil spray and toss together in a bowl to coat. Place in a baking dish and roast for 10–15 minutes, turning midway through the cooking, until tender and browned. Toss with orange juice concentrate and vinegar. Season with salt, pepper, and parsley.

Per serving: 91 calories; 0.4 g fat (3.6 percent calories from fat); 2 g protein; 22 g carbohydrate; 0 mg cholesterol; 35 mg sodium.

Roasted Rosemary Eggplant

MAKES 4 SERVINGS

If you cook eggplant with oil, it soaks it up like a sponge, perhaps more than any other vegetable. But eggplant doesn't need to be cooked with lots of fat since its flesh is soft and juicy on its own. If you prefer, you can use small Japanese eggplants in this recipe rather than the large variety.

    1   **large eggplant, ends discarded, and sliced into ¹⁄₃-inch-thick rounds**
    olive-flavored nonstick vegetable oil spray
    1   **teaspoon dried rosemary**
    salt and pepper to taste
    1   **tablespoon grated Parmesan cheese**

Preheat oven to 425°. Spritz both sides of the eggplant slices with the vegetable oil spray and place in a roasting pan. Sprinkle with the rosemary, salt, and pepper, and roast for 15 minutes. Turn and sprinkle with the cheese. Cook 5 minutes more or until the cheese has slightly melted.

Per serving: 35 calories; 0.6 g fat (13.1 percent calories from fat); 2 g protein; 7 g carbohydrate; 1 mg cholesterol; 27 mg sodium.

Roasted Sesame Green Beans

MAKES 4 SERVINGS

Green beans are my son's favorite—probably because they're great finger food. The sesame seeds in this recipe add a nutty flavor and vitamin E to the dish.

    1   **pound fresh green beans, trimmed and sliced**
    butter-flavored nonstick vegetable oil spray

1   tablespoon poultry seasoning
¹/₂   teaspoon sesame seeds

Preheat oven to 450°. Place the beans in a roasting pan and spritz with the vegetable oil spray. Roast for 10–15 minutes, stirring midway, or until tender. Toss with the seasoning and sesame seeds and roast for another 5 minutes.

Per serving: 40 calories; 0.4 g fat (7.9 percent calories from fat); 2 g protein; 9 g carbohydrate; 0 mg cholesterol; 7 mg sodium.

Salads

"Salad," also known as "rabbit food," is another dirty diet word. But, you guessed it, it doesn't have to be. Instead of thinking of salad as a bunch of greens tossed with dressing, think of it as a combination of cooked and fresh foods—almost anything can go in a salad. I've put together some wonderful fat-free dressing recipes, great no-brainer salads, and a bunch of ways to dress your salads without increasing your dress size.

Fat-Free Salad Dressings

Don't think of salad dressings as just salad dressings. These all go well over fish, chicken, turkey, and baked potatoes. Use them to moisten sandwiches and grain dishes, and as sauté liquid for vegetables, fish, and chicken. There's no fat, just flavor, so put them on *everything*.

Corn Vinaigrettes

MAKES 16 SERVINGS

These two dressings average 40 calories per serving with 0.5 gram of fat per serving.

Corn, Lemon, and Thyme Dressing

1   cup corn juice (see recipe on page 153)
1   teaspoon fresh lemon juice

25 THINGS (YOU MIGHT NOT HAVE THOUGHT OF) TO THROW INTO A SALAD

- water chestnuts
- cooked wild or brown rice
- cooked Kashi
- crumpled flavored rice cakes (a nonfat crouton)
- hearts of palm
- artichoke hearts packed in water
- tuna packed in water
- cooked potatoes
- cooked peas and corn
- grated fat-free cheese
- canned chicken breast
- salsa
- any leftover cooked chicken, turkey, or fish
- crumpled oil-free tortilla chips
- Fakin' Bacon Bits
- chopped pickles
- diced olives
- bamboo shoots
- any kind of sprout—lentil, bean, pea, alfalfa
- sun-dried tomatoes (chopped, not packed in oil)
- raisins
- fat-free cottage cheese
- mandarin orange sections
- chopped apple
- pomegranate seeds

1   tablespoon oil-free Italian salad dressing
2   teaspoons thyme
1   teaspoon minced fresh parsley
1   teaspoon salt
pinch pepper

Combine all ingredients in a cruet or bowl. Chill until ready to use.

Corn Vinaigrette with Lime and Chili

1   cup corn juice (see below)
1   teaspoon seeded and chopped jalapeño
4   teaspoons minced fresh cilantro
1   teaspoon fresh lime juice
1   tablespoon oil-free Italian salad dressing
1   teaspoon salt
pinch pepper

Combine all ingredients in a cruet or bowl. Chill until ready to use.

Corn Juice

MAKES ABOUT 1 CUP

5   ears of corn on the cob, husked

Cut the kernels off the corn with a sharp knife. Pass them through a juice extractor to create juice or process in a blender, then strain through a fine sieve.

Cucumber Dressings

The taste of cucumber is subtle yet refreshing. These four variations all go nicely drizzled over a crisp fresh bowl of greens. They average 30 calories and 0.5 gram of fat per serving.

Buttermilk Cucumber Dressing

1	cup cucumber juice (see page 155)
6	tablespoons nonfat buttermilk
1	tablespoon dried dill
1/2	teaspoon salt
1/2	teaspoon lemon pepper
pinch pepper	

Combine all ingredients in a cruet or bowl. Chill until ready to use.

Lemon Cucumber Dressing

1	cup cucumber juice (see page 155)
4	teaspoons fresh lemon juice
4	teaspoons chopped fresh Italian parsley
1	teaspoon thyme
1/2	teaspoon salt

Combine all ingredients in a cruet or bowl. Chill until ready to use.

Creamy Mustard Cucumber Dressing

1	cup cucumber juice (see page 155)
3	tablespoons plain nonfat yogurt
1	tablespoon Dijon mustard
1	teaspoon crushed caraway seeds
4	teaspoons finely chopped scallions
1/2	teaspoon salt

Combine all ingredients in a cruet or bowl. Chill until ready to use.

Creamy Basil-Garlic-Cucumber Dressing

1   cup cucumber juice (see below)
2   tablespoons plain nonfat yogurt
4   teaspoons finely chopped scallions
2   teaspoons chopped basil leaves
1   clove garlic, minced
$^1/_2$ teaspoon salt
pinch pepper

Combine all ingredients in a cruet or bowl. Chill until ready to use.

Cucumber Juice

MAKES ABOUT $^1/_2$–$^3/_4$ CUP

2   large cucumbers, peeled and sliced

Pass the cucumber through a juice extractor to create juice or process in a blender until pureed, then strain through a fine sieve.

Red-Pepper Juice Vinaigrettes

MAKES 8 SERVINGS

Besides being excellent green salad dressings, these make a fabulous fat-free dip for lobster, and are splendid over a shellfish salad. They average 15 calories and 0.1 gram of fat per serving.

Balsamic Red-Pepper Dressing

1   cup red pepper juice (see page 156)
1   teaspoon balsamic vinegar
$^1/_2$ teaspoon fresh lemon juice
2   teaspoons oil-free Italian salad dressing
$^1/_2$ teaspoon salt

Place ingredients in a blender and blend until smooth. Refrigerate until ready to use.

Cumin Red-Pepper Dressing

1   cup red pepper juice (see below)
1   teaspoon sherry vinegar
1/2 teaspoon almond flavoring
2   teaspoons oil-free Italian salad dressing
1/8 teaspoon cumin
1/2 teaspoon salt
pinch pepper

Place ingredients in a blender and blend until smooth. Refrigerate until ready to use.

Red-Pepper Juice

MAKES ABOUT 1 CUP

3   large red bell peppers, cored, seeded, and chopped
1/2 cup water

Place the peppers and water in a blender and blend until pureed. Strain through a fine sieve and skim off any foam.

Tomato Salad Dressings

MAKES 8 SERVINGS

You can use the juice of two fresh tomatoes or canned tomato juice for these dressings. If you prefer a thicker dressing, add 1–2 tablespoons Italian oil-free salad dressing to either recipe. They average 20 calories per serving and 0.1 gram of fat per serving.

Tomato-Orange-Basil Dressing

1   cup tomato juice
2   tablespoons orange juice
1/2 teaspoon salt
pinch pepper
1/2 teaspoon grated lemon peel
2   teaspoons chopped fresh basil
2   teaspoons chopped scallions

Place the ingredients except basil and scallions in a blender or food processor. Blend until smooth, then pour in a small bowl. Add the basil and scallions and stir well. Refrigerate until ready to use.

Tomato Horseradish Dressing

1   cup tomato juice
2   teaspoons grated horseradish
2   teaspoons chopped fresh Italian parsley
2   teaspoons fresh lime juice
2   teaspoons clam juice (optional)
1   teaspoon salt
pinch pepper

Place ingredients in a blender and blend until smooth. Refrigerate until ready to use.

Creamy Rice Vinegar and Spice Dressing

MAKES 8 SERVINGS

Rice vinegar is underutilized. It has a lovely mellow flavor that complements everything from vegetables to poultry and fish. I like to use this dressing drizzled over a tuna, chicken, or seafood salad. It has approximately 40 calories and 1 gram of fat per serving.

1   cup nonfat yogurt
½   cup finely chopped fresh parsley
2   tablespoons rice vinegar
1   teaspoon poultry seasoning
1   clove garlic, minced
salt and pepper to taste

Combine all ingredients in a cruet or bowl. Chill until ready to use.

Dijon Vinaigrette

This vinaigrette can also be made with tarragon vinegar. To infuse more flavor, add 1 teaspoon of crushed garlic, dill, Parsley Patch Garlic Saltless Seasoning, or capers. This vinaigrette has only 7 calories and 0.1 gram of fat per serving.

1   cup red wine vinegar
1   tablespoon Dijon mustard or herb mustard
1   teaspoon grated Parmesan cheese
1   teaspoon frozen apple juice concentrate
½   teaspoon black pepper

Combine all ingredients in a cruet or bowl. Chill until ready to use.

Thousand Island Dressing

MAKES 8 SERVINGS

Thousand Island? It might as well be Thousand Calorie dressing, and no wonder: The traditional recipe is ketchup, mayonnaise, and pickle relish. This is a much, much lighter version—only 78 calories and 0.2 gram of fat per serving—but with all of the creaminess and flavor left in. Add a few Fakin' Bacon Bits to any dish you serve it with.

1   pint plain nonfat yogurt
½   cup nonfat sour cream
½   cup ketchup
½   cup sweet pickle relish
2   tablespoons apple cider vinegar

Place ingredients in a blender and blend until smooth. Refrigerate until ready to use.

WonderSlim's Basic Fat-Free Honey Mustard Dressing

MAKES 6 SERVINGS

Tastes rich, doesn't have any fat. What could be better to have on hand when you come home from a hard day and just want to throw together a salad? For variety, I like to add 1 tablespoon chopped tarragon to this dressing. Only 22 calories and less than 1 gram of fat per serving.

2 teaspoons honey
2 teaspoons Dijon mustard
4 tablespoons balsamic vinegar
8 tablespoons WonderSlim Fat & Egg Substitute
salt and pepper to taste

In a medium bowl, whisk the honey and mustard together. Add the vinegar, then whisk in the WonderSlim and salt and pepper until the mixture is well blended.

Variations on Hain Dry Package Mix Dressings

MAKES 4 SERVINGS

These dressings come in a variety of flavors, but I like to add to each of them to make them taste richer. All dry package mixes tend to be a little dull when you follow the package directions. I use more vinegar than water, for instance, and add additional seasonings to them all. You can be creative and try your own fresh herbs and dried seasonings. Use the dressings on just about anything. The Caesar is a great marinade for swordfish; the Herb a great marinade for grilled vegetables; and the Thousand Island a great topping for potato salad with some black olives thrown in. These average 20 calories and 0 grams of fat per serving.

Caesar Dressing

1   package Hain Caesar salad dressing mix
½   cup cider vinegar
1   tablespoon water

Thousand Island Dressing

1   package Hain Thousand Island salad dressing mix
$^{1}/_{2}$ cup cider vinegar
1   tablespoon water
1   tablespoon pickle relish
1   teaspoon ketchup

Buttermilk Dressing

1   package Hain Buttermilk salad dressing mix
$^{1}/_{2}$ cup cider vinegar
1   tablespoon water
1   teaspoon Dijon mustard
pinch pepper

Herb Dressing

1   package Hain Herb salad dressing mix
$^{1}/_{2}$ cup cider vinegar
1   tablespoon water
1   teaspoon Parsley Patch Garlic Saltless Seasoning or other garlic seasoning

Disregard the directions on the package and combine all ingredients in a cruet or bowl. Chill until ready to use.

Some other additions you can make to any of these recipes: red pepper flakes; minced onion flakes; capers; Fakin' Bacon Bits; Worcestershire sauce.

Potato Celery Salad with Cucumber Dressing
MAKES 4 SERVINGS

This is a simple, light, delicious potato salad that can be made either with a cucumber dressing made from scratch or with a fat-free bottled variety. If you have time, add chopped apples and/or scallions to jazz it up.

6   red potatoes, cut into 1-inch cubes
1   cup celery, sliced $^{1}/_{4}$ inch thick on the diagonal
$^{3}/_{4}$ cup cucumber dressing (use any on pages 154–155)

Place the potatoes in a saucepan and cover with water. Bring to a boil, simmer until potatoes are tender, about 15 minutes. Drain and let cool. In a medium-size bowl, toss the potatoes, celery, and dressing. Add cherry tomatoes and some sliced black olives, if desired.

Per serving: 138 calories; 0.2 g fat (1.3 percent calories from fat); 4 g protein; 31 g carbohydrate; 0 mg cholesterol; 36 mg sodium.

Turkey Orange Salad

MAKES 4 SERVINGS

A combination of orange and curry gives this salad its unique flavor. Make it with leftover turkey if you have some on hand.

12   ounces skinless turkey breast, cut into ½-inch cubes
salt and pepper to taste
nonstick vegetable oil spray
1   cup sliced celery
8   ounces water chestnuts, drained
¾   cup fat-free Italian salad dressing
¼   teaspoon curry powder
2   oranges, peeled, seeded, pith removed, and cut into 1-inch
        cubes
½   red onion, sliced thin
8   leaves red leaf lettuce

Season the turkey with salt and pepper and place in a medium-size sauté pan spritzed with vegetable oil spray. Cook over medium heat until cooked through, about 10 minutes; set aside. Toss all of the ingredients except lettuce together in a large bowl. Divide the lettuce among four plates and spoon the salad on top. Serve with bagel toasts.

Per serving: 138 calories; 1.7 g fat (10.2 percent calories from fat); 21 g protein; 13 g carbohydrate; 51 mg cholesterol; 83 mg sodium.

Skinny Slaw

This slaw is made with vanilla yogurt to give it a tangy, sweet taste. For a spicier cole slaw, add more vinegar and mustard to the recipe.

16	ounces cole slaw blend (precut vegetables, found in the produce section)
1½	cups nonfat vanilla yogurt
¼	cup cider vinegar
1	tablespoon Dijon mustard
½	teaspoon paprika
1	teaspoon coarsely crushed pepper
¼	teaspoon salt

Place the cole slaw blend in a large bowl. In a separate bowl, combine the yogurt, vinegar, mustard, and paprika. Pour the dressing over the cole slaw; blend and toss until coated. Add salt and pepper, and refrigerate for at least 20 minutes.

Per serving: 59 calories; 0.6 g fat (9.5 percent calories from fat); 4 g protein; 9 g carbohydrate; 1 mg cholesterol; 190 mg sodium.

Matchstick Salad

This is a spicy alternative to cole slaw. I occasionally add cooked wild rice to give it a nutty flavor.

3	cups broccoli slaw*
1½	cups seeded, julienned cucumber
½	cup red bell pepper, julienned
3	tablespoons rice vinegar
2	tablespoons low-sodium teriyaki marinade such as Premier Japan or San-J
1	teaspoon frozen apple juice concentrate
¼	teaspoon chili powder

*Your supermarket's produce section most likely carries this—it's usually a mixture of broccoli, carrot, and red cabbage and comes in a bag. Or you can shred vegetables and make your own mix.

Combine all the vegetables in a large bowl. Combine the vinegar, teriyaki marinade, apple juice concentrate, and chili powder in a small bowl and blend well with a whisk. Pour over the vegetable mixture and chill for about 2 hours.

Per serving: 57 calories; 1 g fat (9.9 percent calories from fat); 4 g protein; 16 g carbohydrate; 0 mg cholesterol; 174 mg sodium.

Kashi Salad with Cumin Red-Pepper Dressing

Kashi is a wonderfully crunchy, nutty mix of grains usually sold in the cereal section of supermarkets. If you like, toss in some cubed leftover chicken or turkey to turn this into a full meal.

3	cups cooked Kashi
1/4	cup white wine
2	shallots, minced
1	cup corn kernels
1	medium zucchini, diced
1	cup Cumin Red-Pepper Dressing (see page 156)
1/2	teaspoon salt
pinch pepper	
1	tablespoon chopped cilantro

Prepare the Kashi according to package directions and set aside in a large bowl. Heat the wine in a nonstick skillet over medium heat. Add the shallots and cook until just tender. Add the corn and zucchini and cook for 2–3 minutes. Toss the vegetable mixture with the Kashi, then add the vinaigrette, salt, and pepper, and toss again. Top with the chopped cilantro. Serve warm.

Per serving: 126 calories; 1.8 g fat (12.7 percent calories from fat); 4 g protein; 23 g carbohydrate; 0 mg cholesterol; 189 mg sodium.

Soups

Soups are meals in themselves—they contain just about everything you need in one nutritious dish. Some people are daunted by the misconception that whipping one up from scratch is an arduous task, but soup making doesn't have to be a complicated, all-day chopping affair, particularly with the many great precut veggies sold in produce sections now (frozen vegetables shouldn't be forgotten either). Soups are a no-brainer, and they freeze well, so a little bit of work goes a long way.

Unless they're creamy, soups also have the distinction of being inherently low in fat—at least they should be. Many recipes ask you to sauté the vegetables in oil first, which can add up to 22 (or more) grams of fat. That's really unnecessary, since you can just as easily sauté the vegetables in other nonfat liquids (such as chicken broth or wine). Some of the soups lowest in fat are bean soups, which I'm happy to say are becoming more and more popular. Besides being low in fat, legumes are high in protein and contain a good amount of fiber. Plus, they're satisfying and help you sustain your energy for long periods of time. When pureed, beans make a soup seem creamy even when it doesn't contain a drop of cream.

When you don't have time to cook, rest assured that there are now many healthy, fat-free soups on the market deserving of your attention. They're great to keep at home or in the office, a perfect replacement for the junky 3 or 4 P.M. snack you might otherwise have. Soups, too, will really hold you over until dinner. I know I've already said this, but be on the lookout for healthy, low-fat instant cup o' soups (see Chapter 5) and premeasured soup mixes that come with preblended seasonings. These are the best things to come around in a long time for busy people as well as proof that it's possible to make convenience foods without added chemicals.

Brazilian Black Bean Soup

MAKES 6 SERVINGS

This hearty, fiber-rich soup is made with oranges, orange juice, and sherry, which add a hint of sweetness. Freeze it in individual containers to make a quick cup o' soup. Serve with No-Brainer Cajun Corn Bread (see page 95).

2	cups dried black beans
3⅓	cups water or stock of your choice
1	cup chopped onion
3	cloves garlic, minced
1	large carrot, diced

1	stalk celery, chopped
1	cup chopped green bell pepper
1	teaspoon ground coriander
1½	teaspoons ground cumin
1	cup white wine
1½	cups defatted chicken broth
2	oranges, peeled, seeded, sectioned, pith removed
½	cup orange juice
1	tablespoon dry sherry
¼	teaspoon pepper
¼	teaspoon red pepper flakes
½	teaspoon lemon juice
salt	
4	tablespoons nonfat sour cream for garnish

Rinse the beans. Place them in a bowl and cover them with water; let soak overnight or for several hours. Pour off excess water and transfer them to a deep saucepan. Cover with water or stock. Bring to a boil, cover, reduce heat, and simmer 1½ hours over very low heat. During the last half hour of cooking, sauté the chopped onion, garlic, carrot, celery, green pepper, coriander, and cumin in the white wine. Add broth as you go to steam and cook the vegetables. Cook until the wine has evaporated and the vegetables are soft, about 7 minutes. Add the vegetable mixture to the cooked bean mixture. Continue to cook over low heat for about 10 minutes. Add the remaining ingredients to the soup and stir; cover and let cook for 10 minutes more. If you want a creamier soup, run it briefly through the blender, or let it cook a little longer so it becomes thicker. Serve topped with a dollop of nonfat sour cream.

Per serving, not including sour cream: 271 calories; 1.3 g fat (4.1 percent calories from fat); 15 g protein; 54 g carbohydrate; 0 mg cholesterol; 116 mg sodium.

French Onion Soup

MAKES 4 SERVINGS

This is not a fattening soup, but you'd never know it if you have only ordered restaurant versions. What makes their onion soups so high in fat is that they sauté the onions in tons of oil, then top the whole thing off with a

- Thicken your soups with rice, couscous, quinoa, risotto, orzo, Kashi, or any other grain or pasta.
- Make "cream soups" with nonfat plain yogurt, pureed tofu, fat-free sour cream, or pureed beans.
- Use skim or 1 percent milk, or evaporated skim milk, in all soups that ask for whole milk or cream.
- Puree a baked potato in the blender and add it to soup to thicken the broth.
- Add bean flakes to give broth some body.
- Use defatted chicken or turkey broth instead of the regular kind.
- Look for a defatting pitcher. This kitchen tool separates out the fat from a soup after it's finished cooking.
- Use prechopped or frozen chopped vegetables if you don't have time to chop fresh.
- Look for all of the new healthy soup mixes that have blended the seasonings and premeasured everything for you.

high-fat cheese. Also, they often use fatty beef broth as a base; here I use Health Valley defatted broth. If you don't mind adding a few more fat grams to the soup, forgo the Swiss and top it off with some low-fat Jarlsberg cheese.

2   cups dry white wine
4   cups chopped onion
3   cups chopped leeks, carefully rinsed, white and firm green
     parts only
1   bunch scallions, chopped
4   cups defatted beef broth (Health Valley if possible)
nonstick vegetable oil spray
4   slices sourdough bread
1   clove garlic, peeled and halved
2   tablespoons grated fat-free Swiss cheese
1   tablespoon chopped parsley

Pour ½ cup of wine in a large nonstick saucepan. Add the next three ingredients and cook over medium heat until the vegetables are tender. Add the remaining wine and bring to a boil over high heat. Boil until the liquid is reduced by half, about 5 minutes. Add the beef broth, reduce heat, and simmer until the vegetables are soft, about 35 minutes. Preheat oven to 350°, spray a baking sheet with the vegetable oil spray, and arrange the bread slices on it. Rub each slice of bread on both sides with the garlic clove. Bake until lightly toasted on each side. Sprinkle each slice with the cheese and return to the oven just long enough to melt the cheese. Place the bread slices in individual bowls and ladle the soup over the top. Garnish with chopped parsley. Serve with a green salad.

Per serving: 230 calories; 0.7 g fat (4 percent calories from fat); 8 g protein; 29 g carbohydrate; 1 mg cholesterol; 763 mg sodium.

Gazpacho

MAKES 6 SERVINGS

Gazpacho has become a summer staple, and rightly so: it's cool and refreshing, not to mention low in fat and rich in vitamins and minerals. If you like a milder soup, add another cucumber to the recipe. If you like a crunchy soup, top with some chopped celery.

4	cups V-8 juice
1	small onion, minced
2	cups diced tomatoes
1	cup minced green bell pepper
1	teaspoon honey
1	cucumber, peeled and diced
2	scallions, chopped
1	tablespoon lemon juice
1	tablespoon lime juice
2	tablespoons red wine vinegar
1	teaspoon tarragon
1	teaspoon fresh basil, chopped

pinch ground cumin
¼ cup chopped fresh parsley
¼ teaspoon Tabasco sauce
salt and pepper to taste

Combine all of the ingredients in a large bowl and let chill for at least one hour. If the soup is too chunky, run it through the blender ³/₄ cup at a time. Serve with Nacho Quesadillas (see page 131).

Per serving: 75 calories; 0.6 g fat (6.4 percent calories from fat); 3 g protein; 17 g carbohydrate; 0 mg cholesterol; 702 mg sodium.

Shrimp Gazpacho

MAKES 6 SERVINGS

Here's a variation on the theme, worth the time it takes to chop all the fresh ingredients. It's a meal in itself but also makes a great appetizer or lunch dish. The recipe calls for raw shellfish, but don't worry—you won't be eating sashimi. The vinegar and lemon juice mixture "cooks" the shrimp.

2	cloves garlic, chopped
2	tablespoons red wine vinegar
2	tablespoons lemon juice
¹/₂	pound medium raw shrimp, peeled and deveined
³/₄	pound tomatoes, seeded and chopped
1	green bell pepper, chopped
1	red bell pepper, chopped
¹/₂	large cucumber, peeled and chopped
1	bunch scallions, chopped
¹/₂	bunch cilantro, chopped
¹/₂	large jalapeño, minced
4¹/₂	cups V-8 juice
	salt and pepper to taste
6	lemon wedges

Combine the first three ingredients in a medium bowl. Add the shrimp; cover and marinate for 1 to 2 hours to "cook" the shellfish. In a large bowl, combine the tomatoes, green and red bell peppers, cucumber, scallions, cilantro, and jalapeño. Add the V-8 juice and combine with the shrimp mixture. Season with salt and pepper to taste. Garnish with lemon wedges. Serve with crusty sourdough bread.

Per serving: 103 calories; 1.1 g fat (8.9 percent calories from fat); 10 g protein; 15 g carbohydrate; 58 mg cholesterol; 728 mg sodium.

Sauces

Nonfat sauces may seem like an oxymoron because we've gotten so used to topping our food with creamy, oily concoctions. But the truth is, sauces can be just as rich without added fat. Ladle a nonfat sauce over poultry and fish and they'll taste just as succulent and juicy as the old fatty sauces you're probably used to.

If you open my fridge, you'll see bottles and bottles of fat-free sauces. I used to have to make my own pasta and BBQ sauces as well as any other sauces I wanted to be fat-free. But now there is such a great variety of healthy, fat-free sauces on the market that you can literally pour and cook. To make them even better, you can combine a couple of them or doctor them up with seasonings. I like to mix a little BBQ sauce with a dash of Cajun or red pepper sauce. Teriyaki sauce tastes terrific accented with some light soy sauce and orange juice concentrate.

Hickory BBQ Sauce

MAKES 2 CUPS OR 12 SERVINGS

This is the number one selling sauce in my food business, and it is truly delectable. Double the recipe and store the sauce in jars in the fridge. It gets even better as it sits. Serve on poultry, salmon, and turkey dishes.

16	ounces tomato sauce
2	tablespoons lemon juice
2	tablespoons frozen apple juice concentrate
1	tablespoon onion flakes
1	tablespoon celery flakes
1/2	green bell pepper, diced fine
1	tablespoon Worcestershire sauce
1	tablespoon Dijon mustard
1	teaspoon dry mustard
1	teaspoon poultry seasoning
1	teaspoon liquid smoke
1/4	teaspoon garlic powder

Combine all the ingredients in a large saucepan and bring to a boil. Lower the heat and simmer for about 20 minutes. Let cool.

Per serving: *22 calories; 0.2 g fat (6.7 percent calories from fat); 1 g protein; 5 g carbohydrate; 0 mg cholesterol; 259 mg sodium.*

No-Brainer Tips for Giving Fat-Free Sauces More Zip

- To thicken a sauce, add some oil-free salad dressing made with natural gums like carrageenan and xanthan.
- Cornstarch or arrowroot are other super nonfat sauce thickeners.
- Think of oil-free Italian dressing as a sauce. Drizzle some in the pan when you're sautéing onions and peppers. Likewise, think of mustard as a sauce. Try sautéing a dill-flavored mustard with some capers and garlic, then pouring it over chicken or turkey.
- To give sauces a taste of butter or olive oil, use flavored nonstick sprays when you sauté ingredients.
- Replace cream in sauce recipes with soft tofu, nonfat sour cream, nonfat plain yogurt, or bean purees.
- Make "meat" sauces with ground chicken or ground chicken breast.
- Hain makes a natural gravy mix that's wonderful on its own as well as to thicken gravies made from scratch.
- Puree an assortment of fresh vegetables in a blender, then add them to pasta sauces (you can also stir pureed veggies into chilies).

Ginger Curry Sauce

MAKES 1 CUP OR 4 SERVINGS

Serve this creamy sauce over steamed veggies, baked potatoes, and yams, or use as a sandwich spread. It's also great mixed with tuna or chicken in a salad.

1   cup nonfat plain yogurt
1   tablespoon curry powder
2   scallions, white part only, minced
1   teaspoon frozen apple juice concentrate
¼   teaspoon ground ginger
     salt to taste

Blend all of the ingredients in a blender at high speed. Refrigerate until ready to use.

Per serving: 43 calories; 0.4 g fat (7.1 percent calories from fat); 4 g protein; 7 g carbohydrate; 1 mg cholesterol; 46 mg sodium.

Dijonnaise Sauce

MAKES 1$\frac{1}{2}$ CUPS OR 4 SERVINGS

This sauce is terrific served over chicken (see recipe page 186) as well as over fish and turkey. It even makes a great dip. If you like, add a few capers for extra flavor.

1   cup defatted chicken broth
$\frac{1}{2}$ cup nonfat sour cream
$\frac{1}{4}$ cup Dijon mustard
1   tablespoon arrowroot
1   teaspoon poultry seasoning
pinch pepper

Combine all the ingredients in a saucepan. Cook over medium-high heat, stirring rapidly, until the sauce is well blended, reduced slightly, and thickened, about 7 minutes.

Per serving: 43 calories; 0.7 g fat (12.9 percent calories from fat); 3 g protein; 7 g carbohydrate; 0 mg cholesterol; 213 mg sodium.

Rhubarb Honey Sauce

MAKES 1$\frac{1}{2}$ CUPS OR 6 SERVINGS

Rhubarb looks like red celery and is available mostly in the late spring and summer. Most people know it as a pie ingredient, but the tart stalk also makes a wonderful sauce combined with something sweet—in this case honey. My mother used to make this sauce, mix it with some cooked barley, and serve it over pork tenderloin. It was heavenly! I like to serve it over roasted turkey

---

BOTTLED BRANDS TO LOOK FOR

Annie Chums	Robbie's
Ayla's	San-J
John Troy's	Uncle Bum's
Mr. Spice	Westbrae
Premier Japan	

breast or grilled chicken. To go another direction, you can also use it to top fat-free vanilla- or coffee-flavored frozen yogurt or the Vanilla Yogurt Cream on page 281.

4	stalks rhubarb, cut into 1-inch cubes
1	cup Knudsen apple syrup*
1/4	cup honey
2	teaspoons cinnamon

Preheat oven or toaster oven to 350°. Place the chunks of rhubarb in the middle of a big piece of aluminum foil. Fold up the ends of the foil and crunch together to form a "boat." Pour the apple syrup and honey around the rhubarb, then sprinkle the cinnamon evenly over the top. Bake for 10 minutes, stir, and cook for another 10 minutes, or until the rhubarb is soft.

Per serving: 101 calories; 0.5 g fat (4.2 percent calories from fat); 2 g protein; 24 g carbohydrate; 0 mg cholesterol; 10 mg sodium.

Marmalade Chutney

MAKES 6 SERVINGS

Chutney, a staple of Indian cuisine, is simply a chunky, spicy fruit topping. But it's no longer exotic; it's one of those foreign food items that's become a part of our everyday meals (could pasta once have been eaten only by Italians?). One way to use it is to fill a no-oil whole wheat tortilla with some diced chicken and mix a little chutney in. Or top a baked potato or yam with a dollop. There are no rules, so go wild.

1 1/4	cups pineapple chunks in water, juice reserved
1/4	cup golden raisins
1/2	teaspoon crushed red pepper flakes
2	cloves garlic, sliced
1/4	teaspoon ground ginger
pinch nutmeg	
1	teaspoon low-sodium soy sauce
1/4	cup sugar-free marmalade

*If you can't find Knudsen apple syrup (it's pancake syrup), substitute 1/2 cup maple syrup and 1/2 cup frozen apple juice concentrate.

1 teaspoon honey
¼ teaspoon cornstarch

Place the pineapple chunks and their juice in a medium saucepan. Add the raisins, red pepper flakes, garlic, ginger, nutmeg, soy sauce, and marmalade. Bring to a boil, then reduce the heat and simmer. Add the honey. In a separate dish, allow 2 tablespoons of the liquid to cool to room temperature, then mix in the cornstarch. Add the cornstarch mixture back into the pan and cook one minute at a low boil until syrupy. Let cool before serving. Serve with any spicy chicken dish or curry dish.

Per serving, chutney only: 80 calories; 0.5 g fat (5.3 percent calories from fat); 1 g protein; 20 g carbohydrate; 0 mg cholesterol; 36 mg sodium.

Simple Curry Sauce

MAKES 1 CUP OR 4 SERVINGS

This easy curry sauce gives anything you serve it with a bit of Indian flavor. Try it with tandoori chicken, drizzled on a baked potato, or inside a burrito. It's also a super dressing for chicken salad.

1 cup nonfat plain yogurt
1 tablespoon curry powder
¼ teaspoon ground ginger
1 scallion, chopped
¼ teaspoon honey
salt to taste
1 tablespoon raisins (optional)

Combine all of the ingredients in a medium-size bowl. Stir to blend. Toss in a tablespoon of raisins if you like.

Per serving: 40 calories; 0.3 g fat (7.3 percent calories from fat); 4 g protein; 6 g carbohydrate; 1 mg cholesterol; 45 mg sodium.

Sun-Dried Tomato Basil Sauce

MAKES 5–6 CUPS OR 25 SERVINGS

A lot of food companies make sun-dried tomato sauces now, but they're literally swimming in oil. Take the dive and make this fat-free one instead, another delicious sauce you can make in bulk and freeze. Use it to top grilled or baked chicken and toss it with any type pasta, especially the flavored kinds.

1/4	cup white wine
1/2	cup white onion, minced
10	cups fresh tomatoes, peeled and seeded, or 2 22-ounce cans of whole tomatoes
3	cloves garlic, minced
1	ounce sherry
1/2	cup dry vermouth
1	tablespoon honey
	salt and pepper to taste
1	cup chopped sun-dried tomatoes (dry, not in oil)
1	cup fresh basil, chopped

Heat the wine in a large saucepan and add the onion and garlic. Cook over medium heat until transparent. Add the remaining ingredients, except the sun-dried tomatoes and basil. Cook over medium heat until the sauce comes to a boil. Reduce the heat and cook for 20 minutes on a low boil. Remove 2 cups of the sauce and place in a food processor or blender with the sun-dried tomatoes. Puree and return to the pot. Turn off the heat and add the basil; stir well to combine. Top with grated or shaved Parmesan cheese.

Per serving, not including cheese: *35 calories; 0.3 g fat (9.4 percent calories from fat); 1 g protein; 6 g carbohydrate; 0 mg cholesterol; 65 mg sodium.*

Presto Pomodoro Sauce

MAKES 2 CUPS OR 4 SERVINGS

It's nice to make this flavorful all-purpose tomato sauce with fresh ingredients, and it really doesn't take a lot of extra time to do so. But if you don't have fresh on hand, make the substitutions indicated below.

1   small onion, diced
1   clove garlic, minced
1   green bell pepper, cored, seeded, and chopped
1/4 cup white wine
2   tablespoons lemon juice
8   large tomatoes, seeded and chopped, or 1 13-ounce can of
      chopped tomatoes
3   tablespoons chopped fresh basil or 3 teaspoons dried
1   tablespoon chopped fresh Italian parsley or 2 teaspoons
      pepper to taste
8   ounces tomato sauce

In a medium saucepan, sauté onion, garlic, and green pepper in white wine over medium heat until softened. Add lemon juice and tomatoes and bring to a low boil. Reduce heat and simmer for 10–15 minutes. Add the basil, parsley, ground pepper, and tomato sauce. Cook for another 3–5 minutes. Toss with cooked pasta and top with grated or shaved Parmesan cheese.

Per serving, not including cheese: 97 calories; 1.1 g fat (9.2 percent calories from fat); 4 g protein; 20 g carbohydrate; 0 mg cholesterol; 505 mg sodium.

Light Garlic Pasta Sauce

MAKES 1 1/2–2 CUPS OR 4 SERVINGS

When you get tired of a red sauce and want a light, summery sauce, this is easy and delicious. It goes well over pasta, chicken, and chopped vegetables. Experiment with other fresh herbs and seasonings to give it a twist.

1   cup defatted chicken broth
1/2 cup white wine
1/2 cup oil-free Italian salad dressing
2   tablespoons minced garlic
1   teaspoon garlic powder
1   tablespoon chopped parsley
2   teaspoons lemon juice
1   tablespoon grated Parmesan cheese
salt and pepper to taste

Pour the broth, wine, and salad dressing into a large nonstick sauté pan. Heat over medium heat until sizzling, 1–2 minutes, and add the minced garlic and garlic powder. Bring to a boil, lower heat, and add the parsley and lemon juice. Simmer for about 5 minutes. Add the Parmesan, cook 1 minute more, then add the salt and pepper. Serve over an herb pasta.

Per serving: 42 calories; 0.5 g fat (19.4 percent calories from fat); 2 g protein; 3 g carbohydrate; 1 mg cholesterol; 31 mg sodium.

Hot Oregano Salsa

MAKES 6 SERVINGS

I love salsa over everything. Well, not over chocolate, but most everything else. This one, in particular, is terrific over grilled fish.

6 serrano peppers
2 pounds ripe tomatoes, diced
1 small onion, diced
1 tablespoon fresh oregano, chopped, or 1¹/₂ teaspoons dried
¹/₈ teaspoon fresh lime juice
salt to taste

Wear rubber gloves when you chop the peppers (so your hands don't get spicy, a killer if you inadvertently rub your eye or have a cut). Remove the seeds and ribs and dice the peppers. Combine with the next four ingredients in a medium-size bowl. Season with salt. Let sit one hour.

Per serving: 61 calories; 0.7 g fat (8.6 percent calories from fat); 3 g protein; 14 g carbohydrate; 0 mg cholesterol; 109 mg sodium.

Mango Lime Salsa

MAKES 4 SERVINGS

Now is the time to rethink mangoes. It's not some exotic tropical fruit that you can only get in the summertime—or in Hawaii. You can now buy fresh mangoes year-round as well as frozen or in jars. If the latter versions are packed in sugar, which is generally the case, rinse before you use the mango. I like to use this salsa on grilled fish, chicken, or to top off a taco or tortilla. Don't be afraid to tango with the mango.

3/4   **cup peeled, diced mango**
1/4   **cup diced red onion**
2   **tablespoons chopped fresh cilantro**
1   **tablespoon fresh lime juice**

Mix all of the ingredients in a medium-size bowl. Cover and allow to marinate for at least 1 hour or overnight. Stir occasionally.

Per serving: *28 calories; 0.1 g fat (4.3 percent calories from fat); 0 g protein; 7 g carbohydrate; 0 mg cholesterol; 3 mg sodium.*

Papaya Salsa

MAKES 8 SERVINGS

This is definitely my favorite salsa. It has an unbeatable flavor, and I love it over fish, chicken, or even baked potatoes. Not to mention that between the red onion and the papaya you are getting a nice-size dose of the popular antioxidant beta carotene. But don't tell your kids that, just let them enjoy it.

2   **whole papayas, peeled, seeded, and cubed**
1/2   **red onion, peeled and diced**
1   **bunch fresh cilantro, chopped, stems removed**
8   **ounces (1 cup) frozen orange juice concentrate**
1/2   **cup fresh lime juice**
1/2   **jalapeño, seeded and diced**

Let the orange juice concentrate melt slightly in a separate bowl or glass measuring cup. Peel the papayas and remove the seeds; cut in 1/2-inch cubes and place in a medium-size bowl. Add the diced red onion, chopped cilantro, orange juice concentrate, lime juice, and diced jalapeño. Stir and toss gently so that you don't smash the papaya too much. Let chill for at least 30 minutes.

Per serving: *84 calories; 0 g fat (2 percent calories from fat); 1 g protein; 21 g carbohydrate; 0 mg cholesterol; 4 mg sodium.*

Roasted Tomatillo Salsa

MAKES 12 SERVINGS

Tomatillos, which look like little green tomatoes, are sold in most produce departments and are turning up all over the place; they're quite the fashionable food. You can also find tomatillo salsa sold in jars, but this fresh version has even better flavor.

2   tomatoes
1   pound tomatillos in husks
5   poblano chilies, quartered (available in Hispanic markets and
        some supermarket produce sections)
olive-flavored nonstick vegetable oil spray
1   medium onion, quartered
1   cup fresh cilantro
2   teaspoons fresh lime juice
salt to taste

Place the tomatoes, tomatillos, and peppers on a piece of aluminum foil and turn up the edges. Spritz with vegetable oil spray, and roast in your toaster oven, or under the broiler (or you can do them directly on the grill). Turn them until they're charred on all sides. Peel and core the tomatoes and cut them into quarters. Husk the tomatillos and put them in a food processor or blender with the tomatoes. Peel, stem, and seed the chilies and put them, the onion, and the cilantro in the processor with the tomatoes and tomatillos. Process until everything is finely chopped. Add the lime juice and salt. Stir and let sit for one hour. Use as you would a red salsa. This is particularly good over chicken.

Per serving: 29 calories; 0.5 g fat (13.9 percent calories from fat); 1 g protein; 6 g carbohydrate; 0 mg cholesterol; 50 mg sodium.

Tomatillo Salsa

MAKES 6 SERVINGS

This tomatillo salsa is a little simpler and more mild than the one above. Serve it with Monterey Jack cheese and corn tortillas.

1½   cups defatted chicken broth
12   tomatillos, husked

2	jalapeños, peeled and seeded
5	cloves garlic
3/4	cup chopped onions
1/2	bunch cilantro, stems removed

salt to taste

Pour the chicken broth into a large saucepan, and heat until sizzling, about 1–2 minutes, over medium heat. Add the tomatillos, jalapeños, half of the garlic cloves, and half of the onion, and simmer for 30 minutes. Remove from heat and puree with the remaining ingredients except salt in a blender or food processor on high. Return to the saucepan and simmer until thick, about 45 minutes. Season with salt.

Per serving: *39 calories; 0.8 g fat (15.9 percent calories from fat); 2 g protein; 7 g carbohydrate; 0 mg cholesterol; 77 mg sodium.*

Chapter Eleven

Shall We Dine?

If there's one thing that I've learned after all my years as a diet counselor, it's that respect for mealtimes has gone by the wayside. Sitting down with the whole family for a lovely, leisurely meal has become a thing of the past, or at least an only occasional occurrence.

As I've said before, eating has to fit into your lifestyle. If breakfast doesn't suit you, pass. If you don't have time for a traditional lunch, munch around it. But I take exception to skipping dinner. Dinner marks the end of the day and should be given the respect it deserves. In turn, you'll be giving yourself the respect *you* deserve by feeding your body well and allowing your mind to just shut down and enjoy some gustatory sensations. If you're like most people, you probably eat the bulk of your calories after 3:30 or 4 P.M. and on into the night anyway. So why not work with it? Let's do dinner and do it right. Easy, quick, but good for the body, the mind, and the soul.

Keep in mind, though, that *when* you eat dinner doesn't matter. If you eat late, great. Contrary to what many people say, I don't believe eating after 6 or 7 P.M. has any bearing on how healthy you are. Europeans, particularly Mediterranean people, who are now being held up to us as paragons of health, have been eating late dinners for centuries and have survived quite nicely.

What's important is that you eat well—and I'm very aware that there are any number of obstacles that keep people from doing so.

To be truthful, one of the main reasons I've written this book is because *I* have had to learn how to put together healthy, low-fat meals quickly for my family. I'm not going to lie and tell you that every evening is like dinner with the Waltons, but I have managed to create dinner dishes that are quick, delicious, and easy. It relieves so much of the working mom's guilt (and we have plenty) to know that she's feeding her family well and not just throwing burgers or frozen dinners at them. I get so upset when I see commercials that suggest that moms (they never show dads) stop by a burger joint to bring home dinner. It's not the kind of food you want to feed your family on a regular basis. I'm not saying that you shouldn't order out for pizza, or go to McDonald's occasionally to satisfy the kids. But keep it to that—once in a while.

We talk so much these days about obese people who turn to food for love. Well, there *is* love in food. There is great pleasure in eating and sharing a meal with people you care about. There is love in a meal prepared for you; there's no getting around that. We need to respect that fact a little more in our society. As you can see by the recipes here, giving love to your family through food doesn't mean you have to spend hours in the kitchen, and it doesn't have to mean any excessive chopping or prepping. It just means planning a little better and learning some no-brainer kitchen tricks.

Single people deal with a different dilemma entirely. They often feel like it's silly to take the time to make dinner for one. It's easier to heat up a Lean Cuisine or Weight Watchers frozen dinner, foods with health claims on the label, but many are still loaded with artificial ingredients, fats, salts, and sugar. They may make you feel like you've been "good," but your body is likely to be so dissatisfied by these meals, you'll be starving an hour later. Four bites of a Lean Cuisine and in an hour, Ben & Jerry's, anyone?

If you're single you're also more likely to eat out, so why shop when everything will just go bad before you get to it? But there's a solution. You need to learn how to put your freezer to good use and stock your cabinets well. Great rice mixes, cup o' soup dinners, bags of frozen vegetables—these kinds of foods can be turned into a tasty, healthy meal in minutes.

We all need food that is as easy and convenient as frozen dinners but as satisfying as a gourmet meal, packed with nutrients, and lean besides. Years ago, when I first began experimenting with low-fat and nonfat cooking, recipes that fit that description seemed impossible to make and I became very frustrated. All of the so-called low-fat or fat-free recipes called for oil or some junky fat substitute like fat-free mayonnaise. They weren't really fat free, and they weren't really healthy. Many of them were just pared down, asking for one tablespoon of oil instead of two, for instance, or substituting nonfat yogurt for cream. The result was either that they didn't go far enough in reducing fat or they were tasteless.

I really put my mind (and taste buds) to the task of creating lean dinners with flavor—and it worked. Soon I was teaching Carrie Fisher's great Southern cook, Gloria, how to use some new techniques. I was taking Kate Jackson's chef to the market to help her find the right foods. Actress Mel Harris cooks for her own family, so I helped her plan meals for her husband, Cotter Smith, who needed some help getting his cholesterol levels down. Mel herself wanted to lose weight.

The point is, good food with high health credentials is there for the taking, whether you have the luxury of having a chef or not—I certainly don't!
This is about real-life cooking for people in the 1990s. The dishes here are
the ones I serve to my family and friends, use in my food business, and teach
my clients. They make it easy to bring dinner back into your life—you deserve it!

No-Brainer Dinners

When I say "no-brainer" it has nothing to do with your IQ. As a matter of
fact, it means that you have used your brain all day, and are tired at the end
of it, and don't want to have to think about creating elaborate recipes. Think
of it like moving to a new town. At first you don't have a sense of direction,
and need a map or directions to get around. But once you do, it becomes
automatic. That's what these recipes are going to do for you—make cooking
as easy as being on automatic pilot. Some are a little more lengthy than others, and some are so simple you will think I have no brain for even calling
them recipes.

Chicken Dinners

I bet you sometimes think if you see one more plain baked, broiled, or grilled
chicken breast, you'll go crazy! But with these recipes I aim to give chicken a
new lease on life, a new identity. The trick is having lots of wonderful sauces
around. My refrigerator is half full of bottles of sauces because I love the sim-
plicity of pouring them one minute and serving them the next. So stock your
refrigerator with sauces and your freezer with packages of boneless chicken
breasts. Take the chicken out of the freezer and put it in the refrigerator to
defrost before you leave in the morning; then when you come home, whip
out the sauce, put it all in the oven, and you'll have a luscious chicken dinner
in 15 to 20 minutes.

Chicken Oregano over Garlic Rotelli

Although this recipe involves an odd blending of seasonings, it's absolutely delicious. If you're pressed for time, take a few easy shortcuts: use frozen chopped onions and presliced mushrooms or mushrooms from a bottle instead of fresh. If you can't find garlic-flavored rotelli, use plain rotelli pasta and add 1 teaspoon of chopped garlic or 1 teaspoon garlic powder to the boiling water.

nonstick vegetable oil spray
$1/2$ cup white wine
$1/4$ cup chopped onions
3   cloves garlic, minced
$1/2$ cup lemon juice
$5^1/2$ ounces V-8 juice
1   teaspoon oregano
$1/2$ teaspoon pepper
2   teaspoons poultry seasoning
$1/2$ teaspoon paprika
pinch salt
4   6-ounce boneless skinless chicken breasts
1   cup thinly sliced mushrooms
1   cup garlic-flavored rotelli pasta, cooked according to
          package instructions

RANDOM NOTES ON CHICKEN

- Buy boneless chicken breasts with the skin on, then remove the skin before you cook them—it's less expensive than buying preskinned chicken.

- All the recipes that follow call for boneless chicken breasts, but feel free to use chicken on the bone (some people feel chicken on the bone has more flavor). Just add another 5–7 minutes' cooking time.

- A 3-pound chicken will yield $2^1/2$ cups of meat, shredded or diced.

Spritz a medium sauté pan with vegetable oil spray. Warm the pan over medium heat, then add the wine, onions, and garlic. Cook until the onions are transparent but not brown. Add the lemon juice, V-8, oregano, pepper, poultry seasoning, paprika, and salt to the skillet. Heat until bubbly. Place the chicken, fullest side down, in the pan and cover the pan with a lid. Cook over medium heat for about 15 minutes. Turn the chicken, add the mushrooms (pour in more wine if the pan has become too dry), and cook until done, another 5–7 minutes. Spoon over pasta, top with Parmesan if you like, and serve with a green salad.

Per serving, not including Parmesan: 265 calories; 2.7 g fat (9.2 percent calories from fat); 42 g protein; 17 g carbohydrate; 98 mg cholesterol; 329 mg sodium.

Brazilian Chicken

MAKES 4 SERVINGS

This dish is proof that exotic doesn't have to mean chaotic. So shake up your taste buds and try something new.

nonstick vegetable oil spray
4   6-ounce boneless skinless chicken breasts
1   cup ketchup
20 ounces fresh pineapple, chopped, or 2 10-ounce cans water-
       packed crushed pineapple, drained
2   cloves garlic, minced
1   teaspoon ground ginger
1   teaspoon dry mustard
1   teaspoon poultry seasoning
1   cup coffee

Preheat oven to 375°. Line a shallow baking pan with foil and spritz with nonstick vegetable oil spray. Place the chicken breasts in the pan, fullest side down. In a medium bowl, combine the remaining ingredients and pour the mixture over the chicken. Let sit for 10–15 minutes. Cover chicken with aluminum foil and bake for about 20 minutes. Remove the top foil and turn chicken breasts over; cook for another 10 minutes, or until cooked through. Serve with black beans and rice.

Per serving: 308 calories; 3.2 g fat (8.5 percent calories from fat); 41 g protein; 35 g carbohydrate; 98 mg cholesterol; 831 mg sodium.

Chicken Cacciatore

This doesn't look like a no-brainer on paper, but it really is easy when you put it all together and serve it over your favorite pasta. I prefer the thicker pastas such as penne or spinach fettucine. Like a good spaghetti sauce, this dish is even better the next day, so make a large batch.

¹/₂	tablespoon basil
1	teaspoon oregano
1	teaspoon poultry seasoning (I like Paula's)
¹/₄	teaspoon cinnamon
	pinch red pepper flakes
¹/₄	teaspoon coriander
¹/₄	teaspoon fennel seeds, crushed
¹/₂	bay leaf, broken in half
4	6-ounce boneless skinless chicken breasts
¹/₄	cup whole wheat flour
	olive-flavored nonstick vegetable oil spray
³/₄	cup white wine
2	garlic cloves, minced
2	small onions, chopped
1	medium green bell pepper, chopped
¹/₂	pound mushrooms, sliced
1	14.5-ounce can tomatoes, chopped, with liquid, or 1¹/₂ cups Italian green beans, cut on diagonal
1	8-ounce can tomato sauce
1	tablespoon lemon juice
9	ounces Italian green beans

In a small bowl, combine the spices and herbs and set aside. Dredge the chicken breasts in the flour. Spritz a large nonstick sauté pan with vegetable oil spray. Add three quarters of the white wine, then the chicken breasts and, over high heat, sear the chicken, cooking for about 2–3 minutes on each side. Do not let the flour burn. Remove the chicken and place on a plate. Add the rest of the white wine to the pan, then the garlic, onions, and pepper. Sauté over medium heat until transparent. Add the mushrooms and cook a few minutes more. Add the canned tomatoes in their juice and the tomato sauce. Bring to a boil, then add the spices and lemon juice. Return the chicken to the pan, and cover with the sauce. Reduce the heat, cover, and simmer for at least 35 minutes, adding the green beans in the last 10 minutes.

Per serving: 292 calories; 3.2 g fat (9 percent calories from fat); 45 g protein; 26 g carbohydrate; 98 mg cholesterol; 867 mg sodium.

Chicken Dijonnaise

MAKES 4 SERVINGS

This is a simple dish but elegant enough to impress guests. They'll be particularly impressed when they learn that the sauce has 0 grams of fat. Make extra sauce so you can use it to zip up leftover veggies, potatoes, and rice.

4   6-ounce boneless skinless chicken breasts
1/2   teaspoon thyme
1/2   cup white wine vinegar
2   cloves garlic, crushed
2   teaspoons Dijon mustard
1/4   cup Dijonnaise Sauce (see page 171)

Season the chicken breast with the thyme; set aside. Pour the white wine vinegar into a medium-size skillet. Add the garlic and cook over medium heat for 2 to 3 minutes. Blend in the Dijon mustard, stirring quickly. Place the chicken breasts in the pan and cook covered for 7 minutes. Remove the lid, turn the chicken, and cook uncovered for another 7–10 minutes, or until done. If the liquid evaporates, add more vinegar as you go along. Remove the chicken from the pan and transfer to a serving platter. Top with the Dijonnaise Sauce and serve over wild rice pilaf with steamed asparagus.

Per serving: 188 calories; 2.7 g fat (11.9 percent calories from fat); 40 g protein; 4 g carbohydrate; 98 mg cholesterol; 246 mg sodium.

Citrus Chicken

MAKES 4 SERVINGS

Okay, I admit that this takes a little more time to make than I usually like to spend. But it's one of my favorite dishes and is especially tasty when limes are in season. If they aren't, or are just too expensive, use frozen lime juice concentrate instead, and just spring for one lime for the zest (peel). This dish is really only good when grilled, so if you don't have a grill, skip it.

1/3	cup fresh orange juice (or frozen concentrate)
1/4	cup lemon juice
1/4	cup honey
3	tablespoons fresh lime juice (or concentrate)
3	tablespoons chopped fresh mint
1	tablespoon orange peel
2	tablespoons lemon peel
1 1/4	teaspoons lime peel
1/4	teaspoon cumin powder
1/4	teaspoon cinnamon
pinch white pepper	
4	6-ounce boneless skinless chicken breasts
1/4	red onion, thinly sliced

Heat the first 4 ingredients in a small saucepan until the honey is melted. Add the mint, peel, and spices, then stir to blend. Place the chicken and onion in a shallow baking pan and pour the marinade on top. Cover and marinate a minimum of 1 hour, or overnight. Prepare a grill (medium heat). Remove the chicken from the marinade and pour remaining marinade into a small saucepan and bring to a boil; remove from the heat. Grill the chicken until cooked through, about 5 to 8 minutes on each side. Transfer the chicken to a serving dish and pour the marinade on top. Serve over wild rice with grilled asparagus.

Per serving: 255 calories; 2.3 g fat (7.6 percent calories from fat); 40 g protein; 24 g carbohydrate; 98 mg cholesterol; 118 mg sodium.

Crispy Chicken Parmesan

MAKES 4 SERVINGS

I like to serve this easy baked chicken dish with zucchini and rice pilaf. I presteam the zucchini, then set it around the chicken during the last 10 minutes of cooking so it soaks up the juices.

1 1/2	cups whole wheat bread crumbs
1 1/4	cups grated Parmesan cheese

¼	cup parsley flakes
1	teaspoon Italian seasoning
½	cup white wine
2	cloves garlic, minced
4	6-ounce boneless skinless chicken breasts

salt and pepper to taste

2	egg whites, lightly beaten
6	bay leaves

Preheat the oven to 325°. Mix the bread crumbs, Parmesan, parsley, and Italian seasoning in a shallow dish; set aside. Heat the white wine in a medium-size skillet. Add the minced garlic and cook over medium heat until transparent. Season the chicken breasts with the salt and pepper, then place them in the skillet. Brown the chicken on both sides, then remove it from the pan and dip it into the beaten egg. Dredge the chicken in the bread-crumb mixture to coat. Place the breasts in a rectangular baking dish, pour the wine remaining in the skillet into the dish, and place the bay leaves on the chicken. Bake for 1 hour.

Per serving: 174 calories; 8 g fat (41 percent calories from fat); 13 g protein; 4 g carbohydrate; 20 mg cholesterol; 497 mg sodium.

Crispy Southern-Baked Chicken with Honey Mustard Dip

MAKES 4 SERVINGS

I created this dish about eight years ago for my food business. It's wonderfully crispy and delicious and makes a great picnic dish. If you don't have time to go through the whole process of mixing the batter, here's a great no-brainer shortcut: Take any of the great new fat-free flavored crackers like Hain Fire Crackers or Auburn Farms onion crackers, and put them in a blender to turn them into crumbs. Substitute them for the flour mixture, below.

2	6-ounce boneless skinless chicken breasts
2	skinless chicken thighs
2	skinless chicken drumsticks
2	cups ice water

Coating

³/₄ cup whole wheat flour
¹/₄ cup wheat germ
1 tablespoon garlic powder
1 tablespoon onion powder
¹/₄ teaspoon paprika
¹/₄ teaspoon red pepper flakes
¹/₂ teaspoon cinnamon
pinch chili powder
¹/₄ teaspoon ground cloves
pinch white pepper
3 egg whites, lightly beaten
1 teaspoon Worcestershire sauce
pinch white pepper
nonstick vegetable oil spray
Honey Mustard Dip (see page 190)

Preheat the oven to 400°. Remove the skin from the chicken pieces if necessary, then place chicken in the ice water for about 20 minutes. In a medium-size bowl, combine the flour, wheat germ, garlic and onion powders, and spices to create a flour mixture. In a shallow bowl, combine the egg whites, Worcestershire sauce, and white pepper. Take the chicken out of the ice water and pat dry. Roll the chicken pieces in the egg mixture, let excess drip off, then roll them in the flour mixture until completely coated. Spritz a shallow baking pan with vegetable oil spray and place the coated chicken in the pan. Cover the chicken with a layer of wax paper and bake at 400° for about 20 minutes; remove the wax paper and cook for an additional 10 to 15 minutes or until cooked through and golden brown on top. Serve with Honey Mustard Dip, mashed potatoes, and peas.

Per serving: 356 calories; 8.8 g fat (22 percent calories from fat); 47 g protein; 23 g carbohydrate; 132 mg cholesterol; 207 mg sodium.

Cup o' Soup Chicken Delights

MAKES 4 SERVINGS

This is a winner in the no-brainer category. As I've mentioned throughout this book, I love the new healthy instant cup o' soups by Health Valley, Nile

Spice, The Spice Hunter, Fantastic Foods, and Westbrae. They have no added chemicals, are low in fat, and are not only great meals in themselves, they are great additions to other dishes. You can put any of them over rice, pasta, or just serve with some cooked veggies. Add a crusty loaf of bread or salad and you have a fabulous, well-rounded dinner.

4	6-ounce boneless skinless chicken breasts
1	cup Health Valley Zesty Black Bean cup o' soup or other cup o' soup
1/2	cup defatted chicken broth

Place the chicken breasts in a medium-size sauté pan. Cover with the contents of the cup o' soup mix and add the water they ask for on the package and the defatted chicken broth. Stir to blend slightly around the chicken, then cook over medium heat for about 15 minutes. Turn the chicken and cook until done.

Some other soups you can use in this recipe:

Health Valley Corn Chowder with Tomatoes
The Spice Hunter Savory Fettucini with broccoli
Fantastic Foods Spanish Rice and Beans

Per serving: 196 calories; 2.2 g fat (9.6 percent calories from fat); 41 g protein; 6 g carbohydrate; 98 mg cholesterol; 208 mg sodium.

Honey Mustard Dip

MAKES 4 SERVINGS

1/2	cup sugar-free orange marmalade
2	heaping tablespoons Dijon mustard

Place the marmalade and mustard in a small bowl. Whisk until blended.

Per serving: 70 calories; 0.4 g fat (5.3 percent calories from fat); 0.4 g protein; 17.3 g carbohydrate; 0 mg cholesterol; 94 mg sodium.

Drunken Chicken

MAKES 4 SERVINGS

This works best with flat beer, so don't throw out that half-empty can. Pour it into a jar, refrigerate, and save for this easy marinade.

1   12-ounce can flat beer
4   cloves garlic, minced
2   tablespoons low-sodium soy sauce
3   tablespoons fresh or bottled lime juice, unsweetened
4   6-ounce boneless skinless chicken breasts
nonstick vegetable oil spray

Mix the first 4 ingredients in a small saucepan and heat to a low simmer. Simmer for about 5 minutes to cook off some of the alcohol and blend the flavors. Pour over the chicken breasts and let sit for about 10–15 minutes. Heat the grill and spritz with vegetable oil spray. Place the chicken on the grill fullest side down. While it's cooking for the first 10 minutes, briefly reheat the marinade for about two minutes (or place the saucepan right on the grill to heat). Turn the chicken and grill until cooked through but not tough (about 15 minutes on the first side, 10 minutes on the second). Remove the chicken and put it back in the hot marinade. Let sit for 1–2 minutes before serving. If you prefer to cook in the oven, preheat to 350° and place marinated chicken in a shallow baking pan. Bake for 15–20 minutes or until cooked through, then place under the broiler for 2–3 minutes to brown. Serve with brown rice and snow peas or with Bearitos fat-free baked beans and nonfried fries (see page 144).

Per serving: 217 calories; 2.2 g fat (9.8 percent calories from fat); 40 g protein; 6 g carbohydrate; 98 mg cholesterol; 363 mg sodium.

En Papillote Made Easy

MAKES 4 SERVINGS

The phrase "en papillote" is scary. It reeks of lots of preparation time and complicated procedures. I'm going to show you that that's not true. En papillote—literally "in paper"—is a great way to steam/poach a meal and ensures that your food comes out moist and juicy. Don't worry if you can't find the papillote paper; you can use aluminum foil. I use fresh vegetables in this dish, but frozen work just as well.

4   6-ounce boneless skinless chicken breasts
4   teaspoons coarse-grain mustard
2   leeks, white part only, carefully rinsed and julienned
2   carrots, peeled and julienned
2   teaspoons dried thyme
     salt and pepper to taste

Preheat the oven to 400°. Prepare 4 8-inch squares of parchment paper or aluminum foil (I like to call them aluminum boats) for papillotes. (Or use pre-cut parchment paper squares, 2 chicken breasts per square.) Place 1 chicken breast in the center of each opened paper. Spread the mustard evenly over the chicken, then distribute leeks, carrots, and thyme on top. Season with salt and pepper. Seal the packages by folding them over at the top, and place them on a baking sheet. Bake for about 15 minutes or until the packages are puffed. Crack one of the packages open to test for doneness. Place each package on a separate plate. Open and serve. Goes well with brown rice or mashed potatoes.

Per serving: 228 calories; 2.7 g fat (10.2 percent calories from fat); 41 g protein; 13 g carbohydrate; 98 mg cholesterol; 204 mg sodium.

Georgian Orange Cinnamon Chicken

MAKES 4 SERVINGS

The marinade for this chicken is also great over swordfish. I always like to use fresh gingerroot, but if you can't find it, use ground ginger instead.

4   large oranges
3   lemons
¹/₂ cup white wine
1   medium onion, peeled and minced
3   cloves garlic, minced
1   tablespoon peeled, minced gingerroot
3   tablespoons paprika
1   tablespoon frozen apple juice concentrate

1	teaspoon cracked black peppercorns
1/2	teaspoon salt
1/4	teaspoon ground nutmeg
2	teaspoons ground cinnamon
4	6-ounce boneless skinless chicken breasts

Grate the peel of 1 orange and 1 lemon; set aside. Juice all of the oranges and lemons. Combine the orange juice, lemon juice, and wine in a saucepan and boil rapidly until reduced to 1/2 cup liquid. Let cool. In a small bowl, combine the onion with the minced garlic and gingerroot. Stir in the reduced juice mixture, grated peel, paprika, apple juice concentrate, peppercorns, salt, nutmeg, and cinnamon. Mix well and let sit for at least one hour. Whisk and pour over the chicken breasts. Let marinate for about 15 minutes. Place the chicken on a hot grill and while it's cooking during the first 10 minutes, briefly reheat the marinade for about 2 minutes (or place the saucepan right on the grill to heat). Turn the chicken, brush with the marinade, and grill until cooked through but not tough (about 15 minutes on the first side, 10 minutes on the second). Remove the chicken and put it back in the hot marinade. Let sit for 1–2 minutes before serving. If you don't want to grill the chicken, place the breasts in a shallow baking pan, pour the marinade over the top, and bake at 350° for about 25–30 minutes. Serve over brown rice with slivered green beans.

Per serving: 295 calories; 3.7 g fat (9.3 percent calories from fat); 43 g protein; 37 g carbohydrate; 98 mg cholesterol; 530 mg sodium.

Hawaiian Chicken

MAKES 4 SERVINGS

This is an easy marinade to make and you can add some pineapple slices on top of the chicken before you place it under the broiler to heighten the dish's flavor even more. This is also great grilled—baste the pineapple slices and grill those, too.

1/4	tablespoon apricot jam
1/4	cup low-sodium soy sauce
1/4	cup defatted chicken broth
1/2	teaspoon ground ginger or 1/2 inch fresh gingerroot, grated

2   tablespoons Dijon mustard
4   6-ounce boneless skinless chicken breasts
2   skinless chicken thighs

Preheat oven to 400°. Combine the first five ingredients in a medium-size bowl and mix well. Place the chicken in a foil-lined shallow (2 inches) baking pan. Pour the marinade over the chicken and bake for 15 minutes; turn and bake for another 5–10 minutes. Turn the oven to broil and place the pan under the broiler for 1 minute to brown the top. Serve with brown rice and steamed green beans.

Per serving: 245 calories; 4.4 g fat (15.8 percent calories from fat); 50 g protein; 3 g carbohydrate; 137 mg cholesterol; 856 mg sodium.

Jerk Chicken

MAKES 4 SERVINGS

Jerk Chicken is not a dish to serve to your spouse after an argument. Jerk sauce is a blend of onions, spices, green tomatoes, and chilies that originated in Jamaica and is popular in New Orleans and in the South. It happens to be fat free and is delicious served over fish or chicken. I like the brands John Troy's and Uncle Bum's, but there may be a good local brand in the ethnic section of your market.

½   cup Jamaican jerk sauce
1   tablespoon lemon juice
1   tablespoon frozen apple juice concentrate or papaya or
           mango juice
4   6-ounce boneless skinless chicken breasts
nonstick vegetable oil spray

In a small bowl, combine the jerk sauce, lemon juice, and apple or other juice. Pour mixture over the chicken and let sit for about 15–20 minutes. (If you like it spicy, marinate it overnight; the longer the spicier.) Spritz a grill with vegetable oil spray and heat over a medium fire. Place the chicken on the grill and cook about 10 minutes on one side; turn and cook for about 5–7 minutes on the other side. If you prefer to cook in the oven, preheat oven to 350° and place marinated chicken in a shallow baking pan. Bake for 15–20 minutes or until cooked through, then place under the broiler for 2–3 minutes to brown.

Heat the remaining marinade either by placing it in a saucepan on top of the grill or on the stove for 2 minutes. Remove the cooked chicken and place back in the heated marinade. Serve over brown rice topped with chopped cilantro and mango spears.

Per serving: 182 calories; 2.2 g fat (10.1 percent calories from fat); 39 g protein; 5 g carbohydrate; 98 mg cholesterol; 596 mg sodium.

Luke's Adobe Chicken

MAKES 6 SERVINGS

Southwestern cuisine is here to stay, and it's ideal for fat-free cooking because of the salsas, seasonings, and light spicy sauces. Don't let the sound of the first two chilies on the ingredients list scare you away. Most markets now have sections for Hispanic ingredients, where you'll find these chilies sold in bags or loose. They're easy to work with and this sauce keeps for at least three months. Because it's best with grilled food (grilled fish and turkey as well as chicken), I haven't included an oven-preparation alternative in this recipe.

2	dried ancho chilies
5	dried New Mexico chilies or 2 heaping teaspoons chili powder
2	cups hot water
¹/₂	cup chopped yellow onion
5	cloves garlic, chopped
¹/₄	cup white wine
1	teaspoon dried oregano
¹/₂	teaspoon ground cumin
¹/₂	teaspoon cinnamon
¹/₄	teaspoon ground cloves
¹/₂	cup apple cider vinegar
6	6-ounce boneless skinless chicken breasts

Preheat the oven to 350°. Rinse the dried chilies and place on a baking sheet. Bake for about 10 to 15 minutes, or until toasted. Remove and let cool. Take off the stems and seeds, cover chilies with the hot water, and allow to soak for 15 minutes. In a small sauté pan, cook the onion and garlic in white wine over medium heat until the wine has evaporated. Place the chilies, onion mixture, and remaining ingredients, except the chicken, in a blender and blend on low until smooth. Place the sauce in a container and refrigerate for at least 2 hours or overnight. (This sauce lasts for about three months in the fridge, but it will thicken as it sits. To thin it out, combine ¼ cup of the sauce with ¼ cup defatted chicken broth or white wine.) Spread the marinade over the chicken breasts and let sit for 15 minutes. Place the chicken on the grill and cook about 10 minutes on one side; turn, baste with the marinade, and cook for about 5–7 minutes on the other side or until cooked through. Serve over seasoned rice with Pinto Bean Fiesta (see page 146).

Per serving: 210 calories; 2.4 g fat (9.9 percent calories from fat); 41 g protein; 9 g carbohydrate; 98 mg cholesterol; 124 mg sodium.

Pesto Garlic Chicken

MAKES 4 SERVINGS

Pesto is one of the most delicious sauces ever invented—and one of the most fattening. I use a pesto dip mix made by Fantastic Foods (sold in health food stores) for this recipe. The box contains two packages, and I use both, but I don't use the garnish package, which contains chopped nuts. If you can't find this particular brand, there are plenty of other pesto mixes on the market.

4	6-ounce boneless chicken breasts with skin
2	tablespoons lemon juice
⅓	cup Italian no-oil salad dressing
½	teaspoon chopped fresh basil
1	teaspoon minced garlic
1	box Fantastic Foods Pesto Dip mix (2 packages)
2	tablespoons grated Parmesan cheese
1	teaspoon Dijon mustard
1	cup white wine
½	cup defatted chicken broth
1	tablespoon lemon juice

Preheat oven to 400°. Line a shallow baking pan with aluminum foil and place the chicken breasts with the skin up. Sprinkle 1 tablespoon of the lemon juice on top. Mix the salad dressing, basil, garlic, pesto mix, cheese, and mustard in a bowl or glass measuring cup; gently whisk to blend. Lift the skin of the chicken (do not remove), then spoon the sauce under the skin and onto the chicken meat. Gently massage the sauce into the chicken with your fingers, then place the breast skin side down in the pan. Pour the wine, broth, and remaining lemon juice over the chicken. Cover the pan with a foil tent and bake 20–25 minutes. Remove the foil, turn the breasts, and cook for another 10 minutes, or until cooked through. Remove the skin from the chicken and serve over lemon pepper pasta with crusty whole wheat bread.

Per serving: 192 calories; 3 g fat (13.9 percent calories from fat); 41 g protein; 1 g carbohydrate; 100 mg cholesterol; 180 mg sodium.

Red-and-Yellow Dijon Baked Chicken

MAKES 4 SERVINGS

This dish is very colorful and lovely for entertaining. You can substitute bottled roasted red bell peppers that are not packed in oil for the fresh red pepper.

4   6-ounce boneless skinless chicken breasts
2   tablespoons Dijon mustard
1   tablespoon poultry seasoning
1   red bell pepper, seeded and quartered
1   yellow bell pepper, seeded and quartered
8   regular cap mushrooms, sliced
juice of 1 lemon
1/2   cup defatted chicken broth
1   cup white wine

Preheat oven to 350°. Line a 2-inch shallow baking pan with foil. Smother the chicken breasts with the mustard, then sprinkle the poultry seasoning on top. Place the peppers skin side down in the pan. Place the chicken on the peppers and top with the sliced mushrooms. Pour the lemon juice over the chicken breasts; pour the broth and wine around the edges and into the peppers. Cover with foil and bake 12 minutes. Remove foil and turn chicken over so that the peppers are on top; bake another 15 minutes. If you want the peppers to be crispy, place the pan under the broiler for an additional 2 minutes. Serve over spinach fettucine and accompany with a salad.

Per serving: 259 calories; 3.3 g fat (12.2 percent calories from fat); 43 g protein; 11 g carbohydrate; 98 mg cholesterol; 412 mg sodium.

Roasted Garlic Rosemary Chicken

MAKES 4 SERVINGS

I love the mixture of fresh rosemary and garlic. This is great on the grill, but if you're cooking inside, place the chicken in a shallow baking pan, pour the sauce over the chicken, and place in the oven at 350° for 20 minutes; turn the chicken and place under the broiler for 5–10 minutes or until done.

1/8	teaspoon pepper
4	6-ounce boneless skinless chicken breasts
2	cloves garlic
1	teaspoon dried rosemary
1/2	cup no-oil Italian salad dressing (I like Paula's)
1/4	cup white wine
1	tablespoon lemon juice
1/2	teaspoon poultry seasoning

Rub pepper into chicken breasts and set aside in a shallow baking pan. Wrap the garlic cloves in aluminum foil and roast in a toaster oven for about 10 minutes at 350°. Remove and, when cool, chop into small pieces. In a small bowl, whisk together the garlic and remaining ingredients, then pour over the chicken. Let marinate for 10–15 minutes. Place the chicken on a heated grill and cook about 10 minutes on one side; turn and cook about 5–7 minutes on the other side or until cooked through. While the chicken is cooking, heat the remaining marinade either by placing it in a saucepan on top of the grill or on the stove for 2 minutes. Remove the cooked chicken from the grill and place it back in the heated marinade. Serve with wild rice and grilled asparagus.

Per serving: 187 calories; 2.3 g fat (11 percent calories from fat); 40 g protein; 4 g carbohydrate; 98 mg cholesterol; 124 mg sodium.

Sake Cilantro Chicken

MAKES 4 SERVINGS

This is what I call my "fallback recipe" for entertaining. It's always a knockout, exotic enough to be interesting, and easy enough to let me enjoy the evening. You can grill or bake this simple chicken dish, and enjoy it year-round.

6	cloves garlic
2	tablespoons peeled, chopped gingerroot
2	tablespoons rice vinegar
1	bunch cilantro, stems removed
4	6-ounce boneless skinless chicken breasts
1/2	cup sake
1/4	cup low-sodium soy sauce
1/4	cup lemon juice

Place the garlic, ginger, rice vinegar, and cilantro in a blender and puree until it's a paste. Rub the paste all over the chicken breasts and set aside in a shallow bowl or baking pan. Place the sake, soy sauce, and lemon juice in a medium saucepan and heat until it comes to a boil. Pour over the chicken breasts and turn to coat. Let the chicken marinate for a minimum of 5–10 minutes (or overnight). Place the chicken on a heated grill and cook about 10 minutes on one side; turn and cook about 5–7 minutes on the other side or until cooked through. While the chicken is cooking, heat the remaining marinade either by placing it in a saucepan on top of the grill or on the stove for 2 minutes. Remove the cooked chicken from the grill and place it back in the heated marinade. If you prefer to bake the chicken, place breasts in a foil-lined 2-inch shallow baking pan at 400° for 15 minutes; turn and cook for 5 minutes on the other side. Serve with Papaya Salsa (see page 177), brown rice, and grilled mushrooms.

Per serving: 264 calories; 2.6 g fat (9.6 percent calories from fat); 42 g protein; 13 g carbohydrate; 98 mg cholesterol; 730 mg sodium.

Sicilian Chicken

MAKES 8 SERVINGS

This simple dish makes you look like Julia Child. It's so colorful and flavorful you can entertain with fat-free pride. Many people look at the fennel root (also known as anise) in the market like it's from another planet. However, it has a lovely mild flavor and I like to eat it raw and sliced or marinated in a vinaigrette. Keep a few of the fluffy leaves and use them to cover the chicken before baking. This is a meal in itself.

| 2 | cloves garlic, minced |
| 1/4 | teaspoon coarse cracked pepper |

8	6-ounce boneless skinless chicken breasts
3	ounces frozen orange juice concentrate
1	cup vermouth or white wine
2	ounces capers
1	tablespoon orange zest
1	each: red and green bell peppers, sliced into rings
1	small red onion, sliced into rings
1	fennel bulb, sliced into 1/4-inch rings*
3	ounces pitted black olives
3–4	branches (sprigs) fennel leaves

Preheat oven to 400°. Rub the minced garlic and cracked pepper into the chicken breasts. Combine the orange juice, vermouth, and capers in blender and blend for about 2 minutes or just enough to crush the capers. Place the breasts in a foil-lined shallow baking pan. Sprinkle the orange zest over them, then place the sliced peppers, onion, and fennel on top. Sprinkle the olives over the vegetables, cover with the fennel leaves, then pour the liquid over the top. Cover with a foil tent and bake for about 15–20 minutes. Remove the foil, turn the chicken, and bake for another 10 minutes. Serve over fettucine noodles.

Per serving: 253 calories; 3.5 g fat (13.8 percent calories from fat); 40 g protein; 8 g carbohydrate; 98 mg cholesterol; 388 mg sodium.

Southwestern Baked Chicken

MAKES 4 SERVINGS

This is another variation on Southern-fried chicken. It's easy, crispy, and full of flavor.

2/3	cup yellow cornmeal
1/3	cup homemade bread crumbs
2	teaspoons Italian seasoning
2	tablespoons grated Parmesan cheese
3	teaspoons chili powder
2	teaspoons cumin
2	teaspoons garlic powder

*Fennel can be tricky to cut. First slice the root in half lengthwise, then slice on the diagonal for strips that will bake quickly.

1   teaspoon Sucanat or sugar
$1/2$ teaspoon ground red pepper (cayenne)
4   6-ounce boneless skinless chicken breasts
1   tablespoon Worcestershire sauce
2   egg whites, lightly beaten
nonstick vegetable oil spray

Preheat oven to 400°. Place the cornmeal, bread crumbs, and all the spices in a large plastic bag and shake well. Combine the Worcestershire sauce and egg whites in a small bowl. Dip the chicken breasts one at a time into the egg mixture. Allow the excess to drip off, then place in the bag and shake to coat. Spritz a shallow baking pan with vegetable oil spray, then transfer chicken to the pan. Spritz chicken with the vegetable oil spray. Reduce heat to 350°. Bake for 20–25 minutes or until cooked through.

Per serving: 331 calories; 4.5 g fat (12 percent calories from fat); 46 g protein; 29 g carbohydrate; 100 mg cholesterol; 316 mg sodium.

Spanish Pollo and Pilaf

MAKES 4 SERVINGS

For a quick dinner, this recipe can also be made with one can of boneless chicken breasts, which can be found in the same aisle as canned tuna in your supermarket.

1   box Spanish rice pilaf
$1/2$ cup frozen peas
$1/2$ cup frozen corn
3   plum tomatoes, chopped
2   6-ounce boneless skinless chicken breasts
pepper, to taste
nonstick vegetable oil spray

Make the rice according to package directions, eliminating the oil. Add the frozen vegetables and chopped tomatoes to the rice during the last 10 minutes of cooking. Season the chicken with pepper and place in a sauté pan spritzed with vegetable oil spray. Sauté chicken breasts for 12 minutes over medium heat; turn and cook 5 more minutes. Remove chicken from pan and cut into 1-inch cubes. Fold into rice mixture.

Per serving: 372 calories; 3.9 g fat (9.2 percent calories from fat); 41 g protein; 47 g carbohydrate; 82 mg cholesterol; 127 mg sodium.

Chicken Fajitas

The only thing that might put you off about making a fajita dish for a quick dinner is the thought of chopping. Well, worry no more: the supermarkets have done all the work for our tired, overworked hands. You can buy chicken already cut into strips as well as precut red, green, and yellow bell peppers. You can even use frozen chopped onions. All this makes fajitas a welcome dish to the fat-free no-brainer Hall of Fame. If you like your chicken super spicy, add ¼ teaspoon chili powder when you add the other seasonings.

nonstick vegetable oil spray
¼   cup white wine
1   tablespoon minced garlic
1   teaspoon Cajun seasoning
1   teaspoon garlic powder
2   4-ounce boneless skinless chicken breasts cut into strips
½   cup defatted chicken broth
1   teaspoon frozen apple juice concentrate
1   each: red and green bell peppers, cored, seeded, and cut into
        strips
½   red onion, sliced
4   whole wheat pitas

Spritz a nonstick sauté pan with nonstick vegetable oil spray. Heat the white wine and minced garlic and cook until the garlic is just transparent. Add the Cajun seasoning and garlic powder, stir, then add the chicken and half the chicken broth. Cook, turning until the chicken is cooked through; remove and set aside. Add the apple juice concentrate, remaining broth, bell peppers, and onion to the pan. Sauté until just softened, and most of the liquid is gone. Return the chicken and stir for about 2 minutes. Remove from heat. Serve with pinto beans and salsa.

Per serving: 164 calories; 1.8 g fat (10 percent calories from fat); 18 g protein; 19 g carbohydrate; 33 mg cholesterol; 264 mg sodium.

THE NO-BRAINER CHICKEN WINNERS

The easiest way to soup up chicken is just to marinate it in a tasty fat-free sauce or rub it with a spice blend (see the recipes on pages 191–196) before cooking. You will generally need ½ cup of sauce per four 6-ounce chicken breasts. Simply marinate the chicken with the sauce anywhere from 15 minutes to overnight, then baste frequently while cooking. Some sauces to try:

Ayla's Curry or Cajun sauce
Chef Piero's BBQ sauce
Gorilla's BBQ sauce
John Troy's Mexican Mesquite, Indian Curry, Spicy Szechuan, Oriental Ginger, or Thai sauce
Premier Japan's Ginger Tamari, Garlic Tamari, or regular Tamari
Robbie's Sweet & Sour, Honey BBQ, or BBQ sauce
There are lots of other sauces around, but check to make sure they aren't loaded with sugar or MSG.

Taos Game Hens

MAKES 4 SERVINGS

Just as the idea of having turkey only on Thanksgiving has gone by the wayside, so has the idea of Cornish game hens being only for special occasions. They're available year-round either fresh or frozen, and take less time to cook than a full chicken. I love to take them on picnics because they're great cold and are wonderful finger food.

2	Cornish game hens
2	tablespoons frozen orange juice concentrate
1	tablespoon lemon juice
¼	cup white wine
1½	teaspoons chili powder
5	cloves garlic, minced
2½	teaspoons ground cumin
1¼	teaspoons ground coriander
¼	teaspoon cayenne
	salt and pepper to taste

Preheat oven to 450°. Peel the skin off the body of the hens, then split them in half lengthwise. You can peel the skin off the drumsticks after it is cooked. (Or cook the hens with the skin on, then remove after they're cooked.) Place the split breasts cavity side down in a shallow baking pan. Combine all of the remaining ingredients and pour over the split hens. Cover the pan with a foil tent and bake for 20 minutes. Remove the foil and cook 15–20 minutes more at 350° until cooked through and crispy. Remove the hens and reserve the juices in the pan. Using a baster or spoon, remove any remaining fat from the juices. Pour the juices from the pan over the top of the hens before serving. Serve with black beans and rice.

Per serving: 180 calories; 5.4 g fat (28.9 percent calories from fat); 24 g protein; 6 g carbohydrate; 91 mg cholesterol; 110 mg sodium.

Turkey Dinners

In my first book, *Food Cop,* I mentioned that I wanted my daughter to marry a turkey farmer instead of a doctor, because turkey was going big-time. The poor turkey used to achieve glory only once a year, in November, but now it's loved year-round. Turkey is now sold in the fresh poultry section, separated into parts just like chicken, and it's a blessing.

Turkey Scallopini Piccata

MAKES 4 SERVINGS

You can find turkey breast slices in almost every market today, but if you can't find them, just slice a turkey breast into ¼-inch slices. This particular turkey recipe does double duty: it makes a lovely dinner and is great for sandwiches the following day.

1	pound fresh turkey breast slices
¼	cup lemon juice
½	cup seasoned bread crumbs (see notes on Turkey Florentine, see page 206)
1	teaspoon poultry seasoning
½	cup white wine
½	cup Italian fat-free salad dressing
2	cloves garlic, sliced

RANDOM NOTES ON TURKEY

- Turkey breast cooked without the skin can become especially dry if you overcook it. Always check the middle of the thickest part of the breast to make sure that it's no longer pink, but not so overdone that it's stringy.
- Cooking turkey with the skin on will keep the moisture in without adding fat to the meat, just to the juices in the pan. If you do cook with the skin on, remove it before serving.
- Ground turkey breast without the skin is very low in fat. So when you make burgers or meatballs, it tends to fall apart. To hold it together, add some beaten egg white or use half ground turkey breast and half ground dark turkey meat. The additional fat may be worth the improved texture and flavor.
- Turkey tenderloins are wonderful, but they cook up tougher than turkey breast if you just bake them. So instead, I prefer to cut them on the diagonal (like a flank steak) and use them in stir-fries and on the grill.

2   egg whites, lightly beaten
2   teaspoons capers
garlic-flavored nonstick vegetable oil spray

Rinse the turkey breast slices and set aside. Sprinkle half of the lemon juice over the turkey. Combine the bread crumbs and poultry seasoning on a plate. Heat the rest of the lemon juice, the wine, salad dressing, and garlic in a large nonstick sauté pan. Dip the turkey slices in the egg white, then coat with the bread crumbs. Spritz pan with vegetable oil spray. Place the slices in the pan with the wine mixture and cook for about 5 minutes over medium heat. Add the capers and more wine if necessary. Turn and cook for another 2 minutes, or until done. Remove and serve. Goes well with spinach fettucine dusted with Parmesan cheese.

Per serving, not including pasta and Parmesan: 206 calories; 1.9 g fat (9.4 percent calories from fat); 30 g protein; 10 g carbohydrate; 68 mg cholesterol; 200 mg sodium.

Turkey Florentine

I like to make my bread crumbs from stale bread. I just put the bread in a blender in chunks, blend it, and freeze it for later use. Then I can add the seasoning of my choice. However, if you don't have any crumbs prepared, then make sure that those you buy aren't loaded with preservatives.

1	pound fresh turkey breast slices
1/4	cup bread crumbs
1	tablespoon Italian seasoning
1/4	cup grated Parmesan cheese
1	teaspoon granulated garlic powder
	olive-flavored nonstick vegetable oil spray
1/4	cup white wine
1 1/2	cups fat-free pasta sauce
1/2	cup grated fat-free mozzarella

Rinse the turkey breast slices and set aside. In a small bowl, mix the bread crumbs, Italian seasoning, Parmesan, and garlic powder. Coat the wet turkey with the bread crumb mixture. Spritz a large skillet with vegetable oil spray. Pour in the wine and heat until sizzling. Add the coated turkey breasts and cook 2–3 minutes on each side, or until lightly browned. Transfer to a platter. Heat the pasta sauce in a small saucepan, then pour it over the turkey. Top with the mozzarella. Serve over herb-flavored pasta.

Per serving: 232 calories; 3.4 g fat (14.5 percent calories from fat); 32 g protein; 12 g carbohydrate; 73 mg cholesterol; 387 mg sodium.

Spiced Turkey Tenders with Honey Grapefruit Salsa

This dish takes slightly longer to make than most of the recipes in this book, but it's worth it. Plus, it's easier the second time around if you double the spice mix, then store it in an airtight container so you have it on hand.

Salsa

3 large grapefruits, peeled, sectioned, pith and seeds removed
1/4 cup finely chopped red onion
2 tablespoons chopped fresh cilantro
1 tablespoon chopped fresh mint
1 tablespoon red wine vinegar
1 tablespoon honey

Spice mix

1/4 cup mild chili powder
1/2 teaspoon ground cloves
1/2 teaspoon allspice
1/2 teaspoon cinnamon
pinch salt

1 1/2 pounds skinless turkey tenderloin cut into tenders
nonstick vegetable oil spray
1/4 cup white wine

Preheat oven to 400°. Place the grapefruit sections in a medium bowl with the remaining salsa ingredients; set aside. In a small bowl, combine the spices and salt. Dredge the turkey tenders in the spice mix and shake off excess. Spray a large ovenproof skillet with the vegetable oil spray. Over high heat, sear the turkey for about 1 minute on each side. Add the wine. Transfer the skillet to the oven and bake for 4–6 minutes or until the turkey is cooked through. Top with salsa and serve with brown rice.

Per serving: 281 calories; 3.2 g fat (9.9 percent calories from fat); 38.4 g protein; 26.6 g carbohydrate; 36 mg cholesterol; 141 mg sodium.

Country-Style Turkey

MAKES 4 SERVINGS

This is an easy, hearty dish that makes a wonderful Sunday dinner, and the leftovers can be made into sandwiches during the week. If you don't want to peel and slice the carrots this recipe calls for, use the baby carrots in a bag.

nonstick vegetable oil spray

2   teaspoons poultry seasoning
1   boneless turkey breast, skin removed
1   13-ounce can defatted chicken broth
1   cup white wine
3   packages Hain gravy mix
1   cup frozen broccoli
3   carrots, sliced
8   baby (new) potatoes
6   frozen pearl onions
1   teaspoon dried rosemary
1   teaspoon minced onion

Preheat oven to 400°. Line a shallow baking pan with foil, and spritz with vegetable oil spray. Rub the poultry seasoning over the turkey breast and set breast side down into the pan. Heat the broth and wine in a small saucepan over medium heat; add the gravy mix. Stir with a whisk until just blended and pour over the turkey breast. Place the vegetables around the turkey, sprinkle the rosemary and onion on top, and cover with an aluminum tent. Bake for 10 minutes, then reduce the heat to 350° and bake about 20–30 more minutes, or until the turkey is no longer pink in the middle. Slice the turkey breast on the diagonal, and serve over fettucine noodles (or alone) with the roasted veggies and gravy.

Per serving: 312 calories; 0.8 g fat (2.5 percent calories from fat); 9 g protein; 60 g carbohydrate; 2 mg cholesterol; 423 mg sodium.

Nolina's Turkey Chili

MAKES 4 LARGE BOWLFULS

This is my daughter's favorite—and TV talk show host Leeza Gibbons's. I'm crazy about the Brown Bag chili mix, but you can use any seasoning mix you like. If you prefer your chili extra spicy, add 1/8 teaspoon cayenne pepper during the last 10 minutes of cooking. Try this super dish ladled over a turkey burger.

1/4   cup white wine
1   cup chopped onion (frozen is fine)
1   pound ground turkey breast

1	cup tomato sauce
1	cup water
1	package chili seasoning (I like Brown Bag)
1/4	cup masa harina (tortilla flour)
2	tablespoons water
1/4	cup chopped scallions
2	tablespoons grated low-fat cheddar cheese
1	tablespoon chopped cilantro

Heat the wine in a large saucepan. Add the onion and cook over medium heat until just tender (frozen onion will take less time, only 2–3 minutes). Add the ground turkey and cook, stirring, until browned all over. Add the tomato sauce, water, and chili seasoning; stir until blended. Cook over medium heat for 15 minutes. In a small bowl, mix the harina with the water and blend until smooth, adding more water if needed. Add the flour paste (and some cayenne pepper, if you like) to the chili. Stir and cook for another 10 minutes. Serve with chopped scallions, grated cheese, and chopped cilantro.

Per serving: *191 calories; 2.2 g fat (10.9 percent calories from fat); 28 g protein; 11 g carbohydrate; 68 mg cholesterol; 567 mg sodium.*

Have a Burger Brainstorm

You may have noticed that there's been a revolution, or should I say evolution, in burger making. There are so many great ways to make chicken and turkey burgers (see page 210), that you'll never ask, "Where's the beef?" again. Even an extra-lean beef burger gets more than half of its calories from fat, and 6 of its 14 grams of fat are saturated.

There's no need, however, to limit yourself to chicken and turkey burgers. The "veggie burger" has crept into our burger lexicon and, while those words used to scare lots of people away, they shouldn't anymore. Once a veggie burger was some weird meat substitute made of vegetables ground up with oil—most were pretty high in fat. Well, welcome to the nineties; the veggie burger has hit its prime: The flavor is way up and the fat is way down. Here are some to look for:

• Boca Burger—84 calories and 0 grams fat per 2.5 ounces
• Green Giant Harvest Burger—140 calories and 4 grams of fat per 3.1 ounces

- The Hard Rock Café and T.G.I. Friday's as well as many other restaurants are now making them a staple on the menu. Order away!
- Ken & Robert's Truly Amazing Veggie Burger—130 calories and 1 gram of fat per 2.5 ounces
- Lightlife Lemon Grill Tempeh Burger—140 calories and 5.5 grams of fat per 2.7 ounces
- Lightlife Tamari Grill Tempeh Burger—120 calories and 5 grams of fat per 2.7 ounces
- Morningstar Farms Meatless Garden Vege Patties—110 calories and 4 grams of fat per 2.3 ounces
- Natural Touch Garden Vege Patties—110 calories and 4 grams of fat per 2.4 ounces
- Soy Boy Okara Courage Burger—130 calories and 5 grams of fat per 2.2 ounces
- Wholesome & Hearty Foods Garden Burger—140 calories and 2.5 grams of fat per 2.5 ounces
- Woodstock Whole Earth Foods' The Better Burger—172 calories and 3 grams of fat per 3.5 ounces

Ten Variations on the Turkey Burger

EACH RECIPE MAKES 4 BURGERS

To prepare each variation, follow the instructions for the Worcestershire Burgers. Note: Additional toppings, like cheese, are optional and not included in nutritional breakdown.

Worcestershire Burgers

This is best topped with Lifetime's fat-free Jack cheese, which adds only 40 calories and no fat. After cooking add extra Worcestershire sauce, to taste. Serve with a big slice of red onion.

1	pound ground turkey breast
1/4	cup Worcestershire sauce
1	tablespoon steak sauce
2	tablespoons Dijon mustard
2	egg whites, lightly beaten

Combine all of the ingredients in a large bowl. Pat into 4 to 5 turkey patties. If you're going to grill the patties, it's best to bake them for about 10 minutes at 400° first so they don't crumble on the grill. To grill: Place patties on a heated grill and cook for 7 minutes; turn and cook for 7 minutes, or until turkey burgers are cooked through and no longer pink in the middle. To broil: Place patties on a foil-lined broiler pan and broil for 15 minutes; turn and cook for another 5 minutes or until done. Top with fat-free Jack cheese (optional).

Per serving: 159 calories; 2.1 g fat (12.5 percent calories from fat); 29 g protein; 4 g carbohydrate; 68 mg cholesterol; 421 mg sodium.

Spike Burgers

This is as simple as simple can be. Remember, frozen chopped onions will cook faster and work wonderfully in this recipe because you want to keep cooking time to a minimum: the longer the turkey cooks the drier it becomes. Just make sure you defrost and drain the frozen onions first. Serve with fat-free Jack cheese and tomato.

1	pound ground turkey breast
1	tablespoon Spike seasoning
$\frac{1}{2}$	cup chopped onion
2	egg whites, lightly beaten

Per serving: 143 calories; 1.8 g fat (11.8 percent calories from fat); 29 g protein; 1 g carbohydrate; 68 mg cholesterol; 174 mg sodium.

Turkey Burgers Italian Style

You can serve these open-faced with some warm Millina's pasta sauce over the top, or on an onion bun. For variation, toss in $\frac{1}{4}$ cup chopped sun-dried (but not oil-marinated) tomatoes or $\frac{1}{4}$ cup shredded zucchini with the other ingredients as you combine. Top with a slice of mozzarella and a basil leaf.

1	pound ground turkey breast
1	tablespoon garlic powder
2	teaspoons Italian seasoning
1	tablespoon grated Parmesan cheese
2	egg whites, lightly beaten

Per serving: 138 calories; 2.2 g fat (15 percent calories from fat); 27 g protein; 0 g carbohydrate; 69 mg cholesterol; 95 mg sodium.

Tamari Burgers

These are delicious topped with sliced mushrooms sautéed in the ginger tamari sauce. Serve with wasabi (Japanese hot green mustard) or any hot mustard and bean sprouts on a sesame bun.

1   **pound ground turkey breast**
¼   **cup Premier Japan Ginger Tamari sauce or another brand tamari sauce**
1   **teaspoon powdered ginger**
1   **tablespoon soy sauce**
½   **cup chopped scallions**
2   **egg whites, lightly beaten**

Per serving: 205 calories; 1.8 g fat (9.9 percent calories from fat); 29 g protein; 7 g carbohydrate; 68 mg cholesterol; 627 mg sodium.

Curry Burgers

These are wonderful topped with chutney. If you don't have chutney on hand (you can always make the one on page 172), use a mixture of orange marmalade and Knudsen apple syrup to give this burger its hint of sweetness. Serve with basmati rice.

1   **pound ground turkey breast**
1   **tablespoon curry powder**
2   **tablespoons finely chopped celery**
1   **tablespoon Dijon mustard**
½   **cup diced onion**

Per serving: 143 calories; 2.2 g fat (14.2 percent calories from fat); 27 g protein; 2 g carbohydrate; 68 mg cholesterol; 197 mg sodium.

BBQ Turkey Burgers

Eating these is just as satisfying as eating ribs. Serve some extra BBQ sauce on the side for dipping. Top with fat-free Monterey Jack cheese and red onion.

1	pound ground turkey breast
1/2	cup fat-free BBQ sauce
1	teaspoon liquid smoke
2	egg whites, lightly beaten
1/4	cup chopped onion

Per serving: 176 calories; 1.8 g fat (9.5 percent calories from fat); 29 g protein; 10 g carbohydrate; 68 mg cholesterol; 361 mg sodium.

Dijon Dill Burgers

Instead of just plopping a pickle on top of a burger, try this pickle relish burger, which is infused with the dill flavor. Top with fat-free cheddar or garden vegetable cheese.

1	pound ground turkey breast
3	tablespoons pickle relish
1	tablespoon Dijon mustard
1/2	cup chopped onion
1/2	cup chopped tomato
1	tablespoon prepared mustard

Per serving: 142 calories; 2 g fat (13.3 percent calories from fat); 27 g protein; 2 g carbohydrate; 68 mg cholesterol; 195 mg sodium.

Garlic Burgers

Look for prechopped garlic in plastic containers in the produce section of your market. To give this burger a little extra oomph, I like to add 1 tablespoon of dried rosemary leaves. Top with fat-free Swiss cheese and serve with a breath mint.

2	tablespoons white wine
2	tablespoons chopped fresh garlic
1	teaspoon garlic powder
1	pound ground turkey breast
1/2	teaspoon pepper

Place wine in a small sauté pan. Add garlic and sauté over medium heat until the wine is sizzling. Add the garlic powder, and cook until wine is almost evaporated. Mix with the ground turkey and prepare as you do the Worcestershire Burgers.

Per serving: 145 calories; 1.8 g fat (12.1 percent calories from fat); 27 g protein; 2 g carbohydrate; 68 mg cholesterol; 73 mg sodium.

Fakin' Bacon Burger

A great alternative to the traditional heavy bacon cheeseburger. Top with Lifetime fat-free cheddar cheese and sliced tomatoes.

1	pound ground turkey breast
1	tablespoon Fakin' Bacon Bits
1	tablespoon Dijon mustard
1	tablespoon Worcestershire sauce

Mix all the ingredients together and shape into patties. For the broiler—spritz a broiler pan with vegetable oil spray and place the patties in the broiler 4–5 inches from the flame for about 10 minutes on one side; turn and cook for another 10 minutes until cooked through. For the grill—spray a shallow baking pan with vegetable oil spray, place the patties in the pan, and put in the oven at 400° for 10 minutes—or just until gray. This will bind the burgers so that they don't fall apart on the grill. Remove from the oven and place on the pre-heated grill for 5–7 minutes on one side, turn and cook about 2–3 minutes for grill marks.

Per serving: 151 calories; 3 g fat (16 percent calories from fat); 28 g protein; 2 g carbohydrate; 68 mg cholesterol; 197 mg sodium.

Garden Burgers

This is a great way to get those veggies into your kids (or mate) without their knowing. Top with ketchup and sprouts on a whole wheat bun.

¼	cup white wine
¼	cup shredded carrots
¼	cup shredded zucchini
½	cup diced onion
¼	cup diced green bell pepper
1	pound ground turkey breast
2	egg whites, lightly beaten

1   tablespoon Italian seasoning
1   tablespoon Parmesan cheese
1   teaspoon wheat germ

Heat the wine in a medium-size sauté pan. Add the shredded vegetables and sauté until the onion is transparent. Drain and mix with the ground turkey. Prepare as you do the Worcestershire Burgers.

Per serving: 172 calories; 2.3 g fat (13.4 percent calories from fat); 30 g protein; 4 g carbohydrate; 69 mg cholesterol; 204 mg sodium.

Homestyle Turkey Stew

MAKES 6 SERVINGS

In this recipe I use turkey tenderloins, big almond-shaped slices of turkey peeled away from the breastbone and sold separately. They tend to hold together better than regular turkey breast, but you can use that as well. To make a richer stew, use turkey thigh meat, which is a little more fatty, and hence has more flavor.

1½   pounds skinless turkey tenderloin, cut into 1-inch cubes
1   cup whole wheat flour
¼   cup red wine
1   clove garlic, minced
1   13-ounce can defatted chicken broth
2   10-ounce packages frozen stew vegetables, defrosted and
         drained
2   packages Hain gravy mix
1½   teaspoons poultry seasoning
½   teaspoon dried rosemary
salt and pepper to taste
1   cup frozen peas, defrosted

Dredge the turkey cubes in the flour. Heat the red wine in a large nonstick sauté pan. Add the garlic and turkey. Cook over medium heat until the turkey cubes are browned. Pour in half of the can of chicken broth, and the thawed stew vegetables. Mix the gravy according to package instructions, replacing the water called for with the other half can of broth. Add the gravy to the stew. Sprinkle in the seasonings and salt and pepper to taste. Cook over low heat for about 45 minutes, adding in the peas to cook for the last 10 minutes. Serve over egg noodles (optional).

Per serving: 294 calories; 2.8 g fat (8.5 percent calories from fat); 34 g protein; 32 g carbohydrate; 68 mg cholesterol; 145 mg sodium.

Mediterranean Turkey Falafel with Cucumber Sauce

MAKES 6 SERVINGS

Falafel is generally fried in fat—the reason it's so greasy. Here, the falafel is simply sautéed in wine, a real fat-saver, and the whole recipe is a time-saver. Don't be put off by its daunting name; it's easy.

Falafel

1¼	pounds ground turkey breast
¼	cup chopped onion
1½	teaspoons dried oregano
½	teaspoon fresh mint
½	teaspoon dried parsley
½	teaspoon lemon pepper
1	clove garlic, minced
nonstick vegetable oil spray	
¼	cup white wine

Sauce

½	cup nonfat sour cream
½	medium cucumber, peeled and finely chopped
1½	teaspoons lemon juice
pinch pepper	

1	teaspoon dried dill
3	pitas, sliced in half
6	lettuce leaves, torn
1	medium tomato, chopped

In a large bowl, combine the turkey, onion, herbs, pepper, and garlic and mix well. Shape into 1¼-inch balls. Spritz a medium-size skillet with vegetable oil spray. Add the wine to the pan and cook the balls 8–10 minutes, or until lightly browned all over and no longer pink in the center. Combine the sauce ingredients in a small bowl. Stuff each pita half with 3–4 meatballs, lettuce, and tomato. Top with the sauce.

Per serving: 161 calories; 2 g fat (11.6 percent calories from fat); 25 g protein; 10 g carbohydrate; 57 mg cholesterol; 201 mg sodium.

Seafood Dinners

Eat more fish! Seafood is good for your health—recent studies have shown that consuming as little as one serving of salmon a week can help reduce the risk of heart attack—and it's good for your skin and hair, too. These days, we

RANDOM NOTES ON SEAFOOD

- Make sure when you buy fish the meat is bright white or pinkish in color, a sign that it's fresh. Also, check to see that the flesh is firm, the eyes are clear, not cloudy, and that the fish doesn't smell—trust your nose to tell if it's a quality piece of seafood.
- Ask your local fish purveyor to wrap your fish in freezer wrapper. Fish freezes well, and thaws quickly. Put the wrapped fish in a plastic freezer bag—it will keep up to 6 months.
- If you're using raw fish for sushi, gefilte fish, or seviche, the FDA recommends that the fish first be frozen for 3 days to destroy any possible parasites.
- Always rinse the fish under cool water, and sprinkle some fresh lemon juice on top before using—for flavor and to prevent the fish from oxidizing as quickly.
- The highest-fat fish are: herring, mackerel, sockeye salmon, pompano, and shad.
- One *teaspoon* of caviar has 4 grams of protein, 94 mg of cholesterol, and 2 grams fat! Think before you live it up!
- Look for seafood that's fresh and farm raised—even catfish, which used to be looked down on for being bottom feeders, are now farm raised, clean, and healthy.

all have access to a wider variety of fresh fish, and there are hundreds of ways to cook it with great flavor—the old idea that you have to bread and fry fish to make it palatable is obsolete.

Spicy Sea Bass with Fruit Salsa

MAKES 4 SERVINGS

This is a wonderful salsa for any spicy dish, but especially complements sea bass, swordfish, and salmon. You can use frozen whole strawberries if fresh are out of season; just make sure you thaw and drain them well. The salsa can be made in advance—with more time to sit, it will have more of a kick, and dinner the next day will be a snap.

Fruit Salsa

2	large oranges, peeled, seeded, and pith removed
1	pint strawberries, stemmed and chopped
1/2	jalapeño, seeded and minced
1/2	cup chopped scallions
1/4	cup chopped fresh mint
2	tablespoons lime juice—fresh is best, bottled okay
1	tablespoon lemon juice
2	teaspoons honey
salt and pepper to taste	

2	pounds sea bass, cut into 6 pieces
1/2	cup lemon juice
2	teaspoons Cajun seasoning
nonstick vegetable oil spray	

Prepare the salsa first: Section the oranges and chop into 1/2-inch cubes. Let the oranges drain in a colander. Place the strawberries in a medium-size bowl with the oranges, minced jalapeño, scallions, mint, lime juice, and lemon juice. Season with the honey and salt and pepper, and let chill for at least one hour or overnight. Stir occasionally.

To grill the fish: Rinse the fish and pour the lemon juice over it, then sprinkle the Cajun seasoning on top. Heat the grill and spray with vegetable oil spray. Place the fish on the grill and cook over medium heat. In the meantime, place the lemon Cajun marinade in a small saucepan and either set it on top of the grill to heat, or heat it on the stove for 3–5 minutes. Cook the fish for about 15–20 minutes or until it is no longer transparent. Do not turn. When the fish is done, place it on a dish and pour the heated lemon Cajun marinade over the top.

To broil the fish: Place the fish in a shallow baking pan and cover with the lemon Cajun marinade. Place in the broiler about 4–5 inches from the flame. Cook for about 10 minutes and, using a long metal spatula, lift and turn the fish; cook for another 5–10 minutes (depending on the thickness of the pieces) or until no longer transparent.

To serve: Place on individual plates and spoon the cold salsa over the top. Serve over wild rice accompanied by steamed broccoli.

Per serving: 201 calories; 3.4 g fat (15.1 percent calories from fat); 29 g protein; 14 g carbohydrate; 62 mg cholesterol; 177 mg sodium.

Baked Halibut with Roasted Red Bell Pepper Sauce and Fettucine

MAKES 4 SERVINGS

This has always been the best-selling fish entree in my catering business and it looks very haute cuisine: a strip of white halibut placed against a green fettucine background with a diagonal strip of the red bell pepper sauce on top. Sprinkle a few capers on the fish for garnish, too.

1	pound halibut fillet
1/4	cup lemon juice
8	ounces roasted red peppers
1	tablespoon Dijon mustard
1	tablespoon capers
1/4	cup white wine
	salt and pepper to taste
	nonstick vegetable oil spray
4	cups cooked spinach fettucine
	capers for garnish

Preheat oven to 350°. Rinse the fish and pat dry. Cut into 2-inch strips and place in a dish. Sprinkle half of the lemon juice over the top and set aside.

Using a blender or food processor, process the red peppers, mustard, and capers. Blend for about one minute or until smooth—but not too long or the mixture will get watery. Set aside. Spritz a shallow cooking pan with vegetable oil spray and place the strips side by side in the pan. Pour in the white wine, season the fish with the salt and pepper, and bake for 10–15 minutes or until opaque all the way through. While the fish is cooking, prepare the fettucine according to package directions. Divide the cooked fettucine among four plates, place a slice of the halibut on top of each, then spoon a diagonal strip of the red bell pepper sauce across the top. Sprinkle with capers and serve.

Per serving: *337 calories; 4.4 g fat (12.2 percent calories from fat); 31 g protein; 39 g carbohydrate; 36 mg cholesterol; 135 mg sodium.*

Blackened Ahi Tuna

MAKES 4 SERVINGS

Ahi Tuna is great with just some peppercorns and lemon, cooked rare on the grill. However, this spice mix—a basic Cajun combo—gives the fish real zest. You can also use this mix of spices for any other Cajun dish, or try Chef Paul Prudhomme's blackened redfish seasoning.

16 ounces tuna steaks (4 4-ounce steaks)
1   tablespoon lemon juice
1   tablespoon cayenne pepper
1   tablespoon paprika
1   teaspoon dried thyme
1   teaspoon dried rosemary
2   teaspoons granulated garlic
4   teaspoons finely crushed bay leaves
2   teaspoons white pepper
pinch salt
olive-flavored nonstick vegetable oil spray

Rinse the tuna steaks, pat dry, place in a shallow dish, and sprinkle with lemon juice. Mix the seasonings in a small bowl until well blended. Cover the tuna steaks with the seasonings. Spray a nonstick sauté pan with vegetable oil spray and heat until very hot. Sear the tuna until the spices are blackened, about 3 minutes; turn and sear the other side until the fish is cooked but rare inside.

Serve over Wild Rice Bell Pepper Pilaf (see page 147).

Per serving: 184 calories; 6.1 g fat (30.3 percent calories from fat); 27 g protein; 4 g carbohydrate; 43 mg cholesterol; 79 mg sodium.

Caesar Swordfish

MAKES 4 SERVINGS

The dry packaged salad dressing mix this recipe calls for makes a great marinade. If you can't find Hain, try Très Classique oil-free Caesar, or another dry package mix without oil. One of the best things about this swordfish dish— any swordfish dish, for that matter—is that the fish has natural (good for you) fat of its own, so you'd have to really overcook it to dry it out. This marinade also tenderizes the swordfish, so it makes an excellent marinade for defrosted frozen fish.

4   6-ounce swordfish steaks
2   tablespoons lemon juice
$^1/_2$ cup Hain Caesar salad dressing mix
nonstick vegetable oil spray

Rinse the swordfish, pat dry, and place in a shallow dish or baking pan. Pour the lemon juice over the fish, then sprinkle the salad dressing mix on top. Turn to coat both sides. Let the fish sit for at least $^1/_2$ hour. Spritz a grill with vegetable oil spray, and cook the fish over medium heat for 5 minutes. In the meantime, place the marinade in a small saucepan and either set it on top of the grill to heat, or heat on the stove for 3–5 minutes. Turn the fish and cook for another 1–2 minutes, depending on the thickness. Remove the cooked fish from the grill and place back in the heated marinade. Serve with wild rice pilaf and steamed baby carrots.

Per serving: 208 calories; 6.9 g fat (31.1 percent calories from fat); 34 g protein; 1 g carbohydrate; 66 mg cholesterol; 154 mg sodium.

Swordfish Vinaigrette

MAKES 4 SERVINGS

For those of you who don't like the unsubtle taste of Caesar dressing, here's a slightly milder swordfish dish. I love swordfish rare, but add a few minutes of cooking time if you like it more well done. The leftover swordfish from this dish is excellent cut into 1/2-inch strips and served over a bed of fresh greens with the Italian salad dressing.

1	teaspoon garlic powder
1/2	teaspoon pepper
4	6-ounce swordfish steaks
1	cup oil-free Italian salad dressing
1	teaspoon dried tarragon
2	tablespoons lemon juice

Preheat broiler and set oven rack 4–5 inches from the heating element. Rub the garlic powder and pepper evenly into the fish; set aside. Combine the salad dressing, tarragon, and lemon juice in a shallow baking pan. Add swordfish and marinate for at least 20 minutes, turning every 5 minutes. Place the pan in the broiler and broil for 3–5 minutes; turn and broil 2–3 minutes more or until it reaches desired doneness. Transfer the fish to a platter and place the pan on a stove burner. Warm over medium heat, rapidly stirring the marinade, for about 2 minutes. Pour over the fish when you serve. Serve over steamed spinach with baked potatoes.

Per serving: 219 calories; 6.9 g fat (29.6 percent calories from fat); 34 g protein; 3 g carbohydrate; 66 mg cholesterol; 167 mg sodium.

Mrs. Yolanda's Low-Fat Fish Sticks

MAKES 4 SERVINGS

These are so tasty, they can trick your kids into eating fish. You can do variations with the seasonings as well. I use poultry and Italian seasonings in this recipe, but for variation you can try Mr. Spice blends or just some garlic powder and pepper.

3/4	cup homemade bread crumbs
3/4	cup wheat germ

¹/₂   teaspoon poultry seasoning
¹/₂   teaspoon Italian seasoning
1¹/₂   pounds cod fillet, skin removed
olive-flavored nonstick vegetable oil spray

Preheat the oven to 400°. Mix the crumbs, wheat germ, and seasonings in a shallow dish or bowl. Rinse the fish and pat dry; cut crosswise into 2-inch strips. Spritz the fish strips all over with vegetable oil spray, and dredge thoroughly in the bread crumb mix. Spritz a baking sheet with the oil spray and place the breaded fish strips on the pan. Bake until the fish is opaque in the center, about 10 minutes. Serve with Herbed Yogurt Cream (see page 281) for dipping.

Per serving, not including Herbed Yogurt Cream: 268 calories; 3 g fat (10.3 percent calories from fat); 37 g protein; 22 g carbohydrate; 73 mg cholesterol; 222 mg sodium.

Pineapple Ginger Teriyaki Fillets

MAKES 4 SERVINGS

This is a quick-to-make marinade that you can use for many types of fish. If you can't find orange roughy for this recipe, sole or tilapia will work just as well (fresh or frozen). Also, if you don't have fresh ginger, substitute 1 teaspoon ground ginger.

3   tablespoons sake, sherry, or mirin (a sweet rice wine)
3   tablespoons low-sodium soy sauce
2   teaspoons dark brown sugar or Sucanat
1   teaspoon grated gingerroot
¹/₄   teaspoon garlic powder
¹/₈   teaspoon red pepper flakes
8   ounces fresh or canned pineapple spears, drained
nonstick vegetable oil spray
1¹/₂   pounds orange roughy fillets, defrosted if frozen

In a large, shallow dish, combine the sake, soy sauce, sugar or Sucanat, ginger, garlic, and pepper flakes. Dip the pineapple spears into the soy mixture to coat, and set aside. Add the fillets to the mixture and coat. Let stand for 10–15 minutes. Preheat the broiler. Spritz a broiler pan or shallow baking pan with vegetable oil spray. Place the fish and the pineapple spears in the pan and broil 4–5 inches from the heat source, until the fish is just opaque through the thickest part, 6–10 minutes. Turn the pineapple spears about halfway through cooking. If the fish is thick, turn it as well. Serve each fillet accompanied by a pineapple wedge. Goes well with brown rice and steamed snow peas.

Per serving: 202 calories; 2.1 g fat (9.4 percent calories from fat); 33 g protein; 12 g carbohydrate; 34 mg cholesterol; 472 mg sodium.

Poached Salmon

MAKES 4 SERVINGS

This is a lovely, can't-fail dish that's great for a sit-down dinner or buffet.

1	pound salmon fillet (4 4-ounce servings)
½	cup lemon juice
1	tablespoon dried minced onion
3	stalks celery, diced fine
2	carrots, diced fine
6	whole peppercorns
½	cup white wine

Preheat oven to 400°. Rinse the fish under cool water, pat dry, and place in a shallow baking pan (or poaching pan) skin side down. Pour the lemon juice on top, then sprinkle the minced onion over the fish. Distribute the celery and carrots around the edges of the fish. Sprinkle the peppercorns on top, then pour the wine around the fish at the bottom of the pan. Cover the pan with aluminum foil and place in the oven for 7 minutes. Reduce the heat to 350° and cook for another 10 minutes. Check the middle of the fish for doneness. Don't let it overcook and become dry (the flesh will be very pale pink if it's overdone). Cook until opaque but not flaky. Serve hot or cold.

Per serving: 207 calories; 4.4 g fat (20.1 percent calories from fat); 25 g protein; 15 g carbohydrate; 59 mg cholesterol; 121 mg sodium.

Simple Salmon in Ginger Lime

The beauty of this dish is the flavor mix of spicy ginger and mouth-puckering lime laced with the zing of cilantro. Fresh lime juice is better than bottled for this recipe, but I find that most store-bought limes are very dry, so use the bottled if necessary. Also, substitute halibut fillets for salmon if you prefer.

1/4	cup chopped fresh cilantro
3	tablespoons peeled and chopped gingerroot
2	tablespoons chopped garlic
1	jalapeño, seeded and chopped
1/4	cup water
3	tablespoons fresh lime juice
1/4	teaspoon turmeric
1 1/2	pounds salmon fillet, cut into 2-inch strips

In a blender (or with a mortar and pestle) grind the cilantro, ginger, garlic, and jalapeño with half the water until it is a paste. Add the lime juice and turmeric and mix well. Coat the fish lightly with the marinade and place on a platter. Add the rest of the water and the remaining marinade to a large skillet and heat briefly. Add the fish to the skillet and cover with the remaining marinade. Cover the skillet and cook over medium heat about 5–10 minutes or until cooked through. Serve over brown rice with steamed snow peas.

Per serving: 220 calories; 6.1 g fat (25.3 percent calories from fat); 35 g protein; 5 g carbohydrate; 89 mg cholesterol; 121 mg sodium.

Garlic Tamari Salmon Fillet

My two favorite sauces for this simple recipe are Premier Japan's Garlic Tamari and John Troy's Oriental Ginger. If you can't find either of these, look for any Asian tamari sauce (made without added oil). Add 1 teaspoon of powdered ginger to the sauce, blend, and use as below. This salmon recipe is delicious with grilled mushrooms soaked in the same marinade.

1 1/2	pounds salmon fillet
1/2	fresh lemon

1   cup Premier Japan's Garlic Tamari or John Troy's Oriental
        Ginger sauce
nonstick vegetable oil spray

Rinse the salmon, pat dry, and place in a shallow dish. Squeeze the ½ lemon over the fish, then cover with the sauce. Turn the fish skin side up so the flesh sits in the marinade, and refrigerate for at least 15 minutes. To grill: Spritz the grill with vegetable oil spray and place the fish skin side down on the grill. Cook over medium heat for 7–10 minutes, on one side—don't turn. (If you are adding mushrooms to the dish, cook them at the same time.) Baste with the marinade as you cook. If you like your salmon rare, remove it while it's still pink in the middle. If you like it well done, cook it until it's no longer transparent in the middle.

To broil: Lay the fish skin side down in a shallow baking pan and place under the broiler 7–10 minutes. (Place mushrooms, if you're using them, around the fish.) Check for doneness as above. Serve with wild rice and asparagus.

Per serving: *203 calories; 5.9 g fat (26.8 percent calories from fat); 34 g protein; 2 g carbohydrate; 89 mg cholesterol; 156 mg sodium.*

Santa Fe Snapper

MAKES 4 SERVINGS

If you can't find the Guiltless Gourmet bean dip called for in this spicy Southwestern dish, use the one on page 137. You can also use any Cajun seasoning in place of Chef Paul Prudhomme's seafood mix, or the one on page 68. Believe me, the blend of these flavors is wonderful!

4   snapper fillets
2   lemons or ¼ cup bottled lemon juice
2   scant tablespoons Chef Paul Prudhomme's Seafood Magic
¾   cup Guiltless Gourmet mild black bean dip
¾   cup salsa

Rinse the snapper and place in a foil-lined shallow (2 inches) baking pan. Squeeze the lemons over the fish and sprinkle the seasoning over both sides. Heat the bean dip in a saucepan until warm, or microwave for 1 minute. Broil or grill the fish 5 minutes on one side, then 3–4 minutes on the other side. Divide the hot bean dip among four plates and place equal portions of snapper over each. Top each with a dollop of salsa. Serve with steamed broccoli and baby (new) potatoes.

Per serving: 350 calories; 7.4 g fat (19.1 percent calories from fat); 50 g protein; 21 g carbohydrate; 82 mg cholesterol; 245 mg sodium.

Mesquite Shrimp Kabobs

MAKES 4 SERVINGS

It seems as if shish kabob is a lot of work, but there are many shortcuts you can use. If you have the time to use fresh shrimp, great. But if you don't have time to peel and cook, use precooked frozen shrimp. You can also find many precut vegetables in the produce department these days. This recipe calls for bottled BBQ sauce; if you can't find one to your liking, check out the recipe on page 169.

20   shrimp, shelled
1   red onion, cut into 1-inch cubes (there will be several layers
        sticking together, making it possible to skewer)
1   each: red and green bell peppers, seeded, and cut into 1-inch
        cubes
10   baby (new) potatoes, steamed and sliced in half
10   mushrooms, stems removed
1   cup fat-free BBQ sauce
nonstick vegetable oil spray

If you're using bamboo skewers, soak them in warm water first, so that they don't burn on the grill. Stack pieces of shrimp, onion, red pepper, green pepper, potato, and mushroom on skewers, repeating until the skewers are full. Marinate the kabobs in the BBQ sauce, and set aside. Spritz the grill with vegetable oil spray. Over medium heat, cook the kabobs until they begin to brown, about 2 minutes. Turn, cook 2 minutes on the other side, then turn again. Cook 2 more minutes on both sides, or until the shrimp are opaque. Don't allow them to char. Baste with more BBQ sauce as you go.

If you don't have a grill, use the broiler: Place the kabobs in a broiling pan. Cook 5–7 minutes on one side, 5–7 minutes on the other. Serve over brown rice with lemon wedges on the side.

Per serving: 170 calories; 1.4 g fat (7.3 percent calories from fat); 15 g protein; 25 g carbohydrate; 99 mg cholesterol; 540 mg sodium.

Spanish Shrimp and Rice

Yes, of course it's ideal to have lovely fresh shrimp and make Spanish rice from scratch, but remember we belong to the "rush-hour, no-brainer" school of cooking. Hence, this recipe is made with frozen shrimp (saving you a trip to the fish store) and rice in a box (quick, quick, quick!). You don't even have to measure the spices, because they're all included in the packaged mix. The dish is delicious, proving once again that good ethnic food doesn't have to be difficult or fattening. Look for Spanish rice pilaf made by Near East, Arrowhead Mills, Lundberg, Casbah, or Fantastic Foods.

16	ounces frozen medium shrimp, defrosted
1	box Spanish rice pilaf
1/4	cup white wine
1	teaspoon minced garlic
1/2	red onion, chopped
1/2	green bell pepper, diced
16	ounces canned tomatoes
1	cup frozen peas
1	can diced green chilies

Rinse the shrimp in a colander and let it drain. Prepare the Spanish rice mix according to directions, eliminating any oil that the recipe calls for. Set aside. Heat the wine and minced garlic in a medium nonstick saucepan for about 2 minutes, or until the garlic starts to become transparent. Add the red onion, bell pepper, and tomatoes. Cook, stirring gently, until the onion and bell pepper are soft but not mushy, about 7 minutes. Add the peas, chilies, and shrimp and continue to stir. Cook about 3 minutes, stirring until the peas and shrimp are cooked, then pour over the rice mixture. If you like, add an 8-ounce can of tomato sauce to make the dish richer. Serve with cold gazpacho and crusty whole wheat bread.

Per serving: 252 calories; 2.5 g fat (9.1 percent calories from fat); 21 g protein; 34 g carbohydrate; 115 mg cholesterol; 265 mg sodium.

Oh So Simple Stir-fry Shrimp

It used to be that Asian stir-fries meant a lot of work. Just watching a Japanese chef chop those vegetables at rapid-fire speed was enough to intimidate anyone! The word "fry" didn't help matters either. But now that we have access to bags of frozen and fresh precut veggies, stir-fries are one of the easiest dishes to prepare. Certainly, go ahead and use fresh vegetables and shrimp if you like, but adjust the cooking times. If you use fresh vegetables, then allow about 5 more minutes' cooking time. If you use fresh shrimp, allow about 2 more minutes' cooking time after you add the shrimp.

2	tablespoons defatted chicken broth
1/4	cup sake
2	cloves garlic, minced
1	tablespoon gingerroot, peeled and minced
1	cup Premier Japan ginger tamari sauce (San-J also makes good tamari sauces)
1	6-ounce package frozen Japanese vegetables, defrosted and drained
1	pound frozen bay shrimp

Heat a wok or large nonstick sauté pan over medium heat. Add the chicken broth, sake, garlic, and gingerroot. Cook on high heat for about 4 minutes, until the mixture is bubbling and most of the sake has burned off. Add the tamari sauce and the vegetables and stir. Cook for about 2 minutes more, then remove the vegetables with a slotted spoon. Add the shrimp. Keep stirring and cook until the shrimp is no longer frozen—about 3 minutes. Remove with a slotted spoon and place on top of the vegetables. If you want to add some bean sprouts or bamboo shoots, do so now and cook for 2 minutes. Serve the shrimp and vegetable mixture over brown rice and pour the leftover sauce over each serving.

Per serving: 360 calories; 2.3 g fat (6.5 percent calories from fat); 31 g protein; 45 g carbohydrate; 172 mg cholesterol; 2,369 mg sodium.

Sole Veracruz

There's nothing worse than the thought of "going on a diet" and living on plain old sole with lemon squeezed over it. Sole *is* a wonderfully low-fat fish, but there's no reason to eat it plain. Here's a great way to jazz it up, and each serving miraculously has only 1 single minuscule gram of fat.

8   Dover sole fillets (which are small, but generally less
        expensive than other types of sole) or 6 large Petrale sole
        fillets
nonstick vegetable oil spray
2   tablespoons lemon juice
1   teaspoon poultry seasoning
1/4   cup dry vermouth
1   large onion, chopped
2   shallots, chopped
4   tomatoes, peeled, seeded, and chopped
1   cup orange juice
2   tablespoons frozen orange juice concentrate
2   tablespoons frozen apple juice concentrate
pinch crushed red pepper flakes
1/2   teaspoon fennel seeds
pinch pepper

Preheat oven to 350°. Place the sole fillets in a shallow baking dish sprayed with vegetable oil spray. Pour lemon juice over the fillets and sprinkle with poultry seasoning; set aside. In a nonstick sauté pan, bring vermouth to a boil. Reduce the heat and add the onion and shallots; sauté over medium heat until transparent. Add tomatoes and simmer for 10 minutes. Add the fresh juice and juice concentrates, red pepper flakes, fennel seeds, and pepper. Simmer for 5 minutes, pour mixture on top of sole, and bake for 25–30 minutes or until fish flakes when touched with a fork. Serve over fettucine with steamed zucchini strips.

Per serving: 170 calories; 1.1 g fat (6.2 percent calories from fat); 22 g protein; 11 g carbohydrate; 0 mg cholesterol; 178 mg sodium.

Spanish Sole

If you like, take a shortcut here: just pour the salsa and stewed tomatoes over the fish before cooking rather than adding all the other ingredients. For more flavor you can also top this with some spicy bean dip—the next day you can fill a corn tortilla with the leftovers for a quick lunch. You can also use other white fish such as snapper, orange roughy, and tilapia.

1/4	cup white wine
1	large onion, halved and sliced
1	red bell pepper, cored, seeded, and chopped
1	clove garlic, minced
2	8-ounce cans stewed tomatoes
3	tablespoons salsa
2	pounds white fish fillets, boned
1/4	cup olives

Preheat oven to 450°. Heat the wine in a skillet over medium heat. Add the onion, bell pepper, and garlic, and sauté until the onion is transparent. Add the tomatoes and salsa to the skillet and simmer, covered, for 10 minutes. Place the fillets in a large baking dish. Pour the tomato mixture over the fish and top with the olives. Bake until the fish is cooked through, about 15–20 minutes. Serve over Spanish rice pilaf with peas.

Per serving: 176 calories; 1.9 g fat (9.8 percent calories from fat); 24 g protein; 15 g carbohydrate; 0 mg cholesterol; 363 mg sodium.

Stuffed Dover Sole Dijon

Dover sole is inexpensive but has a certain cachet. It's very fragile, so treat it delicately and remember that it can dry out quickly. Be careful not to overcook.

	olive-flavored nonstick vegetable oil spray
3/4	cup white wine
2	cloves garlic, minced
1/4	onion, chopped

$^{1}/_{2}$	pound mushrooms, sliced
4	4-ounce Dover sole fillets
2	teaspoons Dijon mustard
1	10-ounce box frozen chopped spinach, thawed
2	tablespoons grated Parmesan cheese

Preheat oven to 350°. Spray a medium-size sauté pan with vegetable oil spray. Add $^{1}/_{2}$ cup of the wine and heat about 1 minute. Add the garlic and cook for 1 minute more, then add the onion and mushrooms. Cook until onion is transparent and set aside. Coat the sole with the mustard. Add spinach and Parmesan to the onion and mushrooms and blend well. Spritz a shallow baking pan with the nonstick spray. Place about 1 tablespoon of the spinach mixture in the middle of each fillet. Roll the fillet around the mixture and place in the pan, edges down. Pour the remaining $^{1}/_{4}$ cup white wine over all the rolls. Cover the pan with foil and bake about 20 minutes or until the fish is cooked through. Serve with Wild Rice Bell Pepper Pilaf (see page 147).

Per serving: 123 calories; 1.7 g fat (14.5 percent calories from fat); 18 g protein; 4 g carbohydrate; 2 mg cholesterol; 183 mg sodium.

Tandoori Shrimp and Scallop Kabobs

MAKES 6 SERVINGS

This dish is one of TV host Leeza Gibbons's number one picks. Make extra kabobs—they're great cold as a midday snack. You can also make these kabobs with chunks of chicken or turkey. Make sure that your vegetables are all about the same size so that they'll all cook in the same amount of time.

1	tablespoon tandoori seasoning
$^{1}/_{4}$	cup unsweetened lime juice
1	teaspoon frozen apple juice concentrate
$^{1}/_{2}$	cup plain nonfat yogurt
12	shrimp, peeled, deveined, and thawed if frozen
12	sea scallops
18	cherry tomatoes
12	mushrooms, stems removed
1	green bell pepper, chopped into 1-inch pieces

If you're using bamboo skewers, soak them in warm water first, so that they don't burn on the grill. In a medium-size bowl, whisk together the tandoori seasoning, lime juice, apple juice concentrate, and yogurt for the marinade. Place the shrimp, scallops, tomatoes, mushrooms and green pepper in the marinade and coat evenly. Stack the mushrooms on the skewers first, then the tomato, green pepper, the shrimp and the scallops, then repeat until the skewers are full. Soak the whole skewers in the marinade and place on a heated grill. Cook for 2–3 minutes, turning occasionally to cook all sides. Heat the marinade on the grill while the skewers cook, then place the skewers back in the marinade when they're done cooking. Serve with Marmalade Chutney (see page 172).

Per serving: 185 calories; 2.6 g fat (11.3 percent calories from fat); 15 g protein; 31 g carbohydrate; 46 mg cholesterol; 136 mg sodium.

Vegetarian Dinners

By now we all know that we should be eating more grains and legumes for their fiber and nutrients. However, many of us think that a vegetarian dish made up of grains and beans has to look dull and brown and have little taste. This simply isn't true. I recommend having a vegetarian dinner at least once or twice a week. They are generally inexpensive to make and very satisfying.

Eggplant Parmesan

MAKES 6 SERVINGS

This traditionally rich and fattening Italian dish has always been a big "no" for anyone interested in eating lean. But not anymore. This recipe is low in fat and still maintains its great flavor. What's more, it's so easy that I taught it to a seventeen-year-old male client so he could make it after school. If a kid can do it, you have no excuse! If you can't find the Millina's pasta sauce called for here, look for any of the new no-oil, fat-free sauces on the market.

1	eggplant, peeled and cut into 1/4-inch-thick slices
1/4	cup white wine
2	teaspoons minced garlic
1	teaspoon garlic powder

- There are many healthy gourmet bean soup mixes sold at all of the markets these days, usually in little brown paper or cellophane bags. Pick one up and you'll be surprised at how easy they are to make and how delicious they taste.
- Take advantage of the wonderful frozen vegetables and seasoned rice mixes available. Just add the vegetables to the cooking water of the seasoned rice mix for a really quick vegetarian dinner.
- Many vegetarian dinners need added protein. If you add nuts or seeds, keep them to a minimum—the fat grams can really add up.
- Tossing in some tofu is a great way to increase a vegetarian dish's protein content. Tofu also has calcium, an added bonus.

nonstick vegetable oil spray
2   cups Millina's or other brand fat-free pasta sauce
1   tablespoon dried basil
1   tablespoon dried oregano
8   ounces fat-free mozzarella, sliced 1/8 inch thick
1/2   cup grated Parmesan cheese

Preheat oven to 350°. Rinse the eggplant and set aside. Heat the wine, minced garlic, and garlic powder in a medium nonstick sauté pan. Add the eggplant and cook about 1–2 minutes on each side until lightly brown. Remove from the stove and set aside. Spritz a shallow casserole or baking pan with vegetable oil spray, then pour in a little of the pasta sauce to coat the bottom of the pan. Place the eggplant slices on the sauce, sprinkle a little of each seasoning on top, then cover with the mozzarella. Sprinkle some Parmesan on top, then add another layer of eggplant. Cover with a layer of sauce, then repeat. End with sauce covering the entire top. Make an aluminum-foil tent over the pan, place in the oven for about 20 minutes. Remove the foil and bake for another 5–10 minutes until it's bubbling slightly around the edges. Garnish with fresh basil and serve with a green salad.

Per serving: *118 calories; 2.6 g fat (19.3 percent calories from fat); 14 g protein; 10 g carbohydrate; 7 mg cholesterol; 430 mg sodium.*

Ratatouille Fresca

As French and exotic as this dish seems, it's really very simple to make. Traditionally, ratatouille is served as a dip, hors d'oeuvre, or antipasto. But I find it so versatile that I use it over pasta, or spooned on top of a toasted baguette or brown rice. Make a huge batch to have on hand for lunch—it's even better the second day. Just toss it in the microwave and sprinkle a little Parmesan cheese on top. If you have any leftover steamed broccoli, green beans, or peas, toss them in during the last few minutes of cooking.

½	cup white wine
½	cup defatted chicken broth
1	onion, cut into ¼-inch slices
3	cloves garlic, minced
1	medium eggplant, diced
1	28-ounce can whole tomatoes
2	teaspoons Italian seasoning
1	zucchini, thinly sliced
1	green bell pepper, cored, seeded, and sliced thin
¼	teaspoon black pepper
¼	cup sliced black olives

Pour the wine and half of the broth into a large nonstick saucepan. Add the onion and garlic and cook over medium heat, stirring until the onion is soft. Add the eggplant, tomatoes, and Italian seasoning. Cook over medium heat for 15 minutes. Add the zucchini, bell pepper, and pepper to the saucepan, and simmer for another 10 minutes. Toss in the black olives during the last 2–3 minutes of cooking. If the ratatouille is too liquidy, drain off the extra liquid and let sit for a while. Serve with grated cheddar or Parmesan cheese (optional).

Per serving, not including cheese: 96 calories; 2 g fat (20.6 percent calories from fat); 3 g protein; 14 g carbohydrate; 0 mg cholesterol; 271 mg sodium.

Red Lentil Chili

This dish is definitely one of my favorites. Not only is it packed with nutrients, vegetables, and fiber, it's scrumptious. Make a large batch and freeze it in individual plastic bags, so you can defrost a serving for lunch.

6	carrots, halved
6	zucchini, halved
6	yellow squash, halved
1	eggplant, quartered
1	yellow onion, quartered
	olive-flavored nonstick vegetable oil spray
1	cup white wine
2	13-ounce cans defatted chicken broth
1½	pounds red lentils
28	ounces canned plum tomatoes
1	teaspoon sea salt
1	teaspoon oregano
1	teaspoon cumin
1	teaspoon chili powder
1	teaspoon cayenne pepper
1½	teaspoons finely chopped garlic
1½	teaspoons nutmeg
¼	jalapeño, minced
	nonfat sour cream for garnish

Put the carrots, zucchini, squash, eggplant, and onion into a food processor and process (it's best to add one vegetable at a time) until well chopped. Spritz a large soup kettle with vegetable oil spray. Add the white wine and processed vegetables and cook over medium heat, stirring frequently, until the vegetables are tender and the onion is transparent. Add the broth, lentils, tomatoes, seasonings, and jalapeño. Continue to cook on medium heat for 1½ hours if you like your chili slightly crunchy; 1 hour and 45 minutes for softer chili. Stir frequently as the chili cooks. Serve in bowls topped with a dollop of nonfat sour cream.

Per serving, not including sour cream: *264 calories; 1.3 g fat (4.2 percent calories from fat); 19 g protein; 48 g carbohydrate; 0 mg cholesterol; 290 mg sodium.*

Sweet Potato Chili

Chili is traditionally served in a bowl, but I say forget the bowl, serve it up in a yam instead. You'll be getting fiber, beta carotene, and a whole lot more flavor. If you don't have time to make chili from scratch, use Health Valley fat-free chili and some fresh salsa to top the potatoes. (Lots of times I just top a microwaved yam or sweet potato with fresh salsa.) If you're a yam aficionado like me, see page 114 for more great ways to use them.

½	cup white wine
2	cups diced red bell pepper
1½	cups chopped onions
1	teaspoon garlic powder
1	tablespoon minced garlic
1	tablespoon chili powder
2	teaspoons ground cumin
1	16-ounce can peeled tomatoes with juice
1	16-ounce can black beans, rinsed and drained
2	cups diced crookneck squash or zucchini
1	tablespoon seeded and chopped jalapeño
4	large yams or sweet potatoes

nonfat sour cream and fresh chopped cilantro for garnish (optional)

Heat the white wine in a large nonstick skillet and add the bell pepper, onions, and garlic powder. Sauté until the onions are golden. Add the fresh garlic and sauté for 2 minutes more. Stir in chili powder, cumin, tomatoes, and beans; reduce the heat and bring to a simmer. Simmer for 20–25 minutes. Add the squash and jalapeño and cook another 6 minutes. Let the chili sit while you prepare the yams.

Prick yams several times all over with a fork and rinse with water. To cook in the microwave: Put the wet yams in a plastic bag and place in the microwave. Cook on high 10–15 minutes (depending on the size of the yam). Poke with a fork to see if they are soft all the way through. To bake in the oven: Wrap the potatoes in aluminum foil and place in a preheated 350° oven. Bake 15–20 minutes or until soft all the way through. Cut in half and mash slightly. Top with the chili, and, if desired, a dollop of nonfat sour cream and sprinkling of cilantro. Or scoop the yam out of its skin, mix with the chili, then refill the skin. Microwave for another 2 minutes and serve.

Per serving: 321 calories; 1.5 g fat (4.3 percent calories from fat); 9 g protein; 67 g carbohydrate; 0 mg cholesterol; 361 mg sodium.

Pasta Dinners

First pasta had a bad reputation. Then it had a good reputation. Then bad, and so forth and so on. There is nothing wrong with a good pasta dinner! If you pour fattening sauces on noodles, then you will have a fattening dinner. Common sense. And if you eat pasta all day, you will develop a pasta belly. Common sense. However, pasta is healthful, inexpensive, and very easy to make. By nature of the fact that you just have to boil the noodles, it's a natural no-brainer.

Artichoke Hearts and Ricotta Penne with Shrimp

MAKES 4 SERVINGS

This sounds like a complicated gourmet dish; in truth, it's a gourmet "no-brainer." If you can't find frozen artichoke hearts, buy canned (packed in water) and drain before using.

9	ounces frozen artichoke hearts, thawed
1	pound penne pasta
1/2	cup defatted chicken broth
1/2	cup white wine
1	small onion, thinly sliced
1	clove garlic, chopped fine
16	medium shrimp
1/2	teaspoon dried oregano
1	teaspoon fresh ground pepper
1/4	cup water
2	tablespoons lemon juice
1/2	cup nonfat ricotta cheese
1	tablespoon grated lemon peel

salt and pepper to taste

Cut all but two of the artichoke hearts into quarters and set aside. In a small bowl, use a fork to mash the 2 remaining hearts into a paste. Cook the pasta according to package directions, but don't add salt to the water. After draining in a colander, rinse the pasta with the broth; set aside. Heat half of the white wine in a sauté pan. Add the onion, garlic, and shrimp. Cook over medium heat, stirring, for one minute. Add the oregano and pepper, stir in the water, and cook until the onion is limp, about 2 minutes. Reduce the heat and add the other $1/4$ cup wine, lemon juice, and the reserved artichoke quarters and artichoke paste. Simmer until heated through, about 1 minute. Add the ricotta and stir until creamy. Toss sauce with the cooked pasta; stir in the lemon peel, and toss again. Season to taste. Serve with a green salad.

Per serving: 533 calories; 3.1 g fat (5.5 percent calories from fat); 29 g protein; 90 g carbohydrate; 80 mg cholesterol; 287 mg sodium.

Curry Apple Stuffed Shells

MAKES 6 SERVINGS

This is a welcome change from the usual tomato- or herb-based pasta dishes. The light sauce looks creamy but is low in fat and calories.

24	jumbo pasta shells
1	cup defatted chicken broth
1	cup white wine
1	onion, chopped
1	green bell pepper, chopped
$1^1/2$	pounds ground turkey breast
2	Golden Delicious apples, cored, seeded, and chopped
$1/4$	cup raisins
1	cup chopped celery
1	tablespoon frozen apple juice concentrate
$2^1/2$	tablespoons curry powder
1	cup skim milk
1	tablespoon cornstarch
$1/4$	cup water
1	pint nonfat plain yogurt
	salt and pepper to taste
	nonstick vegetable oil spray

Preheat oven to 350°. Prepare the shells according to package directions and rinse in a colander. Drain the shells and coat with the chicken broth. Drain again and set aside. Heat half of the white wine in a large nonstick sauté pan. Add the onion and green pepper (if you like, use chopped frozen veggies to save time) and cook until soft; about 5 minutes (less for frozen veggies). Add the ground turkey breast and sauté, stirring until browned. Remove and, in a large bowl, combine the turkey mixture with the apples, raisins, and celery. In the same sauté pan, add the rest of the white wine and apple juice concentrate and bring to a boil. Whisk in the curry powder and milk. In a separate bowl, mix the cornstarch with the water. Alternately add the yogurt and cornstarch mixture to the sauté pan, blending constantly with a whisk as you go. Season to taste with salt and pepper, and stir until the sauce is slightly thick. Spray a shallow baking pan with vegetable oil spray. Stuff the cooked shells with the turkey mixture and place in rows in the baking pan. Drizzle the sauce over the top of each shell until you've used all of the sauce. Cover the pan with an aluminum-foil tent and bake for 10 minutes. Remove the foil and bake for another 5–10 minutes, or until done. Serve with Mango Lime Salsa, page 176.

Per serving: 343 calories; 2.7 g fat (7.8 percent calories from fat); 36 g protein; 36 g carbohydrate; 70 mg cholesterol; 265 mg sodium.

Fettucine with White Clam Sauce

MAKES 4 SERVINGS

Don't be afraid of tofu. It really has no flavor of its own, so it takes on other flavors well and adds the creaminess you look for in a dish like this. The natural fat in tofu is also the kind you want in your diet, much like the natural fats in fish, beans, and poultry. So indulge in a dish that is traditionally fattening, but with this recipe, is guilt-free, good for you, and surprisingly robust.

1	pound fettucine noodles
1/2	cup defatted chicken broth
1 1/2	cups tofu
5	ounces canned clams, with liquid
1/2	cup white wine
1/2	teaspoon minced garlic
1/4	teaspoon salt

pinch white pepper
1   **teaspoon chopped fresh parsley**

Prepare the fettucine according to package directions, rinse with the chicken broth, and set aside. Place the tofu in a blender. Open the can of chopped clams and drain the clam juice into the blender. Process on medium until well blended. Heat a nonstick medium-size saucepan over medium heat. Add the wine, blended tofu, drained clams, garlic, salt, and white pepper. Bring to a low simmer and cook until the sauce is blended and thickened, about 5–7 minutes. Pour over the cooked noodles and top with fresh parsley. Serve with gazpacho and crusty sourdough bread.

Per serving: 457 calories; 6.7 g fat (13.8 percent calories from fat); 22 g protein; 72 g carbohydrate; 9 mg cholesterol; 796 mg sodium.

Garlic Rotelli Pasta Primavera

MAKES 6 SERVINGS

In every market today you can find flavored pastas. One of my favorites is a wonderful garlic rotelli sold in a local Los Angeles market. You can use plain or tricolored rotelli, or try another flavor or another shape pasta. The beauty of this dish is that it's quick and can be served either hot or cold. If you have fresh herbs on hand, substitute a tablespoon of chopped fresh basil for the Italian seasoning.

1   **pound rotelli pasta, garlic or plain (add 1 teaspoon minced garlic to cooking water to flavor the plain)**
16   **ounces frozen mixed vegetables (preferably a mix that has peas, diced carrots, and corn)**
1/2   **cup defatted chicken broth**
1/4   **cup white wine**
3   **cloves garlic, chopped**
1   **teaspoon lemon juice**
1   **tablespoon frozen apple juice concentrate**
28   **ounces canned chopped tomatoes, drained**
1   **tablespoon Italian seasoning**

Cook the pasta according to package directions, adding the frozen vegetables during the last 2–3 minutes of cooking. Drain the pasta and vegetables in a colander, and run cold water over them. Rinse with the defatted chicken broth. In a medium sauté pan, heat the wine, then add the chopped garlic. Cook for 2–3 minutes or until the garlic is transparent. Add the lemon juice, apple juice concentrate, and tomatoes to the pan. Sauté over medium heat for about 3 minutes, then add the Italian seasoning and cook for another 5 minutes, until the liquid has burned partly off. Toss with the pasta and veggies and serve. Top with grated Parmesan and serve with crusty Italian bread.

Per serving, not including Parmesan: 360 calories; 1.8 g fat (4.7 percent calories from fat); 14 g protein; 69 g carbohydrate; 0 mg cholesterol; 373 mg sodium.

Jumbo Stuffed Pasta Shells

MAKES 4 SERVINGS

This is one of the best-selling items in my home delivery service. Everybody loves these attractive shells, and they are undeniably delicious. It's also a great dish for kids because they love the shape of the shells. The dish is easy to freeze, so double the recipe and freeze 4 to 6 servings in individual airtight containers to make your own frozen "lean cuisine." I like to use the Millina's pasta sauce, but you can use your favorite fat-free, no-oil pasta sauce.

32	jumbo pasta shells
1/2	cup defatted chicken broth
16	ounces frozen chopped spinach, thawed and drained
16	ounces fat-free ricotta cheese
4	cloves garlic, minced
2	tablespoons grated Parmesan cheese
2	tablespoons Italian seasoning
1	teaspoon garlic powder
salt and pepper to taste	
2	cups Millina's or other brand fat-free pasta sauce
1/4	cup white wine

Preheat oven to 350°. Prepare the pasta shells according to package directions, drain, then rinse with the defatted chicken broth and set in cold water and broth to stay moist. Squeeze out the excess water from the frozen spinach and, in a medium-size bowl, combine it with the fat-free ricotta. Add the minced garlic, Parmesan cheese, Italian seasoning, and garlic powder. Season to taste with the salt and pepper and mix well. Spread a little of the pasta sauce and white wine over the bottom of the pan to coat. Fill the shells with the cheese-spinach mixture and line them up evenly in the pan. Top with the pasta sauce and cover the pan with a foil tent. Place in a preheated oven and cook for 10 minutes. Remove the foil and cook for another 10–15 minutes or until done. Top with shaved Parmesan and serve with a green salad.

Per serving, not including Parmesan: 305 calories; 1.7 g fat (5 percent calories from fat); 27 g protein; 45 g carbohydrate; 10 mg cholesterol; 390 mg sodium.

Linguine with Zucchini

MAKES 4 SERVINGS

Here we are again: easy, Italian, rich, delicious, and never dull. To make this dish "meatier," sauté ½ pound of ground chicken in ¼ cup of white wine, drain, then add with the sour cream at the end of this recipe.

1	pound linguine noodles
1	cup defatted chicken broth
½	cup chopped onion
1	clove garlic, minced
2	shallots, minced
8	small zucchini, sliced thin
1	teaspoon dried rosemary
pinch pepper	
⅔	cup nonfat sour cream

Prepare the linguine according to package directions, drain, and rinse with cold water. Rinse again with half of the chicken broth, drain, and set aside. Pour the other ½ cup of chicken broth into a skillet and sauté the onion, garlic, and shallots. Cook until the vegetables are just transparent. Add the zucchini, rosemary, and pepper and cook 2–3 minutes more. Add the pasta and sour cream and stir until the noodles are well coated. Remove from heat and transfer to a serving platter. Serve with a green salad and some sourdough rolls.

Per serving: 452 calories; 3.5 g fat (6.9 percent calories from fat); 21 g protein; 87 g carbohydrate; 0 mg cholesterol; 128 mg sodium.

Manicotti

What? Manicotti in a low-fat cookbook? This is another one of those traditional dishes some of us have dropped from our diets due to fat concerns. No more. Check out this skinny version.

¼	cup white wine
4	cloves garlic, minced
1	pound ground chicken breast (ground without skin)
12	manicotti tubes
½	cup defatted chicken broth
1	pound fat-free ricotta cheese
2	tablespoons grated Parmesan cheese
¼	cup chopped parsley
1	tablespoon dried oregano
2	teaspoons dried basil
1	teaspoon garlic powder
1	teaspoon pepper
1	teaspoon salt
1	cup Millina's fat-free Zinfandel flavor pasta sauce or other fat-free sauce

olive-flavored nonstick vegetable oil spray

Preheat oven to 350°. Heat the wine in a large saucepan. Add the garlic and cook over medium heat for about 2 minutes. Add the ground chicken breast and keep tossing in the pan until it's completely browned. Transfer to a large bowl; set aside to cool. Prepare the manicotti according to package directions, drain, and rinse with cold water. Rinse again with the chicken broth, drain, and let the noodles sit in the cold water and chicken broth; set aside. In a large bowl, mix the ricotta, Parmesan, parsley, and remaining seasonings with the cooked ground chicken until blended. Spoon a little of the pasta sauce on the bottom of a baking pan, then spread to cover the bottom. Slit the manicotti tubes down one side and fill with about 3 tablespoons of the filling. If the noodles get too dry and start to tear, spray with the vegetable oil spray. Place the noodles open side down in the pan. Line the noodles up in rows in the pan and drizzle the pasta sauce across the top, zig-zagging back and forth. Leave some of the white of the noodles showing. Cover the pan with an aluminum-foil tent and bake for 15 minutes; remove the foil tent and cook another 7–10 minutes; do not let the noodles brown. Serve topped with Parmesan accompanied by a salad and crusty Italian bread.

Per serving, not including Parmesan: 402 calories; 3.5 g fat (7.9 percent calories from fat); 33 g protein; 57 g carbohydrate; 38 mg cholesterol; 468 mg sodium.

Pasta in a Rage

This pasta dish is usually called Pasta Arrabbiata, which means "in a rage" in Italian. This could refer to the fact that this dish is made so quickly (as if made by a raging cook) or that the red pepper flakes add a fiery, angry quality to the pasta. Ironically, it is quite "the rage" at many trendy restaurants on the East and West coasts. You can adjust the temper or rage of the dish to your taste just by lightening up or going heavy-handed on the red pepper flakes. If you want to reduce the sodium in this pasta, use low-sodium canned tomatoes.

1   **pound penne pasta (or mostaccioli)**
¹/₂   **cup defatted chicken broth**
olive-flavored nonstick vegetable oil spray
¹/₄   **cup white wine**
3   **cloves garlic, chopped**
¹/₄   **teaspoon red pepper flakes, or more to taste**
28   **ounces canned chopped tomatoes, drained**
¹/₂   **cup grated Romano cheese**
¹/₄   **cup chopped parsley**
salt and pepper to taste

Cook the penne according to package directions, drain, and rinse with cold water. Rinse again with the chicken broth, drain, and set aside. Spritz a large nonstick sauté pan with the vegetable oil spray. Add the white wine and bring to a boil. Add the garlic and red pepper flakes; cook over medium heat, stirring until the garlic is golden, about 1 minute. Add the tomatoes and crush them down with a wooden spoon. Bring to a simmer and cook about 5 minutes more. Add the cooked pasta and stir until the pasta sizzles. Remove from the heat and toss with the cheese and parsley. Serve with shaved Parmesan, a green salad, and crusty bread.

Per serving, not including Parmesan: 209 calories; 4.5 g fat (19.6 percent calories from fat); 12 g protein; 29 g carbohydrate; 15 mg cholesterol; 689 mg sodium.

Penne Tonnato with Primavera Sauce

MAKES 6 SERVINGS

Tuna is a very common ingredient in Italian pasta dishes, although we hardly ever think past using it in a sandwich here in the States. Using frozen vegetables cuts down on the time it takes to make this savory dish. The best mix to buy is one that has broccoli, cauliflower, carrots, red bell pepper, and green beans. If you decide to use fresh veggies, add a little more cooking time.

olive-flavored nonstick vegetable oil spray
3   cups canned chopped tomatoes
2   cloves garlic, minced
4   cups mixed frozen vegetables, thawed and drained
1/2 teaspoon dried basil
1/4 teaspoon dried thyme
1/4 teaspoon dried oregano
salt and pepper to taste
1   pound penne pasta
1   6 1/2-ounce can water-packed tuna, drained
1   tablespoon lemon juice

Spritz a medium nonstick sauté pan with the olive-flavored vegetable oil spray. Add the tomatoes and garlic. Cook, covered, over low heat until the tomatoes are softened, about 5 minutes. Add the vegetables, dried herbs, and salt and pepper to taste; stir to blend. Cook covered about 5–7 minutes. In the meantime, cook the pasta according to package directions. During the last few minutes of cooking, spoon out 1/2 cup of the pasta liquid and add it to the sauce. Add the tuna and lemon juice to the sauce, and chop down with a wooden spoon until blended but not mushy. Drain the pasta and toss with the sauce. Top with capers and serve with crusty Italian bread.

Per serving: 400 calories; 3.2 g fat (7 percent calories from fat); 24 g protein; 71 g carbohydrate; 9 mg cholesterol; 350 mg sodium.

Rotelli with Garlic Chicken Marinara

MAKES 8 SERVINGS

This pasta is topped with a basic hearty sauce that I make in batches and freeze. Then when I'm in a rush—which is always—I just defrost the sauce, boil the pasta, open a bag of prechopped salad, and *voilà*—another no-brainer genius meal! You don't have to use rotelli to make this dish, but make sure you use a pasta that is fairly chunky (i.e., penne, shells, or wagon wheels) so that it holds the chicken sauce. A thin pasta like spaghetti or capellini will not hold the sauce.

2	pounds ground chicken breast (ground without the skin)
4	cloves garlic, minced
2	cups red wine
1	teaspoon garlic powder
1	tablespoon Italian seasoning
1/2	teaspoon pepper
4	cups Millina's or other fat-free brand pasta sauce
1	pound rotelli pasta
salt to taste	

In a large nonstick saucepan, sauté the ground chicken breast over medium heat, stirring as you cook. Add the minced garlic and 1/4 cup of the red wine. Stir and chop down the ground chicken breast so that it picks up the minced garlic and browns evenly. Add the garlic powder, Italian seasoning, pepper, and remaining red wine. Let simmer for about 5 minutes, then add the pasta sauce. Continue to stir and cook until evenly blended. Let simmer on low for about 15 minutes while you cook the pasta according to the package directions. Drain the pasta and top with the sauce. Serve with shaved Parmesan and fresh basil.

Per serving, not including Parmesan: *400 calories; 5.1 g fat (13.5 percent calories from fat); 38 g protein; 37 g carbohydrate; 85 mg cholesterol; 287 mg sodium.*

Shrimp and Lemon Pepper Pasta

MAKES 6 SERVINGS

Lemon pepper pasta is fairly common among the flavored pastas these days. If, however, you can't find it, get regular linguine and add 1 tablespoon of lemon pepper to the water as the pasta cooks. This recipe calls for fresh shrimp, but you can also use frozen precooked shrimp—just thaw before you add them to the recipe. Lemon-dill fat-free salad dressing is another ingredient called for here that can be fiddled with: feel free to use regular fat-free Italian dressing instead.

12   ounces lemon pepper pasta
1/2   cup defatted chicken broth
1/2   cup white wine
1   pound medium shrimp, peeled and deveined
1   cup lemon-dill fat-free salad dressing
8   cloves garlic, minced
1/3   cup chopped shallots
2/3   cup clam juice
1/2   cup chopped fresh parsley
1   tablespoon dried dill
1   teaspoon pepper
salt to taste

Cook the pasta according to package directions, drain, and rinse with cold water. Rinse again with the chicken broth, drain, and set aside. Heat 1/4 cup of the white wine in a large nonstick sauté pan over medium heat. Add the shrimp and sauté until just pink, stirring frequently, about 3 minutes. (If you're using frozen, defrost and cook only 1 minute.) Using a slotted spoon, transfer the shrimp to a bowl. Add the dressing, garlic, and shallots to the pan and cook 2 minutes. Add the clam juice and the other 1/4 cup white wine, and decrease the heat to medium low. Return the shrimp to the pan with the clam juice mixture. Add the parsley, dill, pepper, and cooked pasta. Toss to blend. Season with salt to taste. Serve with baked tomatoes and green salad.

Per serving: 308 calories; 3 g fat (9.3 percent calories from fat); 24 g protein; 41 g carbohydrate; 115 mg cholesterol; 137 mg sodium.

Spaghetti and Garlic Chicken Meatballs

MAKES 6 SERVINGS

Yes, it's possible to have a delicious favorite like spaghetti and meatballs and not feel like you have to digest it for days. This is real hearty Italian food without the weight, and a favorite of singer Natalie Cole. If you have time, this dish also goes great with the Sun-Dried Tomato Basil Sauce on page 174, or use your favorite bottled fat-free pasta sauce.

Meatballs

1	egg, lightly beaten
2½	pounds ground chicken breast (ground without the skin)
2	tablespoons Italian seasoning
1	teaspoon salt (optional)
1	tablespoon garlic powder

Sauce

olive-flavored nonstick vegetable oil spray

2	cloves garlic, minced
¼	cup white wine
2	cups Millina's or other fat-free brand pasta sauce
1	pound spaghetti
¼	cup defatted chicken broth

Combine the egg with the ground chicken, Italian seasoning, salt, and garlic powder. Fill a large saucepan with water (4–6 cups), and bring to a low boil. Form the ground chicken mixture into small meatballs, and drop into the water one by one. Cook for 7–10 minutes, or until the meatballs float to the surface and are no longer pink in the middle. With a slotted spoon, transfer to a bowl.

Spray a medium saucepan with the olive-flavored oil and add the minced garlic. Heat on low until the garlic begins to sizzle, then add the white wine. Cook for about 4 minutes, or until the garlic is transparent and the wine is bubbling. Add the pasta sauce and cook about 3–4 minutes, stirring. Turn off heat and set aside. Cook the spaghetti according to package directions, drain, and rinse with cold water. Rinse again with the chicken broth, drain, and serve topped with the chicken meatballs and pasta sauce. Top with grated Parmesan and serve with salad and crusty bread.

Per serving, not including Parmesan: 424 calories; 4 g fat (8.6 percent calories from fat); 53 g protein; 43 g carbohydrate; 144 mg cholesterol; 647 mg sodium.

Spaghetti with Pomodoro Clam Sauce

MAKES 4 SERVINGS

I suppose in an ideal world, this recipe is better with fresh clams and fresh basil, and if you have the time, by all means use them. But we are in the "no-brainer" world here and this recipe tastes scrumptious no matter what.

1/2	cup white wine
1	onion, chopped
1/4	cup V-8 juice
4	Roma tomatoes, seeded and chopped
2	cloves garlic, minced
10	ounces canned whole baby clams, drained, with juice reserved
1	tablespoon dried basil
1/3	cup chopped fresh parsley
1/4	teaspoon pepper
	salt to taste
1	pound spaghetti

Heat the white wine in a large nonstick skillet over medium heat. Add the onion and the V-8 juice and cook until the onion is softened, about 5 minutes. Add the chopped tomatoes and garlic and continue stirring, cooking for about 3 minutes. Stir in the reserved clam juice and basil; bring to a simmer. Cook over low heat for 5 minutes. Add the parsley, clams, pepper, and salt, and heat through. In the meantime cook the spaghetti according to package directions. Drain and toss with the sauce. Top with Parmesan and serve with a crusty whole wheat bread.

Per serving, not including Parmesan: *333 calories; 1.7 g fat (4.7 percent calories from fat); 12 g protein; 64 g carbohydrate; 2 mg cholesterol; 382 mg sodium.*

Sweet Pepper Pasta with Mushrooms

MAKES 4 SERVINGS

The secret to this lovely light pasta is the sauce. The blend of the mushrooms, Dijon mustard, and herbes de Provence make this a gourmet de-"lite."

1 pound linguine
1 cup defatted chicken broth
1 red bell pepper, seeded, cored, and diced
2 tablespoons white wine
nonstick vegetable oil spray
1 pound mushrooms, stems removed and reserved

Mushroom stock and sauce

$1/2$ cup defatted chicken broth
$1/2$ onion, chopped
mushroom stems and pieces
1 cup water
1 cup white wine
4 peppercorns
1 bay leaf
$1/2$ teaspoon dried thyme
1 cup diced fresh tomato
1 tablespoon herbes de Provence
2 tablespoons Dijon mustard

Cook the linguine according to package directions, drain, and rinse with cold water. Rinse again with chicken broth, drain, and set aside. Sauté the pepper in the white wine until softened but not mushy. Spritz the grill or broiler with vegetable oil spray and grill or broil the mushrooms until the juices are running out and they are browned but not burned. Set aside.

To make the stock and sauce: Place $1/2$ cup defatted chicken stock in a sauté pan and add the onion and mushroom stems. Sauté about 15 minutes over medium heat. Add the water, wine, peppercorns, bay leaf, and thyme, and cook for about 25 minutes over low heat. Add the diced tomato and herbes de Provence and cook for 15 more minutes. Add the Dijon mustard and run the sauce through a blender or food processor until blended. Toss the pasta with the peppers, then top with the sauce and grilled mushrooms. Garnish with parsley and serve with salad and French bread.

Per serving: 496 calories; 4.4 g fat (8.6 percent calories from fat); 15 g protein; 86 g carbohydrate; 6 mg cholesterol; 190 mg sodium.

Vegetable Lasagne

Just the word "lasagne" sounds like hard work and high fat. But this is an easy and very low-fat lasagne made with fat-free cheese and lots of vegetables. If you want to make it slightly more indulgent, you can add some grated mozzarella to the layers. This is best made the day before, chilled, then heated. It freezes well, too.

1	package lasagne noodles
1½	cups defatted chicken broth
½	cup white wine
8	ounces mushrooms, sliced
4	zucchini, shredded
4	yellow summer squash, shredded
1	tablespoon Italian seasoning
2	teaspoons garlic salt
2	cups fat-free ricotta cheese
	olive-flavored nonstick vegetable oil spray
1½	cups Millina's or other fat-free brand pasta sauce
½	cup grated Parmesan cheese

Preheat oven to 400°. Prepare the lasagne noodles according to package directions, but add 1 cup chicken broth to the water. Drain, rinse with remaining ½ cup chicken broth, and allow to sit in the cold water and broth to stay moist. Heat the white wine in a medium-size nonstick sauté pan and add the vegetables, Italian seasoning, and garlic salt. Sauté until cooked but not brown, about 15 minutes. Remove vegetables from the heat and drain in a colander until all liquid is drained out. Combine with the ricotta until well blended. Spritz a casserole dish or deep baking pan with vegetable oil spray. Pour a little bit of the pasta sauce in the bottom of the pan and spread around. Put a layer of the noodles side by side, overlapping at the edges on top of the sauce. Add a layer of the ricotta-vegetable mix, then sprinkle ⅓ of the Parmesan on top. Add another layer of noodles. Continue this until you are up to the edge of the pan, then top with the pasta sauce. Cover with foil and bake for 20 minutes. Remove the foil and reduce the heat to 350° and bake another 20 minutes. Let cool. Serve with minestrone soup and Italian bread.

Per serving: *181 calories; 2.7 g fat (14.4 percent calories from fat); 11.9 g protein; 24.9 g carbohydrate; 7 mg cholesterol; 279 mg sodium.*

Pizza

Just like pasta, pizza has had a bad rap. But for good reason: In America it's been made into junk food, topping it with stuff like sausage and pepperoni. The basic ingredients, though, can make a nutritious meal, even better if you make your pizza with a whole wheat crust, some fat-free seasoned sauce, low-fat or fat-free cheese, and vegetable toppings. With the recipes here, you can have your pizza and keep your health, too. Life is good.

Basic Pizza Crust #1

MAKES 4 RECTANGULAR CRUSTS 12 × 16 INCHES OR
4 ROUND CRUSTS 10–12 INCHES IN DIAMETER

Don't be daunted by the idea of making a pizza crust; this one's easy. I make lots of them at the same time, then freeze them so that I can whip up a pizza anytime. If you want to change the flavor of the crust, substitute the same amount of another seasoning (i.e., Italian seasoning or basil) for the popcorn seasoning. If you want to cut back on sodium, substitute water for the soy sauce. This is enough dough for four pizzas, spread to a medium thickness in a pizza pan.

1³/₄	**cups warm water (105–115°F)**
2	**tablespoons yeast**
2	**teaspoons soy sauce**
2	**cups whole wheat flour**
2	**cups white flour**
1	**tablespoon popcorn seasoning**
	nonstick vegetable oil spray

Place the water in a large bowl and pour in the yeast so it dissolves. Add the soy sauce. In a separate large bowl, combine the flours and the seasoning. Add this mixture to the yeast mixture 1 cup at a time, stirring after each addition to combine thoroughly. Cover with a damp towel and set in a warm place to rise for about 2 hours, or until it doubles in size. Roll the mixture onto a floured surface and knead for about 5 minutes, adding white flour as needed to keep the dough from sticking. The dough should be smooth and elastic. Separate into 4 pieces and either use immediately, or freeze stored in plastic bags spritzed with nonstick vegetable oil spray.

Random Pizza Notes

- Make a big batch of one of the Basic Pizza Crust recipes that follow, roll it into balls about the size of grapefruits, and freeze it in zip-lock plastic bags. When you're ready to make a pizza, take out a bag, thaw, and proceed with your chosen pizza recipe.
- If you want that olive oil taste but don't want to add olive oil, spray your pizza crust with olive-flavored vegetable oil spray before baking.
- Granted, fat-free cheeses aren't as flavorful as higher-fat ones. If you want more flavor, top your pizza with half reduced-fat cheese and half fat-free cheese.
- As you're making your pizza dough, flavor it with a seasoning of your choice. You can make a garlic-herb crust, a Cajun crust, a pepper crust . . . be creative.
- After you make the dough, you'll need to prebake the pizza crust (see directions for Basic Pizza Crust recipes). Then, follow the recipe for pizza topping and complete baking.
- In a pinch, split open 4 or 5 pitas and layer them in a baking pan to create a quickie pizza dough.
- Fat-free pasta sauce doubles as a pizza sauce. Use different flavors to give your pizzas variety.
- Try some of the new fat-free or soy-based cold cuts to top your pizza instead of sausage and pepperoni.

To make crust, preheat oven to 350°. Roll one piece of the dough into a rectangle 12 × 16 inches or a circle 10–12 inches. Spritz a baking sheet, baking pan, or pizza pan with vegetable oil spray and place the dough on the sheet or in the pan. Bake 5 minutes. Remove the crust from the oven and follow pizza recipe of your choice.

Per single slice (without toppings): *75 calories; 0.3 g fat (3.9 percent calories from fat); 3 g protein; 16 g carbohydrate; 0 mg cholesterol; 25 mg sodium.*

Basic Pizza Crust #2

MAKES 1 RECTANGULAR CRUST 12 × 16 INCHES OR
1 ROUND CRUST 10–12 INCHES IN DIAMETER

This crust isn't as healthy as number one, but it's a little lighter. If you want to make crusts for later on, double or triple the recipe and freeze the extras.

1	teaspoon active dry yeast
1	cup warm water (105–115°F.)
1²/₃	cups unbleached flour
1	cup cake flour
1	teaspoon salt
	nonstick vegetable oil spray

In a small cup or bowl sprinkle the yeast over ¼ cup warm water; stir until dissolved. In a large bowl combine the unbleached flour, cake flour, and salt. Make a well in the center of the flour mixture and pour in the yeast mixture. With a wooden spoon, slowly work the flour mixture into the yeast mixture, adding ³/₄ cup warm water as you mix. Turn the dough out and knead until very smooth, about 10 minutes. Spray a bowl with vegetable oil spray and place the dough in; cover with a damp towel and let rise for 2–2¹/₂ hours, or until doubled. You can freeze this dough or use right away. If making a crust immediately, preheat oven to 350°. Roll the dough into a rectangle 12 × 16 inches or round 10–12 inches. Spritz a baking sheet, baking pan, or pizza pan with vegetable oil spray and place the dough on the sheet or in the pan. Bake (as above) 5 minutes. Remove the crust from the oven and follow pizza recipe of your choice.

Per single slice (without toppings): 49 calories; 0.4 g fat (2 percent calories from fat); 1 g protein; 11 g carbohydrate; 0 mg cholesterol; 267 mg sodium.

Basic Pizza Sauce

TOPS ONE MEDIUM PIZZA

For a spicier sauce add another ¼ teaspoon red pepper flakes. Make double and triple batches and store in jars in your freezer.

³/₄	cup white wine
1	teaspoon garlic powder
2	cloves garlic, minced

1¼	cups canned, plain tomato sauce
2	tablespoons tomato paste
1	tablespoon frozen apple juice concentrate
1	teaspoon dried basil
½	teaspoon dried oregano
⅛	teaspoon red pepper flakes

Heat the wine and garlic powder in a medium saucepan over medium heat until it boils; add the minced garlic and sauté about 30 seconds. Add tomato sauce and remaining ingredients; bring to a boil. Reduce heat and simmer, uncovered, for 8 minutes, stirring frequently.

Per serving: 34 calories; 0.1 g fat (5.1 percent calories from fat); 1 g protein; 4 g carbohydrate; 0 mg cholesterol; 236 mg sodium.

Pizza Sauce Cruda

TOPS ONE MEDIUM PIZZA

I use canned tomatoes, but you can use fresh plum tomatoes, cut into chunks, if you like. If you are making the Roasted Garlic Pizza (see page 266), add 1 tablespoon of fresh chopped basil.

½	cup white wine
1	teaspoon garlic powder
3	cloves garlic, sliced
1	teaspoon lemon juice
28	ounces canned tomatoes, drained
1	teaspoon salt
1	tablespoon frozen apple juice concentrate

Heat the wine and garlic powder in a large, heavy saucepan. Add the fresh garlic and lemon juice. Cook, stirring, for about 30–60 seconds. Add the remaining ingredients and cook briskly over medium heat, stirring frequently, for 15–20 minutes or until the tomatoes cook down to a thick mass. Remove the sauce and press through a colander with a spoon. (Do not use a blender or food processor as it will crush the seeds and leave a bitter taste.)

Per serving: 34 calories; 0.3 g fat (8.2 percent calories from fat); 1 g protein; 5 g carbohydrate; 0 mg cholesterol; 429 mg sodium.

The Classic Cheese Pizza

MAKES 6 SERVINGS

When it comes to pizza, most of the television commercials show someone taking a bite as the melted cheese pulls away in long, gooey strings. It looks fattening, and it *is* fattening—but this one isn't and it's just as luscious and cheesy. If you don't have time to make pizza crust from scratch (or you haven't frozen one you made earlier), look for a fat-free pizza crust in your freezer section. When buying a pizza sauce, look for one that is not only fat free but has a low sugar content.

1	pizza crust (recipe page 253), prebaked for 5 minutes
1¹/₂	cups fat-free pizza sauce (bottled or see page 255)
¹/₂	cup fresh basil, chopped
6	ounces grated fat-free mozzarella cheese
3	tablespoons grated Parmesan cheese
¹/₈	teaspoon salt
¹/₈	teaspoon cracked pepper

Preheat oven to 350°. Keeping the prebaked crust on the baking sheet (or in the baking pan), spread the sauce on top, leaving a half-inch sauce-free border. Distribute the fresh basil, mozzarella, and Parmesan over the crust. Season with salt and pepper (you may want to eliminate the pepper if this pizza is for the kids). Bake the pizza for 10–15 minutes, or until the cheese begins to bubble but doesn't brown. Let cool slightly and slice into pizza wedges. Serve with a salad.

Per serving: 381 calories; 2.1 g fat (14.7 percent calories from fat); 12 g protein; 15 g carbohydrate; 5 mg cholesterol; 534 mg sodium.

Garden Pizza

MAKES 6 SERVINGS

This is a great meal or appetizer for all of you who work hard, come home tired, and want something tasty *and* easy. Don't limit yourself to the vegetables called for here; be creative and toss your favorites on top. Also try adding some pinto, navy, or black beans.

1	pizza crust (see page 253), prebaked for 5 minutes
1¹/₂	cups fat-free pizza sauce (bottled or see page 255)

$^{1}/_{2}$	cup frozen chopped onions, defrosted and drained
$^{1}/_{4}$	cup frozen chopped green bell pepper, defrosted and drained
$^{1}/_{4}$	cup shredded zucchini
$^{1}/_{4}$	cup shredded carrots
$^{1}/_{2}$	cup frozen corn, defrosted and drained
$^{1}/_{2}$	cup frozen peas, defrosted and drained
$^{1}/_{2}$	cup frozen asparagus spears, defrosted and drained, sliced into 1-inch pieces
6	ounces shredded fat-free Monterey Jack cheese
	nonstick vegetable oil spray

Preheat oven to 350°. Keeping the prebaked crust on the baking sheet (or in the baking pan), spread the sauce on top, leaving a half-inch sauce-free border. Top the pizza first with the onions and bell pepper; then the shredded zucchini and carrots; corn and peas; and finally the asparagus. Scatter the cheese over the pizza (add more if you like). Bake for about 10 minutes or until the cheese bubbles. Don't let the crust get too brown. Let cool slightly and slice into pizza wedges.

Per serving: 167 calories; 2.5 g fat (17.1 percent calories from fat); 11 g protein; 16 g carbohydrate; 3 mg cholesterol; 634 mg sodium.

Mexican Pizza

MAKES 6 SERVINGS

Who said pizza is the sole domain of the Italians? With all of the great new fat-free bean dips on the market you can really jazz up this Mexican-style pizza. If you don't want to go to the trouble of making a crust, try layering oil-free whole wheat tortillas on the pizza pan. Other toppings you can add if desired: pickled jalapeños or canned green chilies.

1	pizza crust (recipe page 253), prebaked for 5 minutes
1	cup fat-free pinto or black bean dip
1	cup frozen corn, cooked
$^{1}/_{2}$	each: red and green bell peppers, chopped
2	ounces grated low-fat mozzarella cheese
2	ounces fat-free mild Mexican or cheddar cheese
$^{3}/_{4}$	cup salsa (I like Pace Picante)
$^{1}/_{2}$	cup sliced black olives

Preheat oven to 350°. Keeping the prebaked crust on the baking sheet (or in the baking pan), spread the bean dip evenly over the top, leaving a half-inch dip-free border. Distribute the corn and chopped peppers over the crust, then the cheeses and salsa. Garnish with the black olives. Bake for about 10 minutes, or until the cheese is melted and bubbly. Let cool slightly and slice into pizza wedges.

Per serving: 164 calories; 3.2 g fat (21.7 percent calories from fat); 10 g protein; 16 g carbohydrate; 2 mg cholesterol; 273 mg sodium.

Roasted Bell Pesto Pizza

MAKES 6 SERVINGS

Roasted red peppers and basil give this pizza pizzazz. And you will enjoy it all the better knowing that you don't have to take the time to roast the peppers yourself (a messy, time-consuming process); the ones in the jar work quite well.

2	cloves garlic
1/2	cup chopped fresh basil leaves, stems removed
1/2	teaspoon pepper
2	tablespoons oil-free Italian salad dressing
1/3	cup fat-free pizza sauce (bottled or see page 255)
1	pizza crust (recipe page 253), prebaked for 5 minutes
1	13-ounce jar water-packed roasted red peppers
10	small black olives, pitted
1	cup grated fat-free mozzarella

Preheat oven to 350°. Place the garlic and basil in a food processor or blender and process until well chopped. Add the pepper, process again to combine, then add the salad dressing; process until a pesto paste forms. Keeping the prebaked crust on the baking sheet (or in the baking pan), spread the sauce over the top, leaving a half-inch sauce-free border. Top with the peppers, olives, and cheese. Drizzle the pesto mixture over the pizza. Bake for 10 minutes or until the cheese is melted and bubbly. Let cool slightly and slice into pizza wedges.

Per serving: 157 calories; 1.5 g fat (12.2 percent calories from fat); 17 g protein; 7 g carbohydrate; 6 mg cholesterol; 614 mg sodium.

Roasted Garlic Pizza

For this pizza, or any Italian-style pizza, you might try replacing the popcorn seasoning in the #1 crust recipe with garlic powder. Also keep in mind that you don't have to use any crust at all: a sourdough baguette split in half will work as a base just as well. It's the combination of the fresh basil and roasted garlic (you can buy garlic cloves already peeled in the market as a time-saver) that give this pizza its great flavor. I find that it's a favorite with kids.

9   cloves garlic, peeled and sliced
olive-flavored nonstick vegetable oil spray
1   pizza crust (recipe page 253), unbaked
1½   cups fat-free pizza sauce (bottled or see page 255)
1   cup whole basil leaves, stems removed
8   ounces grated fat-free mozzarella cheese
¼   cup sliced black olives

Preheat oven to 350°. Place the garlic cloves on a sheet of aluminum foil spritzed with the vegetable oil spray. Fold the aluminum foil up and around the garlic to make a "boat" and seal the edges. Place in a 350° toaster oven for about 10 minutes, or until brown. Remove and set aside. Roll out the pizza dough into a rectangle 12 × 16 inches. Spritz a baking sheet or baking pan with the vegetable oil spray and place the dough on the sheet or in the pan. Bake for about 10 minutes, or until lightly brown but not doughy. Spread the pasta sauce on the crust, leaving a half-inch, sauce-free border, then scatter the roasted garlic on top. Top with the basil leaves, then the mozzarella. Garnish with the olives. Return the pizza to the oven for 5–10 minutes, or until the cheese is melted and bubbly. Let cool slightly and slice into pizza wedges. Serve with a crisp salad.

Per serving: 152 calories; 2.4 g fat (18.2 percent calories from fat); 13 g protein; 11 g carbohydrate; 4 mg cholesterol; 460 mg sodium.

Smoked Chicken Pizza

I created this pizza for a client who had an addiction to the smoked chicken pizza at his favorite restaurant. That one, though, wasn't as low in fat as this one. For a really smoky flavor, marinate the raw chicken in the hickory flavoring, and then grill, shred, and put on the pizza. If you're in a rush and don't have the time to cook the chicken, use canned chicken meat and marinate in the hickory flavoring.

1/4	**cup hickory flavoring**
2	**6-ounce boneless skinless chicken breasts, cooked and shredded into 1/4-inch strips**
1	**pizza crust (recipe page 253), prebaked for 5 minutes**
1	**cup fat-free pizza sauce (bottled or see page 255)**
1	**onion, diced**
1/2	**green bell pepper, diced**
6	**ounces grated fat-free Jack cheese**

Preheat oven to 350°. Place the hickory flavoring in a bowl, then add the chicken. Coat thoroughly and allow to marinate for about 10 minutes. Keeping the prebaked crust on the baking sheet (or in the baking pan), spread the pizza sauce evenly over the crust, leaving a half-inch sauce-free border, then sprinkle on the onion and bell pepper. Place the shredded chicken across the top, sprinkle with cheese, adding more or less to your taste. Bake for 10–15 minutes, or until the cheese melts and is bubbly.

Per serving: *172 calories; 1 g fat (7.5 percent calories from fat); 22 g protein; 7 g carbohydrate; 36 mg cholesterol; 491 mg sodium.*

Chapter Twelve

Help for the Holidays: Feasting Without the Fat

Every year it's the same old story. And I don't just mean seeing your savings account drain or standing in line to return all of those unwanted gifts again. I mean that you inevitably feel stressed out and have the dubious achievement of hitting the national average: a weight gain of seven pounds.

Why do we repeat this cycle year after year? Is there any way around it that doesn't involve just disappearing for the last three months of the year? How can we break the habit of confronting the same old New Year's resolution: "I will lose weight, I will keep it off, and I will spend a fortune on every diet product advertised on television"?

The cycle of holiday bingeing and post-holiday remorse has become so dependable that, come January, the commercial diet industry pulls out all the stops, hoping to sell you everything that ever related to losing an ounce. Have you ever noticed how television ads for toys lead right into television ads for weight-loss aids and diet centers? It's like clockwork.

So, ladies and gentlemen, step this way, and get off the merry-go-round. Stop looking at the holiday season as a chance to make up for all the chocolate, pastries, fat-filled hors d'oeuvres, and circles of Brie that you avoided all year long. Change your attitude, and change your lifestyle. Think of all those people who will be making New Year's resolutions to lose weight and beat them to the punch: Don't gain an ounce over the holidays and spend your money on a new outfit for January (or keep your savings intact) instead of shelling out big bucks to a diet center.

I'm going to be honest with you here (not that I ever mince words otherwise). If there's one thing I can't abide it's when someone who has gained weight feels like a victim. And that's how most people feel during the holidays. They feel "obligated" to munch on every goodie passed around the office. Obligated to chow down on the delights served at their kids' school parties, at cocktail parties, neighborhood celebrations—wherever, they feel like it's their duty to dip into the candies and treats at every stop along the way. Yes, it's the time of year when glorious goodies are literally pushed into our faces. And we don't want to be rude. But do we want to be fat?

Okay, so now you're thinking, Yolanda is Scrooge in disguise! That's not true. I love the holidays. I think it's a wonderful time for giving, treating oneself and others. But that doesn't mean you have to use it as an excuse to indulge in every, well . . . indulgence. Pick and choose the ones that entice you the most, then leave the rest.

My neighbor Sherry and her family are Jewish and we get together each year to celebrate our Christian holidays along with their Jewish traditions. Potentially, this could be a killer to both Sherry's and my figures. However, Sherry has learned to cut the fat from about 85 percent of her holiday dishes; the rest she leaves in their traditionally rich form. I have done the same with my main dishes and desserts. I trim the fat where I can, and keep the flavor and pleasure where they belong.

One year I revised a family of five's Thanksgiving recipes. Left as is, the dishes would have included 6½ sticks of butter. No wonder they couldn't move after dinner! I took the butter out of the main-meal recipes, lightened up the desserts, and allowed sugar and salt to play their part in keeping the food flavorful. They now have a delightful holiday meal that they can repeat year after year and look forward to without guilt—a new tradition.

Healthful, Low-Fat Holiday Recipes

I hope the following recipes will help you create new traditions of your own. Not only were they designed to take the fat out of holiday dining, they were created to address that other holiday dilemma: how to make a great meal without spending hours of time in the kitchen. That's right, these dishes are *easy*. And preparing them will help give you an education on how to cook without added fats.

Every year, my food business prepares Thanksgiving dinner based on these recipes and they're always a hit with clients, among them Clint Black, Lisa Hartman, and their family. My *own* Thanksgiving dinner, a great low-fat feast, has become so famous in Los Angeles that Channel 7 News covered the event last year.

But most important, these recipes and tips are going to allow *you* to take a new stand on the holidays. Determine from October on that you're not going to be a holiday victim. You'll have certain treats, yes, but you're not going to get on a three-month ride and end up in diet land by January. It really is the best gift you can give yourself!

Scallop Mango Seviche

MAKES 10 SERVINGS

This is a healthy alternative to the usual sour cream dips and cheese-and-cracker plates most people put on the table when they're entertaining. It's also a great dish for lunch or a quick snack. While seviche is made from raw fish, it's not like sushi—the acid in the lime juice and vinegar "cooks" the fish. Some notes on the ingredients: Go the antichop route, if you like, by buying bags of frozen sliced red, yellow, and green bell peppers. Thaw and dice. (And some are already diced.) You can also buy mangoes bottled if they're not in season. Be aware, though, that they're packed in sugar, so rinse them under warm water first, then dice.

1	pound scallops, rinsed and quartered if sea scallops (if you're using bay scallops you don't have to quarter them)
1/2	cup raspberry vinegar
1/4	cup bottled unsweetened lime juice
1	teaspoon salt (optional)
1	teaspoon pepper
2	each: red bell peppers, green bell peppers, and yellow bell peppers, cored, seeded, and diced
1 1/2	red onions, diced
2	large mangoes, cut into large cubes
6	plum tomatoes, diced
5	tablespoons chopped fresh cilantro

Place the scallops in a large bowl. Add the raspberry vinegar, lime juice, salt, and pepper. Marinate overnight. Before serving add the diced peppers, onion, mangoes, tomatoes, and cilantro. Add more salt and pepper, to taste. Let the seviche sit in the refrigerator for another 15–20 minutes. Serve with baked no-oil tortilla chips.

Per serving: 116 calories; 1 g fat (6.8 percent calories from fat); 10 g protein; 20 g carbohydrate; 15 mg cholesterol; 298 mg sodium.

Apricot Curried Yams

When you're not going all-out for company you can make an easier version of this recipe for a weekday dinner or lunch. Microwave or bake a yam, split it down the middle, add a little sugar-free apricot jam, a pinch of curry powder, and some raisins, then mash with a fork to blend. Satisfying and quick.

8	yams
1	cup dried apricots, cut into 1/4-inch slices
1/2	cup raisins
1	cup boiling water
1/4	cup white wine
1	onion, chopped
2	teaspoons curry powder
1	teaspoon salt

Preheat oven to 350° if you'll be baking the yams. Prick several times all over with a fork and rinse with water. To cook in the microwave: Put the wet yams in a plastic bag and place in the microwave. Cook on high 10–15 minutes (depending on the size of the yams). Poke with a fork to see if they are soft all the way through. To bake: Wrap the yams in aluminum foil and place in the oven. Bake 15–20 minutes or until soft all the way through. Peel the yams and cut into cubes. Set aside. In a small bowl, combine the apricots, raisins, and boiling water and let sit about ten minutes. In a large saucepan, heat the white wine. Add the onion and cook over medium heat, stirring until softened. Add the curry powder and salt and cook for another 2 minutes. Drain the dried fruit and add it and the cooked yams to the onion mixture. Stir gently over medium heat until warmed through.

Per serving: 210 calories; 0.4 g fat (1.6 percent calories from fat); 3 g protein; 50 g carbohydrate; 0 mg cholesterol; 282 mg sodium.

Baked Orange-Maple Yams

This is my favorite holiday yam recipe, partly because it's so simple, it allows you to concentrate on the hundred other things you have to make for The Big

Dinner. Like everything else about holiday dinners, these get better the next day.

6   yams
1   cup fresh orange juice
¹/₂ cup maple syrup
pinch nutmeg

Preheat oven to 350° if you'll be baking the yams. Prick several times all over with a fork and rinse with water. To cook in the microwave: Put the wet yams in a plastic bag and place in the microwave. Cook on high 10–15 minutes (depending on the size of the yams). Poke with a fork to see if they are soft all the way through. To bake: Wrap yams in aluminum foil and place in the oven. Bake 15–20 minutes or until soft all the way through. Scrape out the meat of the yams and throw away the skins. Place yams in a large mixing bowl. Add the orange juice, maple syrup, and nutmeg, then blend with a whisk until creamy. Transfer to an ovenproof dish and heat. Serve hot.

Per serving: 132 calories; 0.2 g fat (1.4 percent calories from fat); 1 g protein; 32 g carbohydrate; 0 mg cholesterol; 8 mg sodium.

Maple Acorn Confetti Squash

MAKES 8 SERVINGS

Every Thanksgiving, Lisa Hartman and Clint Black order this dish from my food service for their family meal. I, too, love it so much that I often end up eating the mixture before I even stuff the squash. If you can't find the diced dried fruit mix, then dice some dried apricots, apples, figs, and prunes yourself. It's worth the extra trouble.

nonstick vegetable oil spray
3   acorn squash, sliced in half lengthwise (these are large and I
      have found that 3 squash amply serve eight)
2   teaspoons cinnamon
¹/₂ teaspoon nutmeg
1   cup cooked brown rice, cooked with 1 teaspoon poultry
      seasoning
1   cup diced mixed dried fruit

2   tablespoons maple syrup
6   prunes, pitted

Preheat oven to 350°. Spritz a cookie sheet with vegetable oil spray and place the squash open side down on top. Bake for 20 minutes, or until squash is soft all the way through. Scoop out the meat of the squash, leaving about 1/2 inch in the skin. In a large bowl, combine squash meat with the cinnamon and nutmeg. Mix in the rice, diced dried fruit mix, and maple syrup. Fill each squash shell with the mixture and place one prune in the middle of each half. Bake for 15 minutes.

Per serving: 161 calories; 0.6 g fat (2.8 percent calories from fat); 3 g protein; 40 g carbohydrate; 0 mg cholesterol; 8 mg sodium.

Holiday Broccoli Puree

MAKES 4 SERVINGS

You can also make this recipe using carrots, green beans, peas, turnips, or cauliflower. Add other spices, to taste.

1   bunch broccoli, trimmed and sliced
1   tablespoon plain nonfat yogurt
1   tablespoon nonfat sour cream
1/2 teaspoon Dijon mustard
1   teaspoon poultry seasoning
1   pinch red pepper flakes, crushed

Puree the broccoli in a food processor or blender, making sure the mixture doesn't get too sudsy. Add the yogurt, sour cream, and mustard and process for 30 seconds more. Transfer to a medium-size nonstick saucepan and add the seasonings. Heat through and serve hot. Top with a dollop of mustard in the middle.

Per serving: 12 calories; 0.1 g fat (8.9 percent calories from fat); 1 g protein; 2 g carbohydrate; 0 mg cholesterol; 20 mg sodium.

Spinach Parmesan and Mushroom Squares

MAKES 8 SERVINGS

The choice is yours: Serve this as an appetizer or side dish. Either way, it's delightfully fluffy and rich, not to mention low in fat (only 1 gram per square—thank heaven for egg whites and fat-free cheeses).

½	cup white wine
¾	pound mushrooms, sliced
4	scallions, sliced thin
1	teaspoon poultry seasoning
1	tablespoon Worcestershire sauce
3	10-ounce packages frozen chopped spinach, drained
1½	cups whole wheat bread crumbs
1	cup low-fat cottage cheese
½	cup grated fat-free cheddar cheese
6	egg whites
	nonstick vegetable oil spray

Preheat oven to 350°. In a large nonstick skillet, bring the wine to a boil. Add the mushrooms and scallions and sauté over medium heat until tender. Add the poultry seasoning, Worcestershire sauce, and drained spinach. Blend well and transfer to a mixing bowl. Add the bread crumbs, cottage cheese, and cheddar cheese. Blend. Beat the egg whites until stiff and fold into the spinach mixture. Spritz a 13 × 9 × 2-inch baking dish with vegetable oil spray and transfer the spinach mixture to the dish. Bake uncovered for 30 minutes, or until firm. Let cool for ten minutes before serving. Cut into squares.

Per serving: 211 calories; 2.3 g fat (10.1 percent calories from fat); 17 g protein; 29 g carbohydrate; 3 mg cholesterol; 573 mg sodium.

Spinach Soufflé

MAKES 8 SERVINGS

How can a fancy soufflé be in a book of "no-brainer" recipes? You'll see why when you check out this recipe, another of my best-sellers. This dish can also be made by substituting broccoli or cauliflower for the spinach.

10	ounces frozen chopped spinach, drained and excess water squeezed out
1	13.5-ounce package firm tofu, drained
5	egg whites, lightly beaten
1	teaspoon nutmeg
1	teaspoon cinnamon
$1/2$	teaspoon white pepper
2	tablespoons Dijon mustard
2	tablespoons onion powder
$1^1/2$	tablespoons garlic powder

salt and pepper to taste
nonstick vegetable oil spray

Preheat oven to 350°. Place half of the spinach, half of the tofu, and half of the egg whites in a food processor. Process on high speed until blended. Add the rest of the spinach, tofu, and egg whites and blend again. Add the remaining ingredients, except salt and black pepper, and continue to process as you go along, so that all of the ingredients are blended thoroughly. Add salt and pepper to taste; blend once more. Spritz a shallow baking pan with vegetable oil spray and pour the mixture in. Cover with wax paper and bake for 20 minutes. Remove the wax paper and bake for another 10 minutes, or until a knife run through the middle comes out clean. Serve with a dollop of Dijon mustard and a slice of red beet on top.

Per serving: 90 calories; 3.7 g fat (33.6 percent calories from fat); 10 g protein; 7 g carbohydrate; 0 mg cholesterol; 117 mg sodium.

Cajun Maple Corn Bread Stuffing

MAKES 12 SERVINGS

Stuffing is traditionally fat-packed, but you'll never miss the fat in this sweet and savory recipe (undoubtedly, you won't miss the fat on your hips either). This goes well with Cornish game hens, turkey, or roast chicken.

6	cups No-Brainer Cajun Corn Bread (see page 95)
1	cup white wine
1	cup defatted chicken broth
2	cups chopped onion

2   cups chopped celery
2   eggs, lightly beaten
¼   cup chopped fresh parsley
½   cup maple syrup
      salt and pepper to taste
      nonstick vegetable oil spray

Preheat oven to 350°. Cube the premade corn bread into large 2-inch chunks and set side. In a large nonstick skillet heat the white wine and ½ cup broth. Add the onion and celery and cook until softened, about 5 minutes. Transfer to a large bowl and add the corn bread, beaten eggs, and parsley; stir. Slowly add the remaining chicken broth, tossing until the stuffing is moist. Drizzle the maple syrup across the top and stir once more. Season with salt and pepper and stuff the bird. Place the remaining stuffing into a shallow baking dish or casserole spritzed with vegetable oil spray. Cover the dish with aluminum foil or a lid and bake for about 30 minutes. Stir after 15 minutes and check to see if the stuffing is drying out. If so, then add some juices from the poultry-roasting pan, and stir.

Per serving: 187 calories; 2.6 g fat (13 percent calories from fat); 6 g protein; 33 g carbohydrate; 95 mg cholesterol; 249 mg sodium.

Unstuffing Bread Stuffing

MAKES 16 SERVINGS

This stuffing got its name because it won't leave you feeling overstuffed—you'll even have room for dessert. The other great thing about this stuffing is that it stays moist whether you cook it in or out of the bird. Since the bird holds only 4 to 5 servings, much of this recipe actually gets cooked in a pan. Thus, it won't get the benefit of the moistening juices from the bird, but thanks to liberal amounts of gravy and chicken broth—not thanks to added fat, what most classic recipes call for—it still won't dry out. One important thing to note is that, because stuffing does dry out so easily, most stuffing mixes, even the ones that are just bread cubes, have added fat. That's why I think it's best to make your own. And when you do, don't be afraid to add a lot of liquid to make up for the lack of fat; as you bake your stuffing, the liquid will evaporate, so keep pouring in more. For holiday cooking, I keep a can of chicken broth open at all times for that very purpose.

6	cups whole wheat bread crumbs
2	cups white wine, plus extra as needed
4	shallots, minced
1	cup chopped celery, with leaves
1½	cups chopped onion
1	green bell pepper, chopped
1½	cups sliced mushrooms
1	cup oil-free Italian salad dressing
2	tablespoons poultry seasoning

pinch red pepper flakes

| 2 | packages Hain gravy mix |
| 2 | cups defatted chicken broth |

nonstick vegetable oil spray

Preheat oven to 350°. Place the bread crumbs in a large bowl. Heat the wine in a large nonstick sauté pan. Add the shallots and cook over medium heat for about 2 minutes, or until slightly transparent. Add the celery, onion, and green pepper and cook until all are a little soft but still crunchy. Add the mushrooms and cook 5 minutes more, until softened. Keep adding a little white wine as you go if the liquid evaporates. Transfer the cooked vegetables to the bowl with the bread crumbs. Add the salad dressing and seasonings and stir to thoroughly combine. Prepare the Hain gravy mix according to the package instructions, but substitute chicken broth for water. Add half of the gravy to the bread crumb mixture. Mix thoroughly. Stuff your bird with as much of the stuffing as fits. Cook the bird according to directions. When the bird has 20 minutes more to roast, spritz a shallow baking pan with vegetable oil spray and place the remaining stuffing in the pan. Drizzle the remaining gravy mix over the top. Cover with aluminum foil and bake for 20 minutes. Keep checking for moistness and add more broth if it's drying out.

Per serving: 364 calories; 4.8 g fat (13.3 percent calories from fat); 10 g protein; 61 g carbohydrate; 0 mg cholesterol; 895 mg sodium.

Wild Rice Stuffing

MAKES 12 SERVINGS

Frankly, this is my favorite stuffing. I love wild rice and its crunchy, nutty flavor. Mixed with the moist brown rice, this is a lovely stuffing that adds color to the plate. If there is any left over, toss it with chopped fresh vegetables and vinaigrette for a lunchtime salad.

1	**pound wild rice**
2	**cups brown rice**
5¹/₂	**cups white wine**
4	**shallots, minced**
1	**cup chopped onion**
5	**ribs celery, chopped fine**
1	**pound mushrooms, sliced**
2	**tablespoons poultry seasoning**
1	**cup canned sliced water chestnuts, drained**
pinch	**red pepper flakes**
4	**eggs, lightly beaten**
¹/₂	**cup defatted chicken broth**
1	**cup oil-free Italian salad dressing**

Preheat oven to 350°. Cook the wild rice and brown rice according to package directions, omitting any oil the recipe calls for. Set aside in a large bowl. Heat half the wine in a large nonstick sauté pan. Add the shallots, onion, and celery. Cook until soft but still crunchy. Add a little more wine, the mushrooms, and 1 tablespoon of the poultry seasoning. Cook for another 2 minutes. Add the vegetable mixture to the wild rice and brown rice; stir to blend. Add the rest of the ingredients and stir until blended. If it looks too dry, add a little more salad dressing or broth. Stuff the bird, and place the rest in a casserole pan. Cover the pan with aluminum foil and heat in the oven for 15 minutes; stir, then heat for another 5 minutes, or until heated through.

Per serving: 202 calories; 2.4 g fat (15.6 percent calories from fat); 6 g protein; 23 g carbohydrate; 71 mg cholesterol; 96 mg sodium.

Yolanda's Famous Gravy

MAKES 8 SERVINGS

What I've done here is taken a good thing and made it better. As you may have already noticed, I often use Hain gravy mix, a wonderful convenience food. Here I've doctored it up just a bit to make it more fresh tasting and flavorful. While this gravy is terrific for special occasions, it's also a terrific topper for everyday potato, chicken, and vegetable dishes. Make it in batches and store it in jars in the fridge or freezer.

1   cup red wine
1   tablespoon minced shallot
3   cups defatted chicken broth
2   teaspoons poultry seasoning
1   teaspoon rosemary
1   teaspoon minced garlic
$^1/_2$ teaspoon onion powder
4   packages Hain gravy mix
salt and pepper to taste

Heat the red wine in a large saucepan until just bubbling. Add the minced shallot. Cook until the shallot is transparent, then add the chicken broth and seasonings. Stirring with a whisk, add the Hain gravy mix. Season with salt and pepper, and keep stirring until the gravy starts to boil. Remove from heat and transfer to a gravy boat.

Per serving: 64 calories; 0 g fat (1 percent calories from fat); 2.4 g protein; 8.4 g carbohydrate; 0 mg cholesterol; 2 mg sodium.

Bourbon Dijon Brown Sugar Turkey

MAKES 12 SERVINGS

The glaze used in this turkey dish is also wonderful on roast chicken and Cornish game hens. If you don't want to use brown sugar, you can use Sucanat, the natural cane sugar available at health food stores. Honey or maple syrup can work, too. If you have the luxury of roasting your bird on an outdoor grill, this is the way to go. The aroma alone will create long-lasting memories.

nonstick vegetable oil spray
1   12–14 pound turkey
salt and pepper to taste

Glaze

$^3/_4$ cup bourbon
$^1/_4$ cup Dijon mustard

¹/₄	cup packed dark brown sugar plus 1 tablespoon
1	tablespoon Dijon mustard plus 1 tablespoon

Preheat oven to 325°. Spritz a roasting rack with vegetable oil spray and place on the bottom of a roasting pan. Remove giblets and neck from turkey and reserve for stock (discard the liver). Remove any visible fat. Rinse the turkey inside and out with cold water and pat dry. Season with salt and pepper. Stuff the bird with the stuffing of your choice (I recommend Cajun Maple Corn Bread Stuffing, page 269) and secure the neck cavity with a skewer.

To make glaze: In a small bowl, combine ¹/₄ cup of the bourbon, ¹/₄ cup mustard, and ¹/₄ cup of the sugar; stir to blend. With your fingers, gently lift the skin of the turkey and rub half the glaze on the meat. Tie the drumsticks and tuck the wings behind the turkey's back. Place the bird breast side up in the prepared roasting pan. Cover with aluminum foil and roast for 2¹/₂ hours. Remove the foil and baste with the reserved glaze and pan juices. Add the remaining mustard and sugar to the pan juices as you baste. If the liquid is evaporating, also add a little bourbon as you baste.

Per 3.5-ounce serving (breast alone, no skin): 81 calories; 0.6 g fat (11 percent calories from fat); 5 g protein; 6 g carbohydrate; 11 mg cholesterol; 92 mg sodium.

Skinny Pumpkin Pie

MAKES 8 SERVINGS

Pumpkin pie has the advantage of employing a lot of spices, and lots of spices means that the taste buds are busy with every bite—they don't need fat to keep them happy. If you'd like to make this pie more natural, substitute the ¹/₂ cup brown sugar with ¹/₄ cup FruitSource. And if you find that the crust is too dry, add a little applesauce to the mix.

2	cups canned pumpkin puree
1¹/₂	cups evaporated skim milk
¹/₂	cup maple syrup
¹/₂	cup brown sugar
1	teaspoon cinnamon
¹/₂	teaspoon ground ginger
¹/₄	teaspoon ground nutmeg
1	pinch cloves

3   egg whites, lightly beaten

1   Graham Cracker Crust (see page 300)

Preheat oven to 350°. Combine the pumpkin, milk, maple syrup, brown sugar, cinnamon, ginger, nutmeg, and cloves in a small saucepan and heat, stirring constantly, until the maple syrup has melted. Add the egg whites and stir until blended. Fill the cooled pie shell and bake for 1 hour, or until a toothpick inserted in the middle comes out clean. Serve slices with a dollop of Whip It Slim (see page 301).

Per serving, not including Whip It Slim: 184 calories; 2 g fat (9 percent calories from fat); 6 g protein; 37 g carbohydrate; 8 mg cholesterol; 98 mg sodium.

Pumpkin Chiffon Pie

MAKES 8 SERVINGS

I just had to use the word chiffon at least once in this book. I love to use tofu, but I know most people wrinkle their noses at it. As a matter of fact, I always have to camouflage it when I serve it at home. This is the perfect way to do so. The filling has a creamy texture and a great flavor, so along with the Wheat Germ Pie Crust, this is the way to go for a holiday dessert.

1½   cups firm tofu

2   cups canned pumpkin puree

²/₃   cup honey

1   teaspoon vanilla extract

1½   teaspoons cinnamon

¼   teaspoon nutmeg

⅛   teaspoon ground cloves

1   unbaked Wheat Germ Piecrust (recipe page 276)

Preheat oven to 250°. Puree the tofu in a food processor or blender until smooth. Add the remaining ingredients, except the piecrust, and blend well. Pour the pumpkin mixture into the pie shell. Bake for one hour. The filling should be soft but will firm up—chill for 30 minutes before serving.

Per serving: 178 calories; 4 g fat (18 percent calories from fat); 7 g protein; 33 g carbohydrate; 0 mg cholesterol; 12 mg sodium.

Wheat Germ Piecrust

As you know, I'm not a huge fan of margarine, so I feel a bit hypocritical using it in this recipe. But it is nearly (although not totally) impossible to make a piecrust without any fat to hold it together. I love this crust, though, because it adds a slightly nutty flavor to the filling. And wheat germ is a nutritional star that's rich in zinc, selenium, B vitamins, and vitamin E. If you prefer graham cracker flavor to wheat germ, go ahead and use an equal amount of graham cracker crumbs instead.

1	egg white
2	teaspoons water
1½	cups toasted wheat germ
⅓	cup packed brown sugar
1	tablespoon margarine, preferably soybean margarine, chilled
1	teaspoon cinnamon

In a medium bowl, combine the egg white and water and beat until frothy. Add the wheat germ and sugar. Cut the margarine into the wheat germ mixture until the mixture becomes crumbly. Press into an 8-inch pie pan. Cover with aluminum foil until ready to use. Fill with the pie filling of your choice and bake according to pie instructions.

Per serving, crust only: *122 calories; 3 g fat (19 percent calories from fat); 7 g protein; 20 g carbohydrate; 0 mg cholesterol; 17 mg sodium.*

Chapter Thirteen

Desserts You Deserve

Dessert is misunderstood. Most people believe that if you care at all about your weight, you should simply avoid it. They think that any dessert short of plain fruit is just plain bad—nutrient free and packed with all the things, like sugar and fat, we shouldn't be eating.

But let's get to the simple truth here. Number one is that dessert is not a meal; it's not food we look to for vitamins and other nutrients. Dessert is made to be, and supposed to be, sinful. That doesn't mean that it has to be a total bomb to your body, but it should still be delightful. When we eat dessert, we're eating to give pleasure to our palate; we don't eat it to satisfy our appetite. Tell me, do you crave dessert because you're really still hungry after dinner? No, dessert exists purely for pleasure. And it should taste sinful, whether it truly is or not.

Here is another simple truth: Dessert doesn't have to be a diet disaster. It's indeed possible to give dessert the reverence it deserves while giving our figures the reverence *they* deserve at the same time.

When I started making meals for my home delivery service, I happily took on the challenge of creating things like fat-free pesto sauce and skinny enchiladas. But when people asked if I made healthy desserts, I sort of hit a wall. At first I wasn't interested in the challenge of making desserts without butter, oil, or refined sugar. Angelic desserts seemed a little like nonalcoholic wine; since it's stripped of its essential element, you kind of have to wonder, why bother? But after doing some research, I found it was possible to create desserts that bridge the gap between healthy and hedonistic. Now the joy and happiness of eating lean foods is fully rounded out. Nothing is missing.

Which isn't to say that all my desserts are paragons of dietary virtue. I'll admit, when it comes to these sweets, I break some of my own rules—you might even think I sound hypocritical. I prefer to think of it as just being realistic. Do I believe in using natural sugars over refined sugar? Yes. But do I use refined sugar in some recipes? Yup. Although I try to use a fruit juice concentrate, honey, or rice syrup rather than refined sugar, there are some desserts that just don't taste as good when made with these substitutes. And I don't think having a little refined sugar now and then is so bad anyway. It has always been my belief that if you clean up 85 or 90 percent of your daily diet, you can afford to have treats!

Treats, by definition (at least by my definition), are things that you have once in a while. In the land of plenty, we have access to candy bars, ice cream, cookies, and snack cakes whenever we please. We can have them anytime—but that doesn't mean we should. You can have a drink anytime, too, but that doesn't mean you should. It causes problems.

I remember taking a few of my daughter's friends for ice cream after school one day, and one of the girls asked for three scoops on her cone. I said no, I was only buying one scoop for everybody. She whipped out her little purse and said, "I have my own money, I'm buying three scoops!" My daughter gave me a look indicating that she thought I was being the mean, chintzy mom. Even so, I proceeded to buy the other girls one scoop.

Later we discussed what had happened and I explained to her that it wasn't about the money, it was about the fact that no one *needs* three scoops of ice cream after school. This is why people are getting fat. They want, expect, and get too much. I can have it, therefore I *will* have it, and have it whenever I want. They don't respect dessert or see it for what it is: a once-in-a-while thing. No other country serves up desserts, candy, sodas, and other assorted junk foods in such huge sizes. I mean, just think of 7-Eleven's Big Gulp. Does anyone really need a drink that big? (Does anyone really need a Big Gulp to begin with? But that's another story.) Do we need to have our candy bars jumbo size? I think the old cliché "abuse it, lose it" applies here. Eat too many sweets and you'll lose your figure and your health (and, quite possibly, your teeth).

Eat the right sweets in moderate amounts, however, and you'll be happy. I really believe that desserts should be delicious and taste decadent, but not be over the top when it comes to fat and sugar. And thanks, in large part, to the many great new fat-free chocolate sauces and natural fat substitutes on the market today, that's possible. So although many of my desserts are not sugar free, they are all low in fat and calories.

They're also easy. If most of us feel we don't even have enough time to cook meals, how must we feel about the very thought of slaving over a stove to make desserts? Just the very word "baking" sends many of us reeling away from the kitchen. That's why the dessert recipes here are all no-brainers, simple and quick. Plus, once you've made one of these desserts the recipe is so elementary that you will remember it, and probably not even have to look at

Tips, Tricks, and Thoughts on Dessert

Here are a few tips for slimming down the dessert recipes you already use.

- The best thing to happen to desserts are natural fat replacements like WonderSlim Fat & Egg Substitute and Just Like Shortening. These can be used to replace butter, oil, and shortening in recipes, as can applesauce, baby food prunes, and plum puree. You'll be surprised at how they make a traditional recipe just as moist. (See page 96 for measurement equivalents.)

- Unadulterated cocoa is not in itself fattening, but chocolate is because it's made by adding fat and sugar to cocoa to soften its natural bitterness. Some cocoa powders, however, do contain fat—and they are the ones to beware of when you're baking. Try WonderSlim, for instance, which makes a 99 percent fat-free cocoa powder. Check the fat content of your local brand.

- By now you're probably tired of hearing me rave about the new fat-free and natural chocolate sauces on the market, but I can't say enough about them—they taste great! I like Wax Orchards (full line) and Newmarket (two chocolate flavors and one butterscotch). They are based on fruit concentrates and cocoa, or rice syrup and cocoa.

- When a dessert recipe calls for cream, use 1 percent, skim milk, or evaporated skim milk instead.

- To reduce the cholesterol content of a dessert, substitute natural egg replacements like Nulaid for regular eggs.

- The problem with most commercial cake mixes is that they're 90 percent chemicals. And frankly, the cakes taste that way: artificial. But there are now many natural cake mixes put out by natural food companies that contain only wholesome ingredients—all they've done is premix the dry ingredients for you (a great time-saver), leaving you to add the wet ones. In doing so, they allow you to make the choice of whether you prefer to use a fat replacement or oil, whole eggs or egg whites, skim milk or whole milk (you know the choices I recommend).

- Look for Hain gelatin and pudding mixes, great natural alternatives to use in pie and cake recipes.

- Any kind of fat-free cookie can be used to make a pie crust. Let them go stale and become hard, then freeze the cookies, place them frozen in the food processor and process until they become crumbs. (You'll need about 1½ cups crumbs.) Spritz a pie plate with butter-flavored nonstick vegetable spray, mix the crumbs with ½ cup milk and one lightly beaten egg white, then press the mixture into the pan using a little water to make it stick together.

• When a dessert recipe calls for nuts, which are high in fat, you have two healthy options: simply reduce the amount of nuts, or use walnut, almond, or hazelnut extract to keep the flavor in and cut the fat out. Better yet, soak some raisins in the nut extract of your choice and add those to the batter. They'll be chewy and impart the nut flavor to your dessert.

the book the next time around. So be brave and try a few of these healthy wonders. I've scooped the fat out and kept the sin in.

No-Brainer Desserts

These easy and sumptuous desserts can be made at the drop of a hat.

Angel Food Cake Get thee to a market and buy one of the best premade low-calorie desserts around. Do, however, check the ingredients list just to make sure they haven't junked up a naturally benign recipe. Serve the cake topped with frozen, defrosted cut-up fruit, a drizzling of fat-free fudge, berry, or whipped berry topping (see below).

Pureed Frozen Fruit Topping/Sorbet Use the chopped frozen fruit that comes in bags. Place it in a blender or food processor and process until smooth. I like to keep quart bags of different kinds of frozen fruit—berries, peaches, mango—in my freezer at all times, ready to be pureed at a moment's notice. To sweeten the fruit, add ½ cup of sugar or ¼ cup honey to one bag of frozen fruit. Eat the puree by itself or serve over frozen nonfat yogurt or low-fat cake.

Berry Topping Blend with a fork or whisk sugar-free jam and frozen berries (defrosted and drained)—the proportions you use depend on how sweet you want to the mixture to be. Makes a great cake frosting or filling.

Whipped Berry Topping Make Whip It Slim (see page 301) and combine with the berry and jam mixture above, then use it to top baked apples or angel food cake.

Nonfat Tiramisu Cover the bottom of a pie plate with fat-free chocolate cookies. Drizzle with Drambuie or another liqueur (or espresso), then top with the berry, jam, and Whip It Slim mixture above. Repeat alternating cookie, liqueur, and berry mixture layers until you reach the top of the pie plate. (Also see Robin's Tiramisu, page 291.)

Fat-Free Frozen Cookie Sandwich Place banana slices on a caramel or other sweet-flavored rice cake. Drizzle with a dollop of fat-free chocolate sauce, then cover with another rice cake. Place in the freezer until frozen. Or melt 1 cup of fat-free chocolate sauce in a shallow dish and coat the rice cakes on the outside; freeze until frozen.

Vanilla Yogurt Cream This has so many uses. I always have it on hand. Be sure to use natural yogurt instead of one made with gels or starches, which won't drain as well and won't be as creamy. Take a container (8 ounces) of nonfat vanilla yogurt and place it in a paper cone coffee filter that's set in a plastic cone; cover with plastic wrap and let sit for at least 2 hours. (Or use a yogurt strainer, sold at health food and kitchen equipment stores.) The liquid drains out, leaving a dense creamy spread that you can use as an icing or filling. You can sweeten the "cream" by adding 1 teaspoon honey and $1/4$ teaspoon cinnamon. Use on bagels and toast, too! Or, add 1 teaspoon of your favorite herb or spice for "Herbed Yogurt Cream."

Honey Lemon Spread Strain one pint of nonfat lemon yogurt for several hours (as above), then blend with 1 tablespoon of honey. Spread on fat-free blueberry muffins or apple-cinnamon rice cakes.

Strawberry Fluff Icing Strain two pints of nonfat vanilla yogurt for several hours (as above), then blend with 2 tablespoons sugar-free strawberry jam and 1 tablespoon honey. Beat 2 egg whites in a separate bowl until just stiff. Fold into the yogurt mixture and blend until a smooth icing has formed.

Ricotta-Yogurt Cream Combine $1^1/2$ cups nonfat ricotta cheese, 2 cups nonfat vanilla yogurt, and 1 teaspoon cardamom in a bowl. Strain for several hours (as above).

Banana Spread Strain 1 cup of nonfat vanilla yogurt for several hours (as above). Stir in $1/2$ cup dried bananas (available at health food stores) and let soak in the yogurt overnight. Place the yogurt-banana mixture in a blender or food processor and process until smooth. This is a great dessert topping as well as a wonderful spread for toast, bagels, or muffins.

Sweet Tortilla Roll-Ups There's a new line of flavored (honey, blueberry, orange-apricot) whole wheat tortillas on the market now made by Homestyle Kitchens Mexican Foods. For the kids' snacks or breakfast I like to spread the lemon and vanilla yogurt toppings on them, then roll them up. They're delicious.

Chocolate Cheesecake with Chocolate-Kahlúa Sauce
MAKES 1 9-INCH CAKE

Rejoice! Cheesecake is back on the "can have" list. This mocha rendition is made from fat-free cocoa and nonfat yogurt. The cheesecake will come out 2 to 3 inches high. If you'd prefer a thicker, higher one, double the filling recipe.

Crust

2¹/₂	cups fat-free granola
¹/₄	cup warm water
2	tablespoons frozen apple juice concentrate
2	tablespoons honey, melted (place in microwave for 30 seconds)
2	egg whites

Filling

4	cups nonfat Vanilla Yogurt Cream (see page 281)
¹/₂	cup honey
¹/₂	cup sugar
2	teaspoons vanilla
²/₃	cup whole wheat pastry flour
²/₃	cup pastry flour
¹/₂	teaspoon finely grated orange peel
³/₄	cup defatted cocoa powder
4	tablespoons arrowroot
4	egg whites

Chocolate Kahlúa Sauce (see recipe on following page)

To make the crust: Preheat oven to 325°. Place the granola in a food processor or blender and process until fine. In a medium bowl, combine the granola, water, apple juice concentrate, melted honey, and 2 egg whites. Blend with a whisk. Press the mixture into a 9-inch springform pan so it covers the bottom and sides. Bake for 12 to 15 minutes. Let cool, then refrigerate for at least ½ hour.

To make the filling: Preheat oven to 300°. Place the yogurt cream, honey, sugar, vanilla, flours, orange peel, cocoa powder, and arrowroot in a mixing bowl. Beat with an electric mixer on high until well combined. Set aside. In a separate bowl, beat the egg whites into soft peaks and fold into the yogurt mixture. Pour into the chilled crust and bake for 60 to 70 minutes or until firm but slightly jiggly in the center. Loosen edges with a knife and allow to cool for one hour. Refrigerate for 6 hours to set. Slice and drizzle each piece with Chocolate Kahlúa Sauce before serving.

Per serving, cake without sauce: *342 calories; 1.2 g fat (4.2 percent calories from fat); 9.8 g protein; 50.9 g carbohydrate; 2 mg cholesterol; 324 mg sodium.*

Chocolate Kahlúa Sauce

MAKES 1½ CUPS OR 12 SERVINGS

This is wonderful served over fresh or frozen berries, swirled in a cappuccino, drizzled on top of angel food cake, or spooned over poached pears. But it's especially good on top of Chocolate Cheesecake. It's a snap to make—and extremely decadent!

1	tablespoon vanilla
¼	cup Kahlúa
½	cup Wax Orchards Fat-Free Fudge
½	cup skim milk
¼	cup honey
1	teaspoon arrowroot

Combine all ingredients in a saucepan. Cook over medium-low heat, stirring frequently until the mixture forms a light sauce.

Per serving: *57 calories; 0 g fat (0.8 percent calories from fat); 0 g protein; 9 g carbohydrate; 0 mg cholesterol; 6 mg sodium.*

Momma's Grape Juice Pie

As I've mentioned, my mother is a gourmet chef, a great cook, and a dedicated disciple of Julia Child. When she cooks she means business. When we were growing up, she—the last of a dying breed—lived by the rule that when the last cake crumb, or pie slice was finished, it was time to make a new one. Among the sumptuous desserts she made—cheesecakes, Black Forest cakes, walnut brownies, éclairs—this simple pie was our childhood favorite. My mother made it for my daughter, Nolina, recently, and now it's her favorite, too. Trust me, this is an awesome pie!

³/₄	cup sugar
6	tablespoons cornstarch
¹/₄	teaspoon salt
1	teaspoon grated lemon peel
¹/₂	teaspoon cinnamon
2¹/₂	cups grape juice
1	tablespoon lemon juice
1	baked Graham Cracker Crust (see page 300)

Combine the first five ingredients in a medium saucepan. Stir in the grape juice with a whisk and cook over low heat until the mixture reaches a pudding consistency. Add the lemon juice; stir to blend. Let cool. Pour into the baked pie shell, and chill for at least one hour. Top with Whip It Slim (see page 301).

Per serving, not including Whip It Slim: 266 calories; 2.9 g fat (9.8 percent calories from fat); 3 g protein; 57 g carbohydrate; 53 mg cholesterol; 183 mg sodium.

Applesauce Cake

Serve this on any occasion where you might normally serve a pound cake (as in "pound-of-butter" cake). It's a wonderful dessert to serve at Sunday brunch.

1	egg, well beaten
1	cup apple butter

$^1/_2$ cup applesauce
1 tablespoon frozen apple juice concentrate
$^1/_4$ cup sugar
$5^1/_2$ cups flour
2 tablespoons baking soda
$^1/_2$ teaspoon cinnamon
$^1/_2$ cup raisins
$^1/_3$ cup honey
3 egg whites, whipped into stiff peaks
nonstick vegetable oil spray

Preheat oven to 375°. Combine the beaten whole egg, apple butter, apple-sauce, and apple juice concentrate in a large bowl. In a separate large bowl, sift together the sugar, flour, baking soda, and cinnamon. Stir in the raisins. Alternate adding the egg mixture and the honey to the flour mixture. Fold in the egg whites and gently stir to blend. Pour batter into a 9-inch pan spritzed with vegetable oil spray. Bake for 30–35 minutes. Cool before serving. Top this rich cake with frozen fat-free vanilla yogurt.

Per serving: 306 calories; 1.1 g fat (3.1 percent calories from fat); 8 g protein; 67 g carbohydrate; 18 mg cholesterol; 232 mg sodium.

Honey Coffee Cake

MAKES 16 SERVINGS

This is another delicious alternative to a traditional pound cake. It's great plain, with Strawberry Fluff Icing (see page 281), or with Wax Orchards Fat-Free Fudge melted over the top.

3 eggs
$^1/_2$ cup sugar
1 cup honey
1 tablespoon molasses
3 tablespoons WonderSlim Fat & Egg Substitute or 6 tablespoons applesauce or baby food prunes
3 cups all-purpose unbleached flour
1 teaspoon baking powder
1 teaspoon baking soda
$^1/_2$ teaspoon ginger

¹/₂   **teaspoon cinnamon**

¹/₂   **cup cold espresso coffee**

Preheat the oven to 350°. Separate the egg yolks from the whites. Place the yolks in a large bowl and beat well. Add the sugar, honey, molasses, and WonderSlim to the egg yolks. Whisk lightly. In another large bowl, combine the flour, baking powder, baking soda, ginger, and cinnamon. Alternate adding small portions of the dry mixture and small portions of the coffee to the honey-egg mixture, stirring well as you go until all the mixtures are blended. Beat the egg whites until stiff and fold into the batter one quarter at a time. Cut a piece of wax paper the size of the bottom of a 10-inch tube or bundt pan. Place it at the bottom of the pan. Pour the batter into the pan and bake for 1 hour. Allow the cake to cool before removing from the pan, then immediately peel away the wax paper from the top of the cake.

Per serving without icing: 194 calories; 1.2 g fat (5.3 percent calories from fat); 4 g protein; 43 g carbohydrate; 40 mg cholesterol; 115 mg sodium.

Raisin Honey Apple Cake

Makes 8 servings

This simple apple cake is a variation on a Finnish recipe. I like to add some chopped figs (about ¹/₂ cup) for added texture and flavor.

¹/₂   **cup all-purpose unbleached flour**

¹/₂   **cup sugar**

1   **teaspoon baking powder**

1   **teaspoon cinnamon**

pinch nutmeg

¹/₈   **teaspoon salt**

2   **medium apples, cored, peeled, and chopped**

1   **egg, lightly beaten**

1   **teaspoon vanilla extract**

¹/₂   **teaspoon almond flavoring**

¹/₂   **cup raisins**

nonstick vegetable oil spray

¹/₄   **cup honey**

¹/₂   **cup fat-free granola**

Preheat oven to 350°. Combine the flour, sugar, baking powder, cinnamon, nutmeg, and salt in a medium bowl; mix well. Add the apples, stirring lightly to coat. In a small bowl, combine the egg, vanilla, and almond flavoring; add to the apple mixture, stirring until the dry mixture is moistened. Add the raisins and mix until blended thoroughly. Spoon the mixture into a round 9-inch cake pan spritzed with vegetable oil spray. Melt the honey in a glass bowl or measuring cup in the microwave for 30 seconds, or melt on the stove in a small saucepan over low heat. Stir in granola and coat evenly. Spoon this mixture in a thin even layer over the top. Bake for 30 minutes or until lightly browned. Serve topped with nonfat vanilla frozen yogurt or Vanilla Yogurt Cream (see page 281) accompanied by meringue cookies.

Per serving: 182 calories; 1.2 g fat (5.8 percent calories from fat); 2 g protein; 43 g carbohydrate; 27 mg cholesterol; 117 mg sodium.

Chocolate Raspberry Angel Food Cake

MAKES 8 SERVINGS

Not only will company be shocked that this luscious dessert is fat free, they'll think you toiled in the kitchen all day. The truth is, it's the no-brainer of no-brainers.

- 1 whole angel food cake
- 1 cup Wax Orchards Fat-Free Fudge
- 1/2 cup water
- 4 ounces frozen raspberries, thawed and drained
- 2 tablespoons sugar-free raspberry jam
- 1/2 cup fresh raspberries

Slice the angel food cake along its width twice, making three layers. Combine the fudge sauce and water in a small saucepan. Cook over low heat until melted, stirring to blend. (Or place in a microwave-safe container and microwave for 30 seconds.) In a medium-size bowl, combine the thawed raspberries and raspberry jam. Place the bottom layer of the angel food cake on a cake platter. Spread fudge on top, then spread raspberry mixture on top of the fudge. Cover with the middle layer of the cake and repeat. Place the final layer on top, then spread with fudge. Decoratively drizzle 3 teaspoons of the raspberry mixture on top of the fudge. Serve sprinkled with fresh raspberries.

Other fillings to try:

Sliced bananas coated with fat-free chocolate sauce
Whipped Berry Topping (see page 280)
Vanilla Yogurt Cream (see page 281)
Frozen fruit, drained and mixed with honey
Any flavor fruit syrup

Per serving: 249 calories; 0.3 g fat (1 percent calories from fat); 5 g protein; 51 g carbohydrate; 0 mg cholesterol; 382 mg sodium.

Orange Zest Icing

MAKES ICING FOR 1 CAKE

This gives angel food cake some glamour but takes only a few minutes to make.

2   cups confectioners' sugar
2   tablespoons orange zest
1   teaspoon lemon zest
$1/2$ cup fresh orange juice

Place the powdered sugar in a large bowl. Add the orange and lemon zest. Slowly add the orange juice, whisking to combine the mixture. When thoroughly blended and creamy, ice the cake. Refrigerate for 30 minutes before serving.

Per serving: 124 calories; 0.1 g fat (0.5 percent calories from fat); 0 g protein; 32 g carbohydrate; 0 mg cholesterol; 1 mg sodium.

Easy Angel Food Cake Icing

MAKES 1 CUP OR 4 SERVINGS

Call this the ultimate no-brainer! When you need a last-minute dessert, just buy a premade angel food cake, ice it with this icing, and top with fresh or frozen berries. Add some grated orange or lemon peel or almond flavoring to the recipe if you like.

$1/4$ cup skim milk
$1/2$ cup confectioners' sugar
$1/4$ teaspoon vanilla extract

Pour the milk in a small saucepan and heat until warm but not near boiling. Add the other ingredients and whisk until blended. Let cool and ice any angel food cake or cupcakes.

Per serving: 64 calories; 0 g fat (0.6 percent calories from fat); 1 g protein; 16 g carbohydrate; 0 mg cholesterol; 8 mg sodium.

F-U-D-G-E Fudge Cake

MAKES 9 SERVINGS

When I say fudge, I mean fudge! This cake is like a pudding cake: rich, fudgy, and indulgent. Yes, it has sugar, but it's a great low-fat dessert nonetheless. WonderSlim makes a defatted cocoa powder, which I use here, but if you can't find it, look for plain cocoa powder, not one with a lot of coconut oil.

1	cup all-purpose unbleached flour
1/2	cup sugar
1 1/2	teaspoons baking powder
1/4	teaspoon salt
2	tablespoons Wax Orchards Fat-Free Fudge
1/2	cup skim milk
1 1/2	teaspoons WonderSlim Fat & Egg substitute or 3 teaspoons applesauce or baby prunes
1 1/2	teaspoons vanilla extract
1/3	cup sugar
2	tablespoons cocoa powder
1/8	teaspoon salt
1 1/2	cups boiling water

Preheat oven to 350°. Combine the flour, 1/2 cup sugar, baking powder, and salt in a medium bowl and mix well. Melt the Wax Orchards fudge in a glass measuring cup for 30 seconds in the microwave or until melted. Or place in a saucepan and melt over medium heat on the stove. In a separate bowl, combine the skim milk, WonderSlim, vanilla, and melted fudge. Add to the dry ingredients and stir well. Spoon batter into a 9-inch-square baking pan. Combine 1/3 cup sugar with the cocoa powder and 1/8 teaspoon salt in a small bowl, then sprinkle over the batter. Pour 1 1/2 cups boiling water over the batter. Do not stir. Bake for 30 minutes, or until the cake springs back. Serve topped with Vanilla Yogurt Cream (see page 281).

*Per serving, not including Vanilla Yogurt Cream: 135 calories; 0.3 g fat (2.2 per-
cent calories from fat); 2 g protein; 31 g carbohydrate; 0 mg cholesterol; 156 mg sodium.*

Brownies for Your Thighs

MAKES 12 SERVINGS

I feel like I pulled the wool over everybody's eyes this past holiday season. I
made these terrific fat-free brownies as gifts and they were such a hit that I
now make them on demand, and have incorporated them into my food business. Why do I think I pulled a fast one? Because they're so easy. That's right,
a real no-brainer! They're good for your health, good for your soul (chocolate brownies are definite a PMS soother), and good for your thighs, too.

16   ounces Mixed Company brownie mix (1 box)
1/2 cup WonderSlim Fat & Egg Substitute or 1 cup applesauce or
       baby food prunes
1   egg
2   egg whites, lightly beaten
3   tablespoons Wax Orchards Fat-Free Fudge
1/4 cup skim milk
     nonstick vegetable oil spray

This is more than a recipe; this is a lesson. First I want to list the ingredients
of this particular brownie mix so that you understand the difference between
it and other commercial mixes. If you can't find the Mixed Company brownie
mix, your health food store may carry a regional brand that's comparable.
Look for one that has similar ingredients to those in the Mixed Company
brownie mix: *Unrefined cane sugar, organic whole wheat flour, organic unbleached
wheat flour with restored germ, pure cocoa, and natural flavoring.*

Why I like these ingredients: The germ of the wheat is where most of the
nutrients are. Most refined or bleached flours have the germ removed. Unrefined cane sugar retains the nutritional elements, which white sugar loses
during the refining process.

Now, the directions on the back of box mixes make great brownies, but
they have added fat. So let's "Yolanda-ize" the directions as follows:

Preheat oven to 350°.

Where it says to use 1 stick (1/2 cup) butter, margarine, or vegetable oil . . .

Substitute: ½ cup WonderSlim or 1 cup applesauce or baby food prunes.
Where it says to use 2 eggs . . .
Substitute: 1 egg and 2 egg whites, lightly beaten.
Where it says to use 3 tablespoons of your favorite liquid . . .
Substitute: 3 tablespoons of Wax Orchards Fat-Free Fudge, melted for 20 seconds in the microwave, and ¼ cup skim milk.

Combine everything in a large bowl and stir to blend. Spritz a pan with nonstick vegetable spray. Pour in batter and bake for 30 minutes. Top with Vanilla Yogurt Cream (see page 281).

It takes about 7 minutes to blend the batter and 30 minutes to cook these amazing brownies. Life is good!

Per serving: 159 calories; 2.3 g fat (12.9 percent calories from fat); 4 g protein; 30 g carbohydrate; 18 mg cholesterol; 26 mg sodium.

Robin's Tiramisu

MAKES 2 SERVINGS

There's nothing I love more than when clients call me up with great fat-free no-brainer recipes they've created on their own. That tells me they're really eating happily and understand my food philosophy. It makes me even happier when they look as good as the actress Robin Riker. She lost about fifteen pounds four years ago and has kept it off by eating this way. So here's a treat that she created and wanted me to share with you. The recipe is for 2 servings, but you can make it for 6 by increasing the ingredients accordingly and using a 9-inch pie pan. You can also do variations on this by using orange liqueur or marsala wine instead of sherry, or using cocoa mocha cookies or fat-free ladyfingers instead of cocoa cookies.

3   tablespoons Wax Orchards Fat-Free Fudge
10 Barbara's Fat-Free Cocoa Cookies or other brand fat-free
      chocolate cookies
2   tablespoons espresso
2   tablespoons sweet sherry
3   tablespoons Vanilla Yogurt Cream (see page 281)

Melt the chocolate sauce in a microwave for 30 seconds or in a saucepan on the stove over low heat. In single-serving round flat-bottomed dessert dishes, layer 5 of the cookies on the bottom, edge to edge. Drizzle one half of the espresso, one half of the sherry, one half of the yogurt cream, and one half of the chocolate sauce over the cookies in each dish. (At this point, you'll have used up half the remaining ingredients.) Place another layer of cookies on top of each, then repeat the layering, ending with the Vanilla Yogurt Cream on top in a dollop in the middle. Or top with Whip It Slim (see page 301).

Per serving, not including Whip It Slim: 248 calories; 0.6 g fat (2.9 percent calories from fat); 20 g protein; 27 g carbohydrate; 6 mg cholesterol; 297 mg sodium.

Skinny Kisses

MAKES 18 SERVINGS

Can you believe it?! Chocolate kisses this low in fat and calories?! It takes time to make these sweets (actually it's just before-you-can-eat-them waiting time, not slaving-in-the-kitchen time), but it's well worth it. Eating fat-free isn't so bad after all. These make a great holiday gift. Enjoy!

2   egg whites at room temperature
¹⁄₄   teaspoon cream of tartar
¹⁄₂   cup sugar
1   teaspoon vanilla extract
¹⁄₄   cup unsweetened cocoa powder

Preheat oven to 350°. In a large bowl, beat the egg whites and cream of tartar until foamy. Gradually add the sugar and continue beating until stiff peaks form. Beat in the vanilla and cocoa. Using a pastry bag with a star tip (you can get these at your local supermarket), drop dollops of about a heaping teaspoon each onto a baking sheet lined with wax paper. Bake for 1 hour, turn off the oven, and let cool overnight in the oven. Do not open the door or they won't set properly.

Per serving: 26 calories; 0.2 g fat (5.1 percent calories from fat); 1 g protein; 6 g carbohydrate; 0 mg cholesterol; 6 mg sodium.

Baked Chocolate Apples

MAKES 4 SERVINGS

This is the Breakfast Baked Apples recipe with an added fat-free chocolate twist. I like to use Pippins or Rome apples. Try all of the variations of Wax Orchards fudge varieties such as Amaretto Fudge, Orange Fudge, and Raspberry Fudge.

4   apples
4   teaspoons Wax Orchards Fat-Free Fudge
4   teaspoons raspberry jam
1   cup fruit juice (your choice)
1   teaspoon cinnamon

Preheat oven to 350°. Line a medium-size baking dish with aluminum foil. Core the apples, but not all the way through: Leave about one inch uncored at the bottom. Place one teaspoon of the fudge in the core of each apple, then one teaspoon of jam. Pour a cup of your favorite fruit juice in the bottom of the pan, and sprinkle the cinnamon across the tops of the apples. Bake for 20 minutes or longer, depending on the size of the apples. Slide a knife through one of the apples to check for doneness. Be careful not to overcook or you will have applesauce. Serve with fat-free vanilla frozen yogurt.

Per serving: 132 calories; 0.7 g fat (4.3 percent calories from fat); 1 g protein; 32 g carbohydrate; 0 mg cholesterol; 3 mg sodium.

Sotted Apples

MAKES 2 SERVINGS

Don't worry, *you* won't get sotted by eating these lovely apples, but they're a real treat. You can use a liqueur or some whiskey in place of the bourbon if you prefer. Or if you don't want to use an alcohol, replace it with almond syrup. These are decadent!

1/4   cup pitted sour cherries, drained
3   tablespoons brown sugar
1/2   teaspoon cinnamon
1/4   teaspoon grated lemon peel
1 1/2 tablespoons bourbon

2   large Rome apples
¹/₂   cup boiling water

Preheat oven to 400°. Combine the drained cherries, 2 tablespoons of the brown sugar, cinnamon, lemon peel, and bourbon in a small bowl. Stir and set side. Core the apples, but not all the way through: Leave about one inch uncored at the bottom. Peel the top third of the apples. Place them in a baking dish and fill the core with the cherry mixture. Sprinkle the remaining brown sugar along the top. Pour the boiling water into the baking dish. Bake for 45 minutes, or until tender (this will depend on the size of your apples).

Per serving: 170 calories; 0.6 g fat (3.3 percent calories from fat); 0 g protein; 37 g carbohydrate; 0 mg cholesterol; 8 mg sodium.

Bananas Rhumba

MAKES 4 SERVINGS

This scrumptious dessert can easily be turned into frozen bananas for kids. Make the sauce without the rum, dip the whole bananas (put a stick through them lengthwise) in the fudge mixture, and freeze.

2   bananas, peeled and sliced lengthwise
2   tablespoons brown sugar
¹/₄   cup dark rum
¹/₂   cup Wax Orchards Fat-Free Fudge
¹/₂   teaspoon cinnamon
4   fresh whole strawberries

Divide the bananas among four small individual dishes. Heat the brown sugar and rum until the sugar is just melting. Add the fudge sauce and cinnamon, and cook one minute more over low heat until all the ingredients are melted together. Pour over the bananas, and top with a fresh strawberry. Serve over a slice of angel food cake, with some nonfat vanilla frozen yogurt, or just plain.

Per serving: 134 calories; 0.3 g fat (3.3 percent calories from fat); 1 g protein; 18 g carbohydrate; 0 mg cholesterol; 3 mg sodium.

Fruity Clafouti

This light French custard gets its rich taste from evaporated skim milk, one of the great little-known ingredients of our time. It calls for pears and frozen raspberries, but you can use any fruit mixture of your choice.

nonstick vegetable oil spray
1   pear, peeled, cored, and diced
1   cup frozen raspberries
1/3   cup honey
2   eggs
2   tablespoons all-purpose unbleached flour
1 1/2 teaspoons vanilla
1/4   cup sugar
1/3   cup evaporated skim milk
1   teaspoon cinnamon

Preheat oven to 375°. Spritz a 9-inch glass pie plate or other small shallow baking dish with vegetable oil spray. Combine the pear with the raspberries in the bottom of the dish. Drizzle honey over the top and bake for about 20 minutes. Meanwhile, in a medium-size bowl, whisk the eggs, flour, vanilla, and sugar together until smooth. Whisk in the evaporated skim milk. Drain the juices from the baked fruit into a small bowl. Reserve the juice, then spread the fruit evenly across the bottom of the baking dish. Pour the egg mixture over the fruit and bake for 12–15 minutes, or until puffed and set. Sprinkle with cinnamon and serve warm with the reserved juice over the top.

Per serving: 294 calories; 2.9 g fat (8.4 percent calories from fat); 6 g protein; 65 g carbohydrate; 107 mg cholesterol; 58 mg sodium.

French Vanilla Fruit Tarts

French fruit tarts always look like a light dessert, but in reality the fat in the traditional pastry crust is a killer. Using a recipe I picked up from Eleanor Brown, a food consultant to The Palms Spa in Palm Springs, I've taken the fat out of these pretty little tarts. Serve them for dessert, high tea, or to make a brunch more special.

Tart shells

nonstick vegetable oil spray
16   wonton wrappers

Fruit glaze

1   cup frozen apple juice concentrate
4   teaspoons arrowroot

Tarts

2   cups Vanilla Yogurt Cream (see page 281), with 1 teaspoon
**   honey and 1/4 teaspoon cinnamon added**
1 1/2 cups sliced fresh strawberries, peaches, or bananas or a
**   combination of any of them, or 1 1/2 cups frozen fruit,**
**   thawed and drained**
2   cups fruit glaze

Preheat oven to 300°. Spray tins with shell-shaped cups with the nonstick vegetable spray. Press a wonton skin into each shell, pressing it lightly into the grooves with your fingers. Trim off the excess wonton dough at the edge. Spritz a cookie sheet (or use your toaster oven pan) with the nonstick spray, and place the tin upside down on the sheet. Place in the oven and bake for 5–7 minutes, or until the dough is dry but not brown. Remove and let cool, then turn and lift the tin, leaving the formed shells on the cookie sheet.

While tarts are cooking, make the fruit glaze. Whisk the apple juice concentrate and the arrowroot together in a small saucepan. Cook over low heat, stirring, until thickened and clear. To microwave: Whisk the ingredients together in a 4-cup glass bowl or measuring cup. Microwave 1–2 minutes, or until thickened.

To assemble tarts: Spoon about one tablespoon of the yogurt cream along the bottom of the shell (more, if you like). Arrange the fruit on top in a pretty pattern. Drizzle the fruit glaze evenly over the fruit to coat, staying within the edges of the shell. Place in the refrigerator until ready to serve. Serve at room temperature or slightly chilled.

Tart Filling Variations

• Drizzle fat-free fudge sauce on the bottom of each shell instead of (or in addition to) the Vanilla Yogurt Cream.

• Flavor the Vanilla Yogurt Cream with coconut, lemon, almond, or orange flavoring.

• Add a pinch of allspice or pumpkin pie spice to the plain Vanilla Yogurt Cream, then drizzle a little maple syrup on top before you add the fruit to the shell.

• Substitute dried fruit marinated in liqueur (like raisins in Amaretto or dates in Grand Marnier) for the fruit.

• Top the tarts with chopped roasted chestnuts.

• After you spoon in the yogurt cream, lay an edible flower (like nasturtiums or pansies, available at gourmet markets) in the middle of the tart and place the fruit around the edges. Then add the glaze. Even Martha Stewart would be impressed!

Per serving: 103 calories; 0.3 g fat (2.4 percent calories from fat); 3 g protein; 23 g carbohydrate; 1 mg cholesterol; 71 mg sodium.

Lemon Flan

MAKES 8 SERVINGS

Flan is a traditional Mexican custard dessert and as such it's a great capper to a spicy meal. It's usually made with a fair amount of fat, but this one, of course, is not—only 2 grams per serving. If you prefer vanilla flavor to lemon, eliminate the lemon extract and lemon peel from the recipe. Serve after any spicy meal.

1⅓   cups sugar
3   eggs, lightly beaten or ¾ cup WonderSlim Fat & Egg
        Substitute
2   egg whites, lightly beaten
¾   teaspoon vanilla

¹/₄	teaspoon lemon extract
1	teaspoon lemon peel
24	ounces evaporated skim milk (2 12-ounce cans)

Preheat oven to 350°. Place 1 cup of the sugar in a large heavy nonstick skillet and heat over medium heat. Cook about 5 minutes, or until the sugar dissolves (do not stir). After it dissolves, continue cooking until golden, and stir well. Immediately pour into a 9-inch round cake pan. Tip to coat the bottom; set aside. Combine the remaining ¹/₃ cup sugar, eggs, egg whites, vanilla, lemon extract and peel, and milk in a medium-size bowl; stir well. Pour into the prepared cake pan and place the cake pan in a shallow baking pan. Add 1 inch of hot water to the baking pan. Bake for 1 hour or until the middle is set. Remove, let cool, then refrigerate for about 4 hours or overnight. To serve, loosen the edges of the flan with a knife, place a plate on top of the pan, and gently flip over; remove the pan. Serve with fat-free cookies.

Per serving: 228 calories; 2 g fat (8 percent calories from fat); 10 g protein; 43 g carbohydrate; 83 mg cholesterol; 135 mg sodium.

Fat-Free Cookie Banana Ice Cream Sandwiches

MAKES 4 SERVINGS

I like to make these with Vanilla Yogurt Cream, but nonfat frozen yogurt in the middle works just as well. An easy way to make these into coated sandwiches is to melt the chocolate in the microwave, dip the sandwiches in the chocolate, then freeze.

8	teaspoons fat-free chocolate sauce
16	fat-free chocolate cookies
16	teaspoons Vanilla Yogurt Cream (see page 281)
1	large banana, sliced

Spread the chocolate sauce on eight of the cookies and the Vanilla Yogurt Cream on the other eight. Place a slice of banana on a chocolate-topped cookie, then place a yogurt-topped cookie upside-down to make a sandwich. Lightly press the sandwiches together. Continue until all the cookies are used. Freeze.

Per serving: 64 calories; 0.2 g fat (3.9 percent calories from fat); 1 g protein; 8 g carbohydrate; 0 mg cholesterol; 50 mg sodium.

Mocha Ice

In New York and Los Angeles, these cool drinks are hot. They are creamy and wonderful, can be whipped up in no time, and best of all, they're fat free. Serve as a summer dessert with fat-free cookies, or alone as an afternoon treat.

1½	cups chilled coffee, preferably espresso
3	tablespoons Wax Orchards Fat-Free Fudge
1½	cups skim milk
1	teaspoon vanilla
½	cup crushed ice
pinch cinnamon	

Combine the coffee, fudge sauce, milk, and vanilla in a blender. Blend until thoroughly combined. Add the ice and blend until smooth. Pour into tall glasses and sprinkle each with cinnamon. Serve immediately. These can also be frozen for one hour, scooped into a bowl, and served with fresh raspberries.

Per serving: 45 calories; 0.2 g fat (4.6 percent calories from fat); 3 g protein; 5 g carbohydrate; 2 mg cholesterol; 48 mg sodium.

Peach Almond Ice

You can make this refreshing frozen dessert with fresh peaches or, if you use frozen, you can enjoy it year-round. Substitute apricots for peaches if you prefer.

6	cups frozen or fresh peach slices
3	cups water
1	cup sugar
2	tablespoons lemon juice
¼	teaspoon almond extract

Rinse the frozen peaches under hot water until defrosted, and drain. Combine all the ingredients except almond extract in a large saucepan and bring to a boil. Cover and reduce heat to medium and cook until the peaches are soft, about 10 minutes. Press the mixture through a metal sieve; reserve 6 cups of the juice mixture and discard the leftover solids. Add the almond extract to the reserved juice and stir well. Pour into ice cube trays; cover and freeze about 8 hours. Break into chunks and put in a food processor or blender and blend until smooth. Serve with a few fortune cookies on the side.

Per serving: 219 calories; 0.2 g fat (0.8 percent calories from fat); 1 g protein; 56 g carbohydrate; 0 mg cholesterol; 11 mg sodium.

Graham Cracker Crust

MAKES 1 9-INCH PIECRUST OR 8 SERVINGS

This is a very basic graham cracker crust that can also be made with other kinds of fat-free cookies. (I always use the natural food manufacturers' cookies.) If you're not using a hard cookie like gingersnaps or vanilla snaps, then make sure the cookies are stale and hard before you make them into crumbs. Look for graham crackers that are low in fat.

1½ **cups fat-free graham cracker crumbs or cookie crumbs**
½ **cup confectioner's sugar, sifted**
2 **tablespoons WonderSlim Fat & Egg Substitute or**
   4 tablespoons applesauce or baby food prunes
2 **tablespoons skim milk**
2 **eggs**
1 **teaspoon cinnamon**
butter-flavor nonstick vegetable oil spray

Preheat oven to 350°. Place graham crackers or cookies in a food processor and blend until crumbed, but not too fine. Put the crumbs in a large bowl and sift in the confectioner's sugar. Add the rest of the ingredients (except spray) and mix with a fork until the crumbs are moist. Spritz a 9-inch pie plate with the vegetable oil spray. Press the crumb mixture into the pie plate and work into a crust. Keep the crust to a thickness of about ¼ to ½ inch on the bottom and sides, then push the extra crust into an edge along the top. Bake for 10 minutes and let cool. Add your choice of filling.

Per serving, crust only: 121 calories; 2.9 g fat (21.1 percent calories from fat); 3 g protein; 21 g carbohydrate; 53 mg cholesterol; 113 mg sodium.

Whip It Slim

The simple fact is that nothing takes the place of real, rich whipped cream. However, real whipped cream is just plain fattening; anyone who wants to eat healthfully can't have it too often. What you *can* have often, though, is this creamy, guilt-free version. Whip it up and plop it on top of any dessert.

2   cups skim milk
1   teaspoon honey
1   teaspoon vanilla
1   teaspoon nonfat dry milk

Combine all of the ingredients in a medium bowl. Whip until the consistency of whipped cream. Another preparation method: Freeze the skim and dry milk in a bowl until small ice crystals begin to form on top. Add the honey and vanilla and whip until creamy.

Per serving: 26 calories; 0.1 g fat (4 percent calories from fat); 2 g protein; 4 g carbo-hydrate; 1 mg cholesterol; 33 mg sodium.

Chapter Fourteen

Gotta Have It:
Cravings, PMS, and Foods We Just Plain Like

They call your name, they tantalize you, entice you, beckon, seduce, and even haunt you. As ominous as it sounds, these are foods that we crave. And everybody has these cravings.

Cravings. Yearnings. Longings. The fact is there are some foods you simply have to have—and have them *now!* The unfortunate thing about food cravings, though, is that when you give in to them (which is usually the case), you feel worse, not better. That's because the foods we crave are usually fattening or unhealthy (know anybody who craves celery sticks?). And although they may temporarily soothe our needs, they leave guilt and remorse in their wake.

This is particularly true of women who have PMS-induced cravings. As a matter of fact, I know women who would swear that "PMS" and "cravings" are synonyms. PMS cravings can be the worst kind. Years ago, there was a great episode of the TV series *Taxi* where Carol Kane (who played the wife of Latka) is having a bad bout of PMS. She is miserable, has dark bags under her eyes, and is crying one second and screaming the next. When Latka comes home from work he can't find her. He searches the tiny apartment, then finally pulls back the curtain to the closet, where he locates her crying and standing with a huge bag of potato chips in her arms, jamming them into her mouth as the crumbs dribble down her chin. It was the perfect depiction of a PMS food-craving attack.

It was actually a man, my husband, Richard, who got me to accept and live with my PMS chocolate cravings. For the first few years of our marriage, I would have chocolate binges two to three days before my period. Then would come the remorse and guilt. Why couldn't I control myself? Why was chocolate something that I *had* to have monthly? Was I an addict? I really didn't understand it.

One day, my husband put it into perspective. "Don't you see that you go through this every month, and that it obviously has more power than you? So why don't you just accept it, and even enjoy it?" "Enjoying it" was not a con-

cept I ever thought of applying to PMS pig-outs, but he had a good point. After all, here is a cycle that is going to repeat month after month, so why not
accept it—and expect it? In other words, if you know a storm is coming, why
not be prepared so it doesn't do as much damage?

So, I tried it. I kept a better calendar of my cycle, and about a week before
my period I'd go buy a large bag of Taffy Lite chocolate chewy candies, or
make a big bowl of diet junk food chocolate mousse, and *allow*—that's the key
word—myself to indulge when the craving hit. At first there was a certain
amount of guilt because I went through the whole bag of chocolate chewies
or ate the whole bowl of chocolate mousse ("whole" is an important concept
during PMS). Then the next day, I realized that what I'd eaten had been low-
cal and low-fat, and so, even though I'd had a lot of it, it didn't add up to all
that much compared to what it might have been had I dug into a carton of
Ben & Jerry's. I didn't feel so bad. I even started to feel like I was getting away
with it. Getting away with chocolate binges—I felt such relief.

Now, many years later, there are even better low-fat, nonfat, low-sugar,
and low-cal treats available. And I don't even consider eating them a binge
anymore. I just eat them when I feel like it. There are also so many wonderful foods to satisfy salty, crunchy, and carbohydrate cravings. (If you crave
peanut butter, though, you're out of luck. It's still fattening.)

The lesson my husband taught me is to never ignore or resist the cravings
that come naturally to you, whether they're caused by PMS or not. Your cravings should be respected and acknowledged or they will blow up in your face
(or, as the case may be, cause your face to blow up). Even to attempt to pre-
tend that you will never eat chocolate or some other indulgence is ridiculous.
Realize that not only will you eat treats, you deserve them.

How to Quell Your Food Cravings

Whether you get PMS-generated cravings or just the regular old gotta-have-
it kind, the following craving-by-craving guide will help you satiate your
yearnings in the least diet-damaging way. All the items I list are just sinful
enough to make you feel satisfied, but not so indulgent that you'll wake up
feeling remorseful the next morning. You will probably even find that your
cravings actually diminish once you stop trying to make them disappear completely.

Answering the Call of Chocolate

Chocolate has become such a hallowed subject that whole books have been written about it. Just what does chocolate have that, say, vanilla doesn't? Well, almost every ingredient in it has, at some point, been credited with making people feel good. The sugar (carbohydrates) triggers the release of serotonin, a brain chemical that contributes to a sense of calm and well-being. Some believe that sweet tastes also produce an immediate rush of endorphins, natural chemicals that increase one's energy and sense of well-being. Then there's the fat in most chocolate candies, cookies, cakes, and ice cream, which satisfies the primordial urge for quick calories. Chocolate also contains phenylethylamine, a chemical that some researchers say stimulates feelings close to those that people experience while in love. However, cheese and salami also have phenylethylamine and they never have the romance of a good Godiva truffle, so go figure.

University of Pennsylvania researcher Paul Rozin sums it up well: "The craving for chocolate is sensory," says Rozin. "It's the desire for the oral experience of chocolate. The odor, the smoothness, the flavor." In other words—chocolate is just damn good.

These chocolaty treats will give you that wonderful sense of eating a rich candy bar, but without the extra fat or guilt. Each is either fat free or low in fat, but does contain sugar—there's really no such thing as a delicious chocolate treat without some kind of sweetener added. The cookies and snack cakes I recommend here are made with whole grain flours and natural, not refined, sweeteners. In other words, while you're squelching the craving monster within, you can actually get some vitamins and minerals as well.

Remember: If you are craving something like Oreos, by the time you've eaten the third healthy fat-free cookie, your craving will be starting to subside. So don't wrinkle your nose at the new alternatives—pretty soon you will be craving the healthy stuff!

• *Barbara's chocolate mini-bite cookies* (6 cookies have 90 calories and 0 grams fat). These are bite-size cookies that have great hand-to-mouth appeal (sometimes that repetitive motion is soothing). Four of them equal one normal cookie.

• *Fudgets Brownies* (240 calories and 0 grams fat each). High in natural sugars and very sweet.

• *Hard chocolate candies* (about 10 calories and 0 grams fat each). Lots of companies make these, and they impart a lot of chocolate flavor for the price of 10 calories.

• *Health Valley Chocolate Chip Rice Chewy Bars* (90 calories and 0 grams fat each). They're like the good old-fashioned crispy rice bars with chocolate chips.

• *Health Valley Chocolate Sandwich Bars* (110 calories and 0 grams fat each). These come with different fillings and are more like snack cakes than cookies.

• *Health Valley creme-filled chocolate sandwich cakes* (150 worthwhile calories and 0 grams fat each). This one is almost too good to be true. They're like a traditional snack cake and really taste extravagant. They come with vanilla, caramel, chocolate, and Bavarian fillings.

• *Health Valley fat-free fudge cookies* (25 to 50 calories and 0 grams fat each). These come in a variety of flavors, some with jam or creme centers.

• *Jammers chocolate and chocolate mint candies* (about 25 calories and 0 grams fat each). Great flavor and very chewy.

• *Newmarket natural fat-free fudge sauce* (102 calories and less than 1 gram fat per 2 tablespoons). Not quite as thick as Wax Orchards's, but great to pour on a banana or drizzle over a slice of angel food cake.

• *Sweet Nothings chocolate (nondairy) ice creams* (213 calories and 0 grams fat per cup). Black Leopard, Espresso Fudge, and more. See ice cream, page 308.

• *Taffy Lite chocolate fudge chewies* (16 calories and 0 grams fat each). About the size of a quarter, they are chewy like gumdrops.

• *Wax Orchards fat-free fudge sauce line* (90 calories and 0.5 grams fat per 2 tablespoons). I've mentioned these throughout the book because they're so rich and delicious, thick enough to eat off a spoon. Available in flavors like Amaretto Fudge and Raspberry Fudge.

Satisfying Salty/Crunchy Cravings

This is really where the issue of portion size comes in. Many chips or munchies say that they are low-fat or fat free, but that is only if you eat the unrealistic portion size they give nutritional statistics for on the back of the bag. When we're suffering from PMS or other kinds of cravings, most of us aren't in the mood to measure. And by the time you've had a couple of good handfuls of this so-called low-fat food, it can add up to as much as 22 grams fat. So before you plow through a bag of "safe" chips, always check the ingredients. Make sure when the label says "fat free" that there are no added oils (particularly hydrogenated oils) on the list. The only fat should come from the inherent fat—the corn in a tortilla chip, for instance. Once again, though, good news: There are a slew of crunchy-food makers who tell the truth. Their products are salty/crunchy craving-pleasers you can depend on:

• *Apple Chips* (110 cal and 0 grams fat per ¹/₂ cup). Plain dried apples, crispy and sweet.

• *Barbara's and Health Valley fat-free cheese puffs* (average 90 to 100 calories and 0 grams fat per 1-ounce serving). I like the onion-chive flavor the best.

• *Cheddar, popcorn, nacho, and other flavored rice cakes* (large kinds have 35–50 calories and 0 grams fat each; the small ones are about 50 calories and 0 grams fat for 5). These are really terrific, but again, look to the ingredients list, as some do have added oil. Believe me, they have enough flavor to compensate for the fat—you don't need it. And just think, you can be having that oil on a wonderful pasta at your favorite Italian restaurant instead.

• *Good Health Potato Sticks* (100 calories and 0 grams fat per ²/₃ cup). They're crunchy and similar to cheese puffs or French fries—they come in two different flavors.

• *Louise's or Childer fat-free potato chips* (average 90 to 100 calories and 0 grams fat per 1-ounce serving). If you don't like the plain, look for the flavored ones such as Maui onion or mesquite.

• *No-oil baked tortilla chips* (110 calories and 1 gram fat per 1-ounce serving). These are now available in practically every store in America. If you don't like one brand, then try another. Also, try one of the new flavors, like Guiltless Gourmet's nacho or chili lime. Try Barbara's pesto-flavored no-oil chips—I'm addicted. Don't forget all these chips' best accompaniment: salsa, salsa, salsa.

• *Rice puffs* (vary according to manufacturer). There are many brands of these on the market, and most are healthy. However, a lot of them have added oil, so make sure you read the ingredients.

Placating Carbohydrate Cravings

Pasta and bread are soothing. And they're filling because complex carbohydrates take a while to break down and digest, leaving an extended sense of satisfaction. Next to protein, they're one of the most satisfying food groups. You really don't need to put butter, margarine, oil, or other fats on these foods. Try them without the extras—it'll take you about three weeks to lose your taste for the added fat.

• *Baked potatoes* (120 calories and less than 1 fat gram each). Glorious root that it is, a baked potato, skin and all, is very satisfying with a little steak sauce or fat-free sour cream on top. But also think of baby new red potatoes, cooked and refrigerated—a great snack. I like to dip them into Dijon mustard. Steam up a whole bag and keep them in the fridge. You might also try Yukon gold potatoes, which have a natural buttery taste. Purple potatoes are great, too, just for the sheer novelty of their hue. And think of all the calories and fat you'll be saving. Eleven French fries (and there are about 20 to 25 in most small orders) have 14 grams fat and 225 calories. I'd rather have a couple of baked potatoes.

• *Bread* (about 70 calories and 0–1 grams fat per slice). Nothing makes me happier than a good baguette with a chewy crust. All across America, wonderful bakeries are making fresh gourmet breads flavored with rosemary, onion, herbs, and more. (Once again, some are made with olive oil—which can add up to 14 grams of fat per serving—so check your ingredients list or ask at the counter.) On the West Coast, we have La Brea bakery and Il Fornaio, but you undoubtedly have a local baker who's making good breads. There are also many low-calorie fat-free bialys and English muffins around. Or try a toasted bagel with some jam, or an onion bagel with some mustard. (Note, though, that a bagel can have a hefty number of calories, depending on its size.)

- *Crackers*. This used to be one of the worst areas for salt and fat in the food industry. But that's in the past. Now look for:

Auburn Farms Fat-Free Seven Grainers (120 calories and 0 grams fat for 20 crackers). They're small like Wheat Thins and come in seven different flavors.

Edwards & Son's rice snaps (7 calories and 0 grams fat per snap except for the Parmesan flavor).

Hain fat-free crackers (50 calories and 0 grams fat per 5 crackers).

Health Valley crackers in a variety of flavors (50 calories and 0 grams fat per 6 crackers).

Jardine's in a variety of flavors (110 calories and 0 grams fat per 20 crackers).

Premier Japan and San-J rice crackers (60 calories and 1 gram fat per 4 crackers).

Venus fat-free water crackers (60 calories and 0 grams fat per 6 crackers). They come in two flavors.

If You Must Scream for Ice Cream

Ice cream is the great American dessert. But consider that a cup of Ben & Jerry's has anywhere between 30 and 50 grams of fat, and even a classic brand name like Breyers has about 17 grams per *serving*—not per container! The real thing can be enough to make even a slight PMS indulgence seem to warrant a sentence of thirty treadmill hours. You've also got to watch out for some of the low-fat and nonfat ice creams, whose manufacturers play a lot of tricks. For instance, a frozen dessert may have only 13 grams of fat per cup, but still have 300 or more calories because of all the sugar that's been added.

A word here about frozen yogurt, too. Remember that frozen yogurt can be just as fattening as ice cream. The real key to these products is, as always, to read the ingredients list. If you are stopping for yogurt at one of the local stores in your area, and the store has a banner screaming "fat free" in the window, then they should have no problems giving you a list of ingredients to back it up. It may be fat free for a 4-ounce serving size (about 4 large spoonfuls), but most "smalls" are about 11 to 12 ounces. If the yogurt contains any hydrogenated or partially hydrogenated oils, then pass.

Thankfully, those of us concerned about our health and weight can still find variations on ice cream and frozen yogurt to satisfy our cravings. And sorbets of all flavors, as long as they're made without cream, are always a great choice. Read on for some of frozen desserts to look for:

- *Ben & Jerry's nonfat yogurt* (287 calories and 0 grams fat per cup).

- *Breyers fat-free frozen yogurt* (204 calories and 0 grams fat per cup).

- *Dole Fruit Juice Bars* (45 calories and 0 grams fat per bar). Come in assorted flavors.

- *Dole Fruit N' Juice raspberry ice* (70 calories and 0 grams fat per cup).

- *Frozfruit* (100 calories and 0 grams fat per bar).

- *Gise* (averages 15 calories and 0 grams fat per cup). Comes in fruit flavors. This is sold in many malls and local yogurt shops. It is like a soft fruit sorbet.

- *Häagen-Dazs frozen yogurt bars* (100 calories and 1 gram fat per bar).

- *Häagen-Dazs Orange Tango, Piña Colada, and Raspberry nonfat yogurts* (260 calories and 3 grams fat per cup).

- *Healthy Choice Banana Foster ice cream* (220 calories and 3 grams fat per cup).

- *Lucerne nonfat ice cream* (184 calories and 0 grams fat per cup).

- *Mattús low-fat ice cream* (333 calories and 6 grams fat per cup).

- *Stars nonfat frozen yogurt* (220 calories and 0 grams fat per cup).

- *Sweet Nothings* (213 calories and 0 grams fat per cup). This is the best nondairy ice cream around, and comes in a great variety of flavors. This company also makes ice cream bars.

- *TCBY classic vanilla yogurt* (220 calories and 3 grams fat per cup).

- *Weight Watchers Chocolate Mousse ice cream bars* (35 calories and 1/2 gram fat per bar).

- *Weight Watchers vanilla sandwich bars* (160 calories and 3.5 fat grams per sandwich).

Satiating Sex Cravings

Oops, sorry. Wrong book.

Chapter Fifteen

Kids! What's the Matter with Kids' Food Today?

As you know by now, I have two little darlings myself. As of this writing, my daughter, Nolina, is fifteen and my son, Rylan, is four. That's right, I had to deal with puberty and the terrible twos all at once. I should get a lot of sympathy for that.

In *Food Cop* I devoted a whole chapter to my ideas about feeding children right. I can't stress strongly enough how important it is to teach kids about eating well. No child is too young to be schooled about good food. The sooner you start educating your kids, the greater the chance that they'll be happy with food—and their bodies—in years to come.

We all feel that we owe our children the best. We don't want them to suffer the same problems that we have and we hope the world will be a better place when they come of age. Unfortunately, much of what happens in the world is beyond our control—but we can focus on what *is* under our control. You have the power to make a strong impact on your kids' relationship with food.

Stop and think for a moment about how many of your favorite childhood memories involve food. Probably a lot of them. Now stop and think of how food has become a problem and often a source of guilt today. Obesity, heart disease, high cholesterol, diabetes, and certain forms of cancer, which are all affected by food, are just a few of the things that we'd like our children to live without. Even a minor weight problem can damage a child psychologically and, in a worst-case scenario, can grow into an eating disorder. So for both their physical and mental health, begin to make some changes in the way you feed your kids.

Before we get to my keys for kid-food happiness, I want to mention how much my fifteen-year-old daughter has taught me about feeding a child. My four-year-old son is easy: When he doesn't like what I give him, he spits it out on the floor and tries to dance on it. I get the message quickly. Nolina, on the other hand, is the queen of mixed messages when it comes to food; she changes her mind on a daily basis. The dinner she adored last week is dog food to her this week. (Then again, my four-year-old loves the dog's food.)

It's frustrating and challenging. Unfortunately, some moms and dads just throw in the towel and let their kids consume what they wish, just to keep peace in the house. They just want to see their children eat, so they don't make an issue over whether they're having a bowl of Froot Loops or a bowl of Grape-Nuts. But believe me, there is a huge, important difference between the two.

My daughter is at a point where she is very aware of her body and consumed with fitting in. In our society, that means eating junk food; soda, pizzas, fast food, chips, and candy are the mainstay of a teenager's diet. The teenage years also happens to be the time that kids (particularly girls) start to gain weight. So what's a parent to do? Well, when it comes to kids, actions speak louder than words. Remember, you are the gatekeeper of the family's foods and, by extension, their health. You lead.

Five Keys to Kid-Food Happiness

1. *Keep home base clean.* If you want your kids to eat good food, provide them with nothing but good food when they are home. Children's meals should be all natural and low in fat, sugar, and salt—just like adults'. By all natural I mean not made from processed foods laden with additives. By low in fat I mean not greased up with butter and oils, particularly saturated ones. Kids will want sugar (the phrase "like a kid in a candy store" was born of an enduring truth), and they should be able to have sweets. But sweetness doesn't belong in meals, it belongs in treats, snacks, and desserts, and then in moderation. Salt is something older people tend to worry about because of high blood pressure, but a taste for salt is something we develop when we're young. There is nothing wrong with having a salt shaker on the table, but don't buy products high in sodium and then let your kids pour the salt on top of their food, too.

2. *Don't allow your children to be ostracized from their social world.* Since your kids are eating nutritious food at home (right?), you can allow them to take part in social (and usually not so healthy) eating with their peers. Let them go to a party and have treats. If all their softball teammates are going to a fast food joint after the game, let them go. I don't know anyone who permits their kids to eat all of the candy they get on Halloween at once, but do allow them to have a daily allotment of it. At least for a while. On all major holidays, kids

should be able to enjoy the festive offerings. Don't make an issue of their indulgences and they won't resent you for making home base a healthy zone.

In fact, you might encourage your older kids to have their friends over to your house instead of hanging at the local fast food place. At home, you can make sure that healthy treats like baked chips and salsa are available to them.

3. *Lunch isn't someone else's responsibility.* A recent USDA report of 545 schools showed that the average school lunch gets 38 percent of its calories from fat. Worse, 15 percent of the fat was saturated and the salt level was double what is considered healthy by most experts. In response, the USDA announced that school lunches must now comply with the 1990 Dietary Guidelines. But while that sounds like good news, the schools have until 1998 to comply. By the time someone else gets around to feeding your kids right, they'll be in college. Believe me, I know how hard it is even to think about going into the kitchen at night to make lunches after you've just come home after a long day of work, taken care of dinner, homework, baths, and everything else. My only response, though, is do it. Do it because it makes a difference to your child's health. Starting on page 112, I have listed so many easy ways to pack those lunches that you can practically do it in your sleep. It makes a difference to your children.

4. *Educate your kids.* I'm not referring to the three R's; I'm talking about teaching your kids how food affects their health. I did a consultation with a single mom and her nine-year-old daughter. The daughter was a little plump and heading toward becoming a fat teen. I sat with both of them and discussed the importance of reading labels and searching out natural products. At one point, the little girl went to the fridge and took out a loaf of Webber's white bread. I had brought with me a loaf of all-natural whole wheat bread. She asked me if the Webber's bread was good or not so I had her read the ingredients. As she read, I explained what they meant. She had no trouble understanding what I was talking about. Later, we did a supermarket tour and I explained the different kinds of food in each aisle.

I respected this girl's mother for attempting to educate her daughter. Actually, the mom lost twenty pounds and the daughter is doing great, too. Don't underestimate your children's ability to comprehend food matters or their desire to know more about what they're eating. Many of my daughter's friends have asked me to lecture at their school (and I have) and are very curious about what our family eats.

You can give your own kids the information they need to eat well. Talk about which foods are good for their health and necessary for their bodies. Teach them that certain foods may taste wonderful but don't have the nutrients they need to help them be strong and healthy. Let them know that those foods are okay once in a while, but they need the healthy foods to grow strong.

We need to have the same attitude toward nutrition that we do toward childhood safety. Don't talk to strangers, cross at the light, don't do drugs, and eat good food—it's very important. Junk food is not *cute*.

5. *Have patience.* Need I say more? Eating (along with sleeping) is one of the few things that kids absolutely don't want to do when they're told to. And they exercise their need for independence, power, and control by confronting us on these matters. So work with them, but don't give in completely. Just as you wouldn't let your children stay up until two in the morning, neither should you allow them to eat junk food all the time. Be aware that they know how to push your buttons with statements like "I hate this," "I have to have white bread," "There's never anything to eat in this house," "I'm not hungry." They'll turn up their noses at the expensive sea bass dinner you've prepared.

Have patience and keep introducing new foods to your children. Let them make choices in the produce section and other areas of the market that offer an array of healthy foods so they feel they have some control over what they eat. Most of all, establish your standards and stick to them.

Kid Food: No-Brainers and Recipes

Life is so complicated for parents today; you hardly need advice that's difficult to implement. What follows are easy answers, food that will make both you and your children happy, not to mention ease your guilt about having no time to slave over a hot stove in the name of good parenthood.

No-Brainer Lunches

These are items that you can load into those Power Rangers and Barney lunch boxes. See Chapter 8 for great easy lunch alternatives, then read below for six super alternatives to traditional peanut-butter-and-jelly sandwiches. Sometimes I make five of each of these sandwiches or roll-ups, then freeze them in plastic bags. Pop one into your child's lunch sack in the morning and it will be thawed by lunchtime.

Mini Fat-Free Cheese Pitas Stuff mini hors d'oeuvre–size pitas with shredded fat-free cheddar cheese, a squirt of mustard, and a slice of dill pickle. If you're serving them at home, place them in the toaster oven to melt the cheese and, *voilà*, healthy grilled cheese sandwiches.

Apple Sandwiches Slice a large apple, then squeeze a little lemon over the slices to keep them from turning brown. Spread peanut butter, low-fat cream cheese and walnuts, or jam and a sprinkling of raisins on top of half of the apple slices *or* place a slice of Jack cheese on top. Cover with the other half of the apple slices.

Cold-Cut Roll-Ups Wrap sliced turkey or tofu-based cold cuts around a piece of string cheese. Secure with a toothpick.

Pasta and Cheese Salad Place leftover pasta in a container, then add chunks of fat-free cheese. Throw the mixture in the microwave for a few minutes to melt it à la macaroni and cheese.

Cracker or Tortilla Sandwiches To keep things interesting, use whole grain crackers, no-oil tortillas, or chapati bread instead of regular bread. Spread with peanut butter or low-fat cream cheese or place a slice of fat-free cheese between them. (Also, see pages 116–119 for healthy tuna and chicken salad ideas.)

Mini subs I like to buy whole wheat hot dog buns and make mini sub sandwiches with a combination of different fillers. Try low-fat cheese or chicken breast or low-fat cold cuts topped with pickles, lettuce, and tomato. Or let your kids stuff them with their favorite sub fillings. A few additional add-ons: onions, sauerkraut, tuna, canned beans, leftover salad, sliced olives.

Dinnertime Delights for Little Darlings

If you want kids to eat nutritiously—if you want kids to eat period!—it helps if you make their meals fun. The kid stuff that follows is just that: A joy for children to eat, plus seriously defatted so that you don't have to worry about their health.

Chicken Nuggets

MAKES 4 SERVINGS

This, too, is a best-seller from my food service in Los Angeles—and it's not just kids who are eating them! Nonetheless, children do love this healthy take on McDonald's Chicken McNuggets. Adults will appreciate them, too; serve them when you're having people over for a game, movie, or card party. Easy to make ahead of time, they're a great finger food.

3	6-ounce boneless skinless chicken breasts
1	cup whole wheat bread crumbs
1/2	cup wheat germ
1	teaspoon garlic powder
1/8	teaspoon red pepper flakes
2	eggs
1	egg white
1	tablespoon Worcestershire sauce

nonstick vegetable oil spray

Preheat oven to 350°. Rinse the chicken breasts and cut into 1/2-inch cubes. Mix the bread crumbs, wheat germ, garlic powder, and red pepper flakes in a shallow bowl. Lightly beat the eggs and egg white (or use all egg whites) in a shallow bowl with the Worcestershire sauce. Spritz a baking sheet with vegetable oil spray. Dip each chicken chunk in the beaten egg, then in the bread crumb mixture, and place in a row on the baking sheet. Spritz all over with the nonstick spray and place in the oven. Cook for 10 minutes on one side; turn and cook 5–10 minutes on the other side, or until golden brown. Serve with Honey Mustard Dip (see page 190).

Per serving, not including dip: *223 calories; 4.9 g fat (19.4 percent calories from fat); 35 g protein; 10 g carbohydrate; 180 mg cholesterol; 254 mg sodium.*

Chicken Tacos

MAKES 2 SERVINGS

If you're short on time, use canned chicken breast meat—it's great for a multi-ingredient dish like this. Really use your imagination with this dish. Just about anything can be used to fill the tacos: various kinds of salsas, pinto beans, bean dip, corn, olives, onions. Make a taco bar and let the kids make their own.

¹/₄ cup defatted chicken broth
1 teaspoon taco seasoning mix
1 6-ounce boneless skinless chicken breast, cut into strips
2 no-oil corn tortillas
1 ounce fat-free cheddar cheese, grated
¹/₂ cup shredded lettuce
¹/₂ cup salsa
2 tablespoons nonfat sour cream

Heat the chicken broth in a medium nonstick sauté pan. Add the taco seasoning and the chicken. Cook over medium heat, stirring, until the chicken is cooked through. Drain and set aside. When cool enough to handle, shred the chicken even more. Fill the tortillas with the chicken, cheese, and lettuce. Top with salsa and sour cream.

Per serving, not including salsa and sour cream: 189 calories; 2.5 g fat (14 percent calories from fat); 27 g protein; 8 g carbohydrate; 51 mg cholesterol; 438 mg sodium.

Ghost Eye Eggs on Rice

MAKES 2 SERVINGS

Believe it or not, this was my absolute favorite dish when I was nine. My mother was an incredible cook, but with four kids there were days when even she wanted to cop out on kitchen duty. This dish has the protein, carbs, and veggies a child needs. It's fun for kids, easy on Mom. Use a few of the peas to make a smile across the rice. When I make this recipe, I like to use Arrowhead Mills quick-cooking brown rice in the box, and add a little poultry seasoning to the water while it cooks.

³/₄ cup frozen diced vegetables
1 cup cooked brown rice
nonstick vegetable oil spray
4 eggs

Add the frozen vegetables to the rice during the last five minutes of cooking. Drain and set aside. Spritz a nonstick sauté pan with vegetable oil spray and fry the eggs sunny side up (don't turn over). Divide the cooked rice and vegetables between two plates, or two shallow bowls. Place two fried eggs on top of each plate of rice. Let the kids mash the eggs into the rice. Serve with ketchup or soy sauce.

Per serving: 258 calories; 10.8 g fat (38.5 percent calories from fat); 15 g protein; 24 g carbohydrate; 425 mg cholesterol; 127 mg sodium.

Hidden Veggie Dogs

MAKES 6 SERVINGS

I came up with this little trick for my four-year-old son as I was writing this book. He became obsessed with Smart Dogs soy-based hot dogs and wanted to eat nothing but. The dogs weren't *bad* for him, but he needed foods other than soy. My desire, like so many moms', was to see vegetables go down his gullet at least once a day. So I decided to replicate the hot dogs and hide some veggies inside. You can vary this recipe with either ground turkey or ground chicken. Let the kids dip these dogs in some ketchup—so you really have a mess.

¹⁄₂	**pound ground turkey breast**
2	**carrots, shredded**
2	**zucchini, shredded**
1	**egg, lightly beaten**
1	**tablespoon poultry seasoning**
	salt and pepper to taste
¹⁄₄	**cup bread crumbs**
1	**tablespoon grated Parmesan cheese**
	nonstick vegetable oil spray

Preheat oven to 350°. Combine all of the ingredients in a medium-size bowl with your hands. Shape the mixture into little hot dog shapes. Spritz a baking sheet with vegetable spray. Lay the dogs in a row and cook for about 15 minutes; turn and cook for another 10–15 minutes until cooked through. Remove, let cool, and chill in the refrigerator. Serve as finger food or on a hot dog bun.

Per serving: 105 calories; 4.4 g fat (37.3 percent calories from fat); 9 g protein; 7 g carbohydrate; 66 mg cholesterol; 101 mg sodium.

Hot Dogs and Beans

Okay. It's late, the kids are hungry, you're stressed, they want food—now! So you smile, take a deep breath, and follow this great fallback recipe. This is the 1990s version of an American favorite, only—dare I say it—healthy! But please, don't tell your kids. If you can't find the Smart Dogs, look for another version of soy-based hot dogs or a healthy, low-fat turkey or chicken dog. The Bearitos baked beans are fat-free, healthy, and delicious without the unnecessary added sugars. If this sounds too easy, remember that this is a very nutritious meal. The soy dogs are high in protein (with no added junk), the sauerkraut and tomato are two great vegetable servings, and the baked beans deliver fiber and protein—just keep an eye out for low-sodium pickles and sauerkraut. Plus, kids like it. It's as simple as that.

4	**Smart Dogs or other soy-based hot dogs**
1	**cup Bearitos baked beans or other fat-free beans**
1	**cup sauerkraut**
1/4	**cup dill pickles**
1/2	**tomato, sliced 1/4 inch thick**

Boil the hot dogs and heat the baked beans, either in the microwave or in a small saucepan over medium heat. Divide the dogs, beans, sauerkraut, pickles, and tomato between two plates. Or put the hot dogs in whole wheat hot dog buns. Serve with ketchup.

Per serving: 214 calories; 0.8 g fat (4.9 percent calories from fat); 7.2 g protein; 27 g carbohydrate; 0 mg cholesterol; 55.7 mg sodium.

Little Chickens for Little Fingers

Cornish game hens are not only tasty, they're cute—which makes them perfect for kids. And with this recipe, they're also easy to fix, making your life easier all around. Plus, at about $2.50 per bird, Cornish hens make good economic sense. They make a terrific at-home meal and are great to take cold on a picnic too.

2	**medium Cornish hens, giblets removed, cavity rinsed with water**

1   apple, seeded and quartered
1   onion, quartered
2   teaspoons poultry seasoning
olive-flavored nonstick vegetable oil spray
1   13-ounce can defatted chicken broth

Preheat the oven to 400°. Place the hens on a roasting rack in a shallow baking pan or in a roasting pan. Stuff the cavity of each hen with chunks of apple and onion. Sprinkle each hen with poultry seasoning, then lightly spritz with the olive-flavored vegetable oil spray all over. Pour half of the broth into the bottom of the pan. Cover the pan with an aluminum-foil tent. Cook at 400° for the first ten minutes, then lower to 350° for the next 20 minutes. Remove the foil and continue cooking for 10 to 15 minutes or until the hens are golden brown and the leg wiggles loosely in its joint. I don't recommend basting more than twice or else the skin may blacken. Add more broth as you cook so that there is always about an inch of liquid in the bottom of the pan. If you want to reduce your kids' fat intake, peel off the skin before serving. If you like, add some baby new potatoes and baby carrots to the pan (in the broth around hens) during the last 20–25 minutes of cooking.

Per serving: *195 calories; 2.3 g fat (10.8 percent calories from fat); 28 g protein; 15 g carbohydrate; 66 mg cholesterol; 325 mg sodium.*

Macaroni and Cheese

MAKES 4 SERVINGS

This is a great take-off on an all-American unhealthy classic. Kids are crazy about the taste and you'll feel a lot happier knowing they're eating mac and cheese without lots of preservatives and fat—and with some vegetables tucked in while the young ones weren't looking.

2   cups macaroni
1/2   cup frozen peas
1/2   cup frozen carrot slices
1/2   cup skim milk
4   ounces fat-free mozzarella, grated
1/2   cup nonfat sour cream
2   tablespoons grated Parmesan cheese
salt and pepper to taste

Prepare the macaroni according to package directions; during the last five minutes of cooking add the frozen peas and carrots to the pot. Drain and set aside. In a medium saucepan, heat the milk and add the grated mozzarella, sour cream, and grated Parmesan cheese. Cook 7–10 minutes over medium-low heat, stirring constantly with a whisk to blend. Don't let the mixture come to a boil or scald. Season with salt and pepper, and stir for one more minute. Toss with the macaroni and serve.

Per serving: 297 calories; 2 g fat (5 percent calories from fat); 20 g protein; 50 g carbohydrate; 6 mg cholesterol; 341 mg sodium.

Slimmer Sloppy Joes

MAKES 4 SERVINGS

The traditional sloppy Joe goes healthy! This version calls for lean ground turkey breast instead of fatty ground beef. And for those of you who never even dare to dream that your kids will eat green bell peppers—or onions—this is a great way to sneak them in.

> nonstick vegetable oil spray
> 1   pound ground turkey breast
> $^1/_2$ onion, chopped
> $^1/_2$ green bell pepper, chopped
> 2   stalks celery, chopped
> 4   tablespoons chili sauce (such as Heinz)
> 2   tablespoons tomato sauce
> $^1/_2$ cup water

Spritz a large nonstick sauté pan with vegetable oil spray. Sauté the ground turkey over medium heat, stirring to brown all over. Add the onion, green pepper (even sneak in some sliced mushrooms if you like), celery chili sauce, tomato sauce, and water. Stir to blend. Cook covered for about 10 minutes, stirring frequently, then cook uncovered another 5–10 minutes until the vegetables are softened and the mixture is slightly thick. Serve spooned over whole wheat buns accompanied by Skinny Slaw (see page 162).

Per serving: 143 calories; 1.8 g fat (12.1 percent calories from fat); 27 g protein; 3 g carbohydrate; 68 mg cholesterol; 206 mg sodium.

South-of-the-Border Tortilla Casserole

MAKES 4 SERVINGS

Sort of like a Mexican quiche, this is a great summer meal. Serve it hot or cold.

1	cup frozen chopped onion
1	cup frozen chopped green bell pepper
1/4	cup defatted chicken broth
2	cloves garlic, chopped
1/2	cup sliced mushrooms
1	cup nonfat sour cream
1	tablespoon Mexican seasoning (I like Spice Hunter's Mexican seasoning, or see page 67)
8	ounces canned diced green chilies
2	6-ounce boneless skinless chicken breasts, cooked and diced
	nonstick vegetable oil spray
1	package no-oil corn tortillas
2	tablespoons grated fat-free cheddar cheese

Preheat oven to 375°. Run the frozen onion and green bell pepper under warm water in a colander until just thawed. Pour the broth in a nonstick medium saucepan. Sauté the chopped garlic in the broth until just bubbling, then add the onion, pepper, and mushrooms. Sauté until the onion and garlic are transparent, and most of the liquid has been soaked up. Remove from the heat and place the vegetables in a bowl with the sour cream, Mexican seasoning, and diced chilies. Add the cooked diced chicken and stir until blended. Spritz a shallow casserole dish with vegetable oil spray and place three of the tortillas on the bottom. Spoon one third of the chicken mixture on top of the tortillas. Place three more tortillas on top, then the chicken mixture: Continue layering until the tortillas are gone (3–4 layers). Sprinkle the grated cheese on top and bake for 35–40 minutes. If you want the casserole to be a little thicker, add 1 tablespoon of grated mild Mexican cheese on top of each tortilla layer. Serve with a crisp salad dressed with a cucumber dressing (see pages 154–155).

Per serving: *227 calories; 2 g fat (8 percent calories from fat); 32 g protein; 19 g carbohydrate; 69 mg cholesterol; 199 mg sodium.*

Tuna Potato Chip Casserole

Is it really possible that this childhood favorite is in a book about healthy low-fat eating? Yes, thanks to all of the great new low-fat products on the market, in particular fat-free potato chips (such as Louise's in various flavors, including Maui onion). You may notice that I left out herbs and spices in this recipe since children tend to hate them. However, a little poultry seasoning couldn't hurt—or be creative and add your own herbs and spices. If you want to make a super-quick version of this dish, prepare Health Valley instant creamy potato cup o' soup by adding boiling water, then combine with noodles and tuna. Transfer to a casserole dish and top with crushed fat-free chips. A great shortcut!

³/₄   **pound egg noodles**
2   **6-ounce cans water-packed tuna, drained**
2   **cups nonfat sour cream**
1   **teaspoon poultry seasoning (optional)**
salt and pepper to taste
nonstick vegetable oil spray
1¹/₂   **cups crumbled fat-free potato chips**

Preheat oven to 350°. Prepare the noodles according to package directions, drain, and toss with the tuna, sour cream, poultry seasoning, and salt and pepper. Transfer mixture to a medium-size casserole dish sprayed with vegetable oil spray. Top with the crumbled potato chips. Bake for 15–20 minutes. Serve with a salad.

Per serving: 348 calories; 2.9 g fat (7.3 percent calories from fat); 28 g protein; 55 g carbohydrate; 70 mg cholesterol; 263 mg sodium.

Chapter Sixteen

The Bottom Line:
What It Takes to Lose Weight Once and for All

*I am tired of theory. I want to hear how we must act
to have a happier and more glorious world. . . .
Reform needs to be the watchword. And somebody
must preach it, who does not depend on the popular
nod for his dinner.*
—Susan B. Anthony, 1848

When I travel around the country and speak at seminars or appear on television shows, I can hear the frustration of millions of men and women who just want to know "How do I lose weight once and for all? What can you tell us that we don't already know? How can you help me?" My first instinct is to stand up and say, "Listen to me! Get rid of your diet sodas, your highly processed fat-free cookies, your fat-free mayonnaise, your packaged meals and shakes. If you want to achieve and maintain your optimal weight, then you can't be living on 'diet' foods." Even though that sounds like a contradiction of sorts, these foods won't get you where you want to go.

"What?!! Yolanda, are you crazy? You can't say that!! You can't tell Americans that these foods won't help them." That's the response I always get from friends and business associates. What I feel that they're saying, though, is "You can't tell the truth. You'll never be successful if you tell people they should get rid of that stuff. That's what the diet industry is built on."

Exactly. And, in some ways, my friends and associates are probably right. Perhaps I would have a more "brilliant career" if I toed the diet-industry line. But I can't and I won't. When it comes to weight loss there are so many ways to sell out. If you like money, and who doesn't, it's easy to get a gig promoting products you don't really believe in or to back a program that isn't healthy. But I'd be lying if I said that I thought these things work or are good for you. I prefer to teach weight-loss tactics that I believe can help you succeed, tactics that I practice myself. Tactics that are sound, healthy, and realistic.

That isn't to say that I've never been a spokesperson for a product before. I have. But only for companies that sell products I think are credible. Those who've asked me to represent them but don't meet my standards I've turned down.

The Bottom Line, Lose-it-for-Good Diet

What you've read in this book up to now has been information designed to help you be lean and healthy. But maintaining weight and losing weight are two entirely different things. I am not big on prescribed diets, particularly those that require you to count calories and fat grams or that prescribe a set menu that may or, more likely, may not, suit your individual tastes. But having worked with hundreds of people and spoken with thousands more, I understand that many individuals feel the need for some kind of set guidelines, a pattern to follow, in order to be successful.

So, I'm going to give you some guidelines, but let me add a few caveats. The six-week Bottom Line Diet that follows is just meant to give you some eating-for-weight-loss specifics and guidelines. It includes numbers (calories and fat grams), but it doesn't include a set menu plan, because I want you to learn to make wise choices on your own. That's what the information in this book is designed to help you do. Besides, I can't predict what you'll feel like eating on a given day—no one can. If you were to have to follow my menus for six weeks, you'd probably give up long before those weeks were up. I don't want you to feel you have to follow rules, but I am telling you the *bottom line truth* when I say that the only way to achieve success is to stick to low-fat and nonfat natural foods. *Stick to*—those are the operative words.

The good news is that every recipe and eating idea in this book is suited to the Bottom Line Diet. Of course, I don't expect you to live solely on the recipes you find here, but you can nonetheless rest assured that anything you do make from these pages is diet appropriate. What's more, since each recipe gives a calorie and fat breakdown, these dishes will make it easy for you to keep track of your intake.

You will, of course, have to reduce the amount of fat you eat if you want to lose weight. If you're really serious about taking weight off, you've got to make some sacrifices. *That's* the bottom line. Don't let anyone tell you it isn't. You simply cannot go on eating whatever you like if you want to shed pounds. As Joan Rivers might say, "Grow up!" But also understand that, while you may think cutting back on fat and calories is going to be tough, I'm here to tell you and show you that it really is easy. And it's worth it.

A Six-Week Plan

Before I tell you the specifics of this plan, I want to tell you the truth once more. As much as I'd love to say, "You'll lose ten pounds on this six-week plan!" the fact is that everyone is different. How many pounds you'll drop will depend on your individual body, how much you were eating before, and how much you're exercising now.

One basic fact, though, may help you gauge what kind of progress you'll make: To lose one pound you must achieve an average calorie deficit of 3,500 either by burning more calories through exercise or by eating less food—or by doing both, the preferable strategy.

You may shed pounds slowly—but don't let that put you off. It's actually *good* news because it means you're not going to be starving, and you're going to be eating healthfully. Plus, everyone should know by now that you're more likely to keep the weight off if you lose *slowly*. Lose quickly, and the weight will probably come back just as fast. Start by following the initial six-week plan here, letting your body adjust, and then, if you want to lose more weight, repeat it from the top to knock your weight down more.

I also want to talk about something that I work very hard on with my clients. Plateaus. It's the nature of the body to stop losing at some time during a weight-loss program. It's part of the process! The more you accept and understand this, the more success you will have. When you eat fewer calories, the body's survival mechanism kicks in and it slows your metabolism, causing your weight loss to cease. Your body is telling you that it wants—needs—to be a certain weight. If you realize this, you can accept a weight that should vary no more than four to five pounds up or down. Allowing your body to adjust to its plateaus is crucial to permanent weight loss. It's all part of finding the weight your body is comfortable with. When you accept that weight, you'll attain real weight loss, not a temporary quick fix.

With that in mind, here are eleven guidelines that will help you get to your goal.

Eleven Absolutes for Everybody

No matter if you're a man or a woman, if you have to lose ten pounds or fifty, these are the basics that can't be ignored.

1. Keep the amount of fat in your daily diet between 20 to 25 grams while you're trying to lose body fat. This applies to both men and women. When you stabilize, you can go a bit higher.

2. Eat only natural foods that your body can use—none of that over-processed, chemical- and preservative-laden, artificially flavored junk (including junk that has "diet" on the label).

3. Move, move, move.

4. Add no oils or other fats to your cooking.

5. Cut red meat down to two servings a week and make sure those servings are lean.

6. Use nonfat or 1 percent milk and other nonfat dairy products; if you can't make the adjustment to either one, start with low-fat 2 percent and work your way down.

7. Cut out nuts, seeds, and avocados.

8. Eliminate mayonnaise, butter, and margarine—even the reduced-calorie kinds.

9. Eat sweets only in low-fat and fat-free forms, and in moderation. Don't eat products with more than 10 grams of sugar per serving.

10. Drink, in moderation, only wine, light beer, or hard liquor. Skip mixed drinks.

11. Use the recipes in this book to help you lose. Every single one of them works into this plan because they are all low-calorie and made with a minimum of fat.

The Plan

Mark these instructions on your calendar so you know what you'll be doing each day. Plus, seeing the days fly by on your calendar will help you realize that six weeks go by in no time.

For Women

Weeks 1 and 2
Calories: Stick to 1,200 to 1,300 calories per day during the week, then allow yourself 1,400 to 1,500 on the weekends. These days are interchangeable. If, for instance, you have a weeknight out where you eat more than usual, then simply cut back on the weekend.

The Exercise Extra: On any day that you do an aerobic workout for a steady or combined time of at least twenty-five to thirty minutes, add 200 fat-free calories to your daily total.

Weeks 3 and 4

Calories: Stick to 1,300 to 1,400 calories per day during the week, then allow yourself 1,400 to 1,500 on the weekends. These days are interchangeable.

The Exercise Extra: On any day that you do an aerobic workout for a steady or combined time of at least twenty-five to thirty minutes, add 250 fat-free calories to your daily total.

Weeks 5 and 6

Calories: Stick to 1,400 to 1,500 calories per day during the week *and* on the weekends. So you'll be eating the same amount of calories every day of the week.

The Exercise Extra: On any day that you do an aerobic workout for a steady or combined time of at least twenty-five to thirty minutes, add 300 fat-free calories to your daily total.

Week 7

Switch to maintenance. See "Continued Success" on the following page.

For Men

Weeks 1 and 2

Calories: Stick to 1,500 to 1,600 calories per day during the week, then allow yourself 1,700 to 1,800 on the weekends. These days are interchangeable.

The Exercise Extra: On any day that you do an aerobic workout for a steady or combined time of at least twenty-five to thirty minutes, add 200 fat-free calories to your daily total.

Weeks 3 and 4

Calories: Stick to 1,600 to 1,700 calories per day during the week, then allow yourself 1,700 to 1,800 on the weekends. These days are interchangeable.

The Exercise Extra: On any day that you do an aerobic workout for a steady or combined time of at least twenty-five to thirty minutes, add 300 fat-free calories to your daily total.

Weeks 5 and 6

Calories: Stick to 1,800 to 1,900 calories per day during the week *and* on the weekends. So you'll be eating the same amount for each one of these days.

The Exercise Extra: On any day that you do an aerobic workout for a steady or combined time of at least twenty-five to thirty minutes, add 350 to 400 fat-free calories to your daily total.

Week 7

Switch to maintenance. See "Continued Success" below.

What if you reach Week 7 and haven't lost all the weight you wanted to?

If you haven't reached your final goal by the end of six weeks, repeat the plan for weeks 3 and 4 for four weeks, then weeks 5 and 6 for four weeks. If you need to continue, repeat weeks 3 and 4 for four weeks. Although you'll be lowering your calories again, the caloric change shouldn't be enough to make your metabolism slow down.

Remember that these guidelines are not strict rules. They are designed to help you shed pounds while also impressing on you that cutting calories doesn't have to mean starvation. If you want to knock your weight down a little faster, you can repeat weeks 1 and 2 instead of weeks 3 and 4. Or, just try to find the calorie count that you are comfortable with that doesn't interfere greatly with your lifestyle.

Continued Success

When you reach that weight and want to maintain it, live on the calories prescribed in weeks 5 and 6. Let yourself have your splurges on the weekends or at special events, then clean up your diet the next day. This is a plan for life. If you get lost along the way, reread Chapter 1, and stick to the recipes in this book. Not only will you achieve your goal, you will be healthy to boot.

About the Authors

YOLANDA BERGMAN is a nationally celebrated authority on healthful eating, as well as fitness and nutrition coach to many actors, musicians, executives, and families. For the last fourteen years, her home-delivery food service has prepared healthy, gourmet meals for clients in Los Angeles. Yolanda has published articles on healthful eating and nutrition in *Glamour*, *Self*, *Vogue*, *Allure*, *Elle*, *Woman's World*, *Ladies' Home Journal*, and *Redbook*, and she has been named to the advisory board for *Shape Cooks*, a new cooking magazine to be published in conjunction with *Shape*. The bestselling author of *Food Cop*, Yolanda lives with her children in Los Angeles.

DARYN ELLER is a Santa Barbara, California-based freelance writer who specializes in health issues. She has written for many national magazines including *American Health*, *Health*, *Good Housekeeping*, *Redbook*, *Self*, *Fitness*, *Women's Sports & Fitness*, and *Parenting*.

Index